DEDICATION

All that is contained within these pages is dedicated to the following individuals who have been the most important influences upon me. With love and appreciation I dedicate this book to:

Mrs Irene May Arnold

My mother in whose strength, wisdom and insights I have always relied. She is a woman who has instilled in me the power of positive thinking and giving truly of oneself. She is more than my mother, for she is also my example, confidante, inspiration, and adviser. She is a woman born before her time and yet rooted in the strengths of her generation. A true Christian woman.

Moss Mohine Arnold Snr

My father and namesake. I owe him a great debt that can never be repaid, for he gave me the greatest gift of love that any can give another.

Susan Silverstone

My former spouse and friend, without her love and influence I never would have studied Reflexology in the first place. She has given me more than words can express, and I thank her for all that she has done for me. A brilliant person and astrologer, who one day will discover the positive potentials that lie within her.

I also dedicate this work to all those questioning souls who are searching for a deeper understanding of a nature of the universe, no matter what field of endeavor they are currently engaged in.

Finally I dedicate this current work to the evolution of humanity and to future generations. May your journey along your path be brightened in some small way by what lies within these pages.

REFLEXOLOGY

Published by Brolga Publishing Pty Ltd
ABN 46 063 962 443
PO Box 12544
A'Beckett St
Melbourne, VIC, 8006
Australia
email: markzocchi@brolgapublishing.com.au

National Library of Australia Cataloguing-in-Publication entry

Arnold, Moss M.
Reflexology : basics of the middle way
9781921596483 (pbk.)
Includes bibliographical references and index.
Reflexology (Therapy).
615.822

Printed in Hong Kong
Cover Design by David Khan
Typeset and designed by Diana Evans

REFLEXOLOGY
Basics of the Middle Way

Moss Arnold

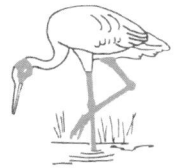

ACKNOWLEDGEMENTS

No work stands in isolation. All works to varying degrees are based at least in part on what has come before. To this extent this current work is based on all that has come before, including Reflexology theory and practice as developed by Eunice Ingham and promoted by Dwight Byers, for this is the basis of all Reflexology currently in the world today.

Receivers of Reflexology and Chi-Reflexology over many years also need acknowledging as they have in many ways, been my teacher. It is through them, through my thirst for understanding and the taking of risks and using my clients as 'guinea-pigs' that much that follows has developed. For this I thank each and every one of them; for each in their own unique way have added to the sum of my knowledge and understanding.

Also worth acknowledging are my students, seminar participants and graduates, both here in Australia and around the world, who like my clients have helped me formulate and expand my understanding of the science and art of Reflexology. Those skeptical Reflexologists who have critically questioned me have been of most value. To all of them I extend a heartfelt thank you.

I have been blessed by many of my students and graduates who have contributed in so many ways to my journey and this current work. Special thanks to Jody and Phil Morrison whose friendship, honest advice and forthrightness are here acknowledged. Both have always been there. Others have contributed through the process including Maurice Federici, Maria Vaccaro, Kellie Mangan, Vera Payne and especially Sharon and Paul Hartley. I acknowledge their contribution and efforts as well as their support and friendship.

A special thank you to all the organizers and organizations around the world that have invited me to present. Special thanks to Palvi Hannonen and Merja Pennanen from Finland; Audrey Scully from Sheffield, England (my UK representative), Jacqueline Munroe from Edinburgh, Scotland, and Samantha Langridge (my Victorian Representative and great mate) for their support and friendship.

A very special thank you to my illustrator, Annette Kyle, who knows nothing of Reflexology, and yet has always supported me, even when I asked for the impossible, which she duly produced. She is amazing for she has the talent, persistence and skills to translate my thoughts into shape and form: a truly amazing gift. She is a true Christian woman, who calls me "her little brother". I cannot speak highly enough of her personally and professionally. I also thank her for her friendship and advice, and for tolerating me.

I would also like to thank those that have edited the manuscript – Anne Fell, Audrey Scully (England) and Lila Mueller (Wisconsin, United States) and others. Thank you for your guidance and words of wisdom. A special thank you to Anne Fell who not only did the editing once, but actually did it a second time.

There are three Reflexologists I would like here to acknowledge for their contribution to this work, and they are:

Chris Stormer of South Africa, who was the first to 'step out of the box' and so by her very nature and actions, have paved the way for this work. To Chris, one of the most beautiful souls I have met on my journey, I acknowledge her contribution and support, in ways she will never completely understand.

Suzanne Enzer, who got the ball rolling. It was Suzanne

who, although not necessarily provided the answers to the multitude of questions I had, at least guided me towards the answers. In the beginning of this journey, she encouraged me to search. For this I am eternally grateful.

Last but not least, Russell McAllister, an Australian, publisher of the only independent international Reflexology magazine, *Reflexology World*. He has encouraged and aided me along the way. He is an inspiration through his limitless passion for the art and science of Reflexology. I thank him for his support, encouragement and friendship.

There are two Foot Charts that I wish to mention here. They are Chris Stormer's (the first attempt at understanding the feet accurately) and the Western Australian School of Reflexology Foot Chart. These two charts are significantly different from others, as they have begun analysing the premises and basics of Reflexology. These two Foot Charts are important, for they have questioned the original and begun the process of attempting to understand Reflexology. Ironically, both of these foot charts have evolved from a non-physical and energy-type approach which is ironic. To these two I acknowledge a debt as they helped me to understand Reflexology better.

Finally I would like to acknowledge my former-wife Susan Silverstone who was the one who introduced me to Reflexology, for she was the one who wanted to study it; not me. If it wasn't for her, I would never have studied Reflexology in the first place.

I also thank God however you define the Supreme Being, for my journey. It may be fraught with challenges and is never dull, but…

"The Journey is worthwhile."

CONTENTS

SECTION ONE:
Reflexology Theory

SECTION TWO:
Reflexology PracticalTechniques

SECTION THREE:
Systematic Approach to Reflexology

SECTION FOUR:
Receivers of Reflexology

APPENDICES

LIST OF ILLUSTRATIONS

FOREWORD

I first met Moss about four years ago when he came to Napier University to do an evening talk. One of his opening lines was something like 'Whatever you think you know about Reflexology throw it out the window…' and I knew instantly that I was going to like him. I went on to organize and attend Chi Reflexology training with him and I would be lost professionally without knowledge of his work and his ethos.

What I love most about Moss is his ability to speak passionately about Reflexology and its application, his dedication to giving only the best treatment and the respect that he affords everyone while being pragmatic enough to say 'if you don't agree with me then throw it out'. He is also extremely generous with his information and has given much of his work and knowledge away for free.

This book goes back to basics but is in no way a basic book. Moss has an honest approach to everything and this book tells it like it is. Starting at the beginning is always helpful and this book looks at the client approach in terms of spiritual, mental, emotional and physical but goes further and also explains why. This, for me, is something that can often be left out of other books and is the one question I am always left asking: but why am I doing it like this?

Each section takes a straightforward look at the approach, techniques and rationale behind what is being taught and this makes for an extremely comprehensive reflexology book which will prove hard to put down and essential to pick up.

Moss not being a man to mince his words also tells you here clearly what he does not believe in and that is an important part of what makes this book so powerful. Having the courage of your convictions as a Reflexologist is one of the most important lessons we have to learn and it is not something that can easily be taught, but by seeing it here in this book we can at least start to look at our own beliefs and practice and see if we really agree with everything we are doing.

Knowing Moss, I know there is more to come than is in this book but I also know that this book will be one of those on my treatment room bookshelves that will be instantly recognisable from the fact it is dog eared and well thumbed as it becomes a useful resource to my professional practice and teaching. We need to always be challenging ourselves as therapists and be willing to question and expand our practice for the benefit of our clients and ourselves; this book will help you do that.

So pick this book up, but do so with an open mind and an open heart and there will be something you find is new information or is useful to you as a Reflexologist and be prepared to throw some of what you already know out.

In conclusion I would like to say that without Moss and his work in my life I would not be the Reflexologist I am and for that I am grateful.

Jacqueline Munro
Reflexologist

ABOUT THE AUTHOR

Moss Arnold, *BA Dip Ed, Dip FR, Dip OM, Dip TCM*, Natural Therapist, Reflexologist, author and international presenter, has been an educator for his whole professional life and a therapist for more than twenty years. He is Principal and founder of the **Australian College of Chi-Reflexology**. He lives and has a clinic in Winmalee in the Blue Mountains area of New South Wales, Australia.

Awakening to the fascination of natural therapies, he studied various fields including Reflexology, Shiatsu, Acupressure, Touch for Health, and Aromatherapy, with an obvious emphasis on the Orient, and its philosophical as well as medical theories. Through these studies and his own experiences, he has developed what he calls *Chi-Reflexology*, a combination of the Chinese philosophy, including Traditional Chinese Medicine (TCM) and acupressure techniques, with Reflexology, a predominantly western modality.

Falling in love with the feet as a reflection of the human condition, Moss began to specialise in Reflexology, which led to his examination of the basics of the science and art of Reflexology, the development of Chi-Reflexology and ultimately this current work. For Moss has to understand what he does. His thirst for knowledge and understanding is insatiable and infectious. He challenges and motivates others to understand what they do, how and why.

Moss is an international presenter on Chi-Reflexology and author of his first self-published book "Chi-Reflexology:

Guidelines for the Middle Way", and has produced an accompanying Chi-Reflexology video (and now DVD) on the practical aspects of Chi-Reflexology covered in his book, as well as a Chi-Reflexology Foot Chart. Moss is a prolific writer, writing on a range of subjects including various aspects of health, well-being, Reflexology, Chi-Reflexology, and the Four Poison Points, which have been printed and reproduced around the world. For more information see the College's website at www.chi-reflexology.com.au

Further plans include a DVD to accompany this work, as well as one or two further books on advanced Chi-Reflexology with accompanying DVD/s, and an acupressure book. Another of Moss' passion is for Numerology, the science of numbers, which is introduced in this work, and is an integral component of working with the human being. So another planned project is a detailed Numerology text called "Wholistic (Soul Growth) Numerology".

Moss has dedicated the rest of this life to helping people as he believes life is all about giving, for as you give, you receive. His motivation is a strong desire to help others, through his practice, his teaching, and in all that he does. Moss has a strong desire to help and through sharing, challenging and motivating others to expand themselves and Reflexology, both as a science and an art form, he can help more human beings than he can by doing it himself.

Reflexology, from his perspective is a science, but like any tool it is what you do with it that is most significant: 'to make the tool fit your hand' so to speak. This is the art,which is the most significant and challenging aspect of Reflexology or any therapy. The task, therefore, is for you to develop Reflexology into your own tool or art, to bring it alive, let it live and grow, for yourself and for those you work on. To allow the magic to flow, and miracles to happen.

FEET FIRST – I TOUCH. I FEEL. I THINK. I AM.

ABOUT THE ILLUSTRATOR

Annette Kyle has worked professionally as a Show card and Ticket writer for fifteen years during which time she has practiced a wide range of artistic mediums including displays, screen printing, airbrush, banners and drawing illustrations. She was also a Technical and Further Education (TAFE) instructor in Show card and Ticket writing.

She has had a lifetime of experience of various art forms and continues a long family tradition of commercial art. Her father who was a commercial artist has passed on his knowledge and experience to his daughter.

Annette's passionate dream has always been to illustrate books and she would like to take this opportunity to thank Moss Arnold for giving her the opportunity to follow her dream. He is a talented lateral thinker. Combine his genius with Annette's ability to draw the spoken thoughts of others, and the result is Moss's books: 'Chi-Reflexology: Guidelines for the Middle Way' and this current work 'Reflexology: Basics of the Middle Way'. Through this combination of talents and abilities, both works come alive with new ideas and new ways of practicing the healing arts of Reflexology and Chi-Reflexology.

NO TASK TOO SMALL. NO TASK TOO BIG.

Annette Kyle can be contacted via: Moss Arnold
www.chi-reflexology.com.au
Email: moss.arnold@chi-reflexology.com.au

INTRODUCTION

When I studied Reflexology many years ago I had questions for which I could find no answers. In fact the basics of Reflexology were so poorly espoused both in written and verbal forms that I dismissed Reflexology as a serious therapy and as a profession. However, in my own Clinic I found I had fallen in love with the feet and was doing this thing called Reflexology. As I am a person who has to understand what he does, once I admitted to myself that I was a Reflexologist I then had to begin the process of discovering answers to the questions I had. This book is the consequence of that journey. I have attempted to answer the questions I had as well as answer the unanswered questions many qualified Reflexologists have. This then is the aim of this work: to begin the process of putting Reflexology on a more solid base; or to fill in the gaps, if you like.

One rule I started with was that when working on the feet I work intuitively (the yin aspect of the therapeutic situation). But the other side of the coin was that I would never re-use a new technique (or later share a new technique) until I had worked it out (the yang aspect of the therapeutic situation). This was my way of combining the yin (intuitive) and yang (logical) aspects as well as getting confirmation. It led to intuition (yin) and knowledge (yang) working together.

This current work has come about for other reasons also. First and foremost is the lack of detailed analysis of the basic premises upon which Reflexology is based. This book is a beginning to the process of self-examination of Reflexology theory and practice, as the most modern of all natural therapies has lacked a solid foundation upon which to stand.

It is also designed for those interested in or studying Reflexology. The purpose here is to give a solid foundation to the exploration of this wonderful therapy. It provides the foundations and explanations of the practice and theory of Reflexology as a science.

Lastly, it is designed for the Reflexology community, from beginner to student to professional, to fill in the gaps that I perceive currently exist in the body of knowledge of Reflexology.

For any profession to progress and grow it needs a solid foundation upon which to stand. Reflexology around the world has put effort into promoting itself rather than understanding this fascinating science and art. As a result there is little since its inception that is actually new in the field. This book attempts to rectify that situation.

My first work was "Chi-Reflexology: Guidelines for the Middle Way" which is an advanced Reflexology approach, but I quickly discovered that many Reflexologists lack the basic practical and theoretical understanding of their own therapy, which made it extremely difficult to understand an advanced approach without this solid foundation, so again this work is an attempt to rectify this situation.

As to the structure of the book, there are four sections as follows:

- Section One: Reflexology Theory
- Section Two: Reflexology Techniques (The Practical)
- Section Three: Systematic Approach to Reflexology
- Section Four: Receivers of Reflexology

Section One (Reflexology Theory) examines the theories that have been proposed for the science of Reflexology, critically evaluating these and proposing an explanation of Reflexology: 'The Anatomical Reflection Theory' offering a detailed analysis of aspects of Reflexology such as the Solar Plexus Reflex, divisions of the feet, landmarks, referral and helper areas, and concluding the theory of Reflexology with a new detailed physical chart of the Reflexes of the body through the feet.

Section Two (Reflexology Techniques) outlines and explains in detail the practical aspects of a basic Reflexology treatment sequence and concludes with two 'Summaries of the Basic Practical Sequence':

1. Verbal, for those who learn best reading the written word
2. Visual, for those who learn best looking and seeing.

Section Three (Systematic Approach to Reflexology) outlines the physical aspects of the feet, introduces Biomechanics and reflects each system of the body accurately through the feet based on the 'Anatomical Reflection Theory'.

Finally, the Appendices includes a Glossary of terms used in this work (Appendix A), Consultations sheets (Appendix B), an outline of the significance of Numerology to Reflexology (Appendix C), Recommended Reading and Reflexology Resources (Appendix D), and Reflexology around the world (Appendix E), which provides a place to begin to search for Reflexology in different parts of the world.

There is certain terminology which I have consciously chosen to use in this book, requiring explanation. Firstly, I have deliberately chosen the term "Western Industrial medicine", or simply "Industrial medicine" to describe western medicine as opposed to 'traditional', which Industrial medicine has adopted and yet is not actually traditional at all. Industrial medicine is the major medical model currently pervading in the world and yet is increasingly being challenged by traditional, natural and complimentary medical fields, including the body therapies and Reflexology.

All health care approaches have their strengths and weaknesses, and no approach has all the answers, including Reflexology. This is one aspect that needs acknowledging by all involved. Neither the Natural Therapies, including Reflexology, nor Western Industrial medicine have all the answers. Each one brings strengths that should be combined for the betterment of the whole system, but this is sadly not the case at the moment. I do not here wish to get into the issue of the current state of changes that are occurring in Industrial medicine, except to say that there are basically three models that pervade the question of combining different health care practices, and these models are:

- Industrial medicine and natural therapies as separate entities, which was the case historically and up until fairly recently;
- Industrial medicine taking pieces of the natural therapies and including these pieces in the health care system, excluding many of the very strengths of said therapies, resulting in the sanitation and thus the watering down of said therapies, in essence destroying their strengths;
- The Natural Therapies, including Reflexology entering as equals in professional collaboration, working together for the betterment of the patients, the clients and the whole health care system.

Which of the above scenarios is the best option? The choice is now being made and the future will be strongly influenced by that decision. So I hope it is a good one.

Next is the question of the term "Natural Therapies". I avoid using such terms as 'alternative' or 'complementary'. Instead I use 'Natural Therapies' or 'Body Therapies' throughout this work, but are natural or body therapies 'alternative' or 'complimentary'?

Of these two choices I would choose 'complimentary' which implies the third point above rather than the first, which is implied by the word 'alternative'? To this end then 'natural therapies', 'body therapies' and 'Reflexology' are used extensively throughout this work, and these therapies are viewed as complimentary rather than alternative.

Before beginning the Reflexology journey that awaits one other term that is used throughout this work needs explaining: the term "dis-ease". This is not a misprint as I have consciously chosen to use "dis-ease" rather than its more common 'disease', due to the fact that I want to emphasize the meaning of the word and that is:

- 'dis' is of Latin origin meaning "not",
- 'ease' meaning "freedom from annoyances of any kind" as in 'at ease', rest, comfortable and secure.

Therefore the very word used for "imbalances" is not at ease, or lack of equilibrium or out of balance. Thus dis-ease is deliberately used through this work to replace the concept of disease with the concept of dis-ease or imbalance.

I also consciously chose to use the word 'wholistic' and 'Wholism' rather than 'holistic' and 'holism'. The reason for this is I want to emphasize the concept of the **whole** rather than the possible misinterpretation of a **hole**.

Lastly, to simplify matters, through this work the terms 'inside', 'outside', 'back', 'ball of the foot' and 'sole' will be used, rather than the medical terms of medial, lateral, dorsal, metatarsal pad and plantar. So you need to realise that when talking about the foot that:

- The inside of the foot is called the medial foot;
- The outside of the foot is called the lateral foot;
- The back (or top) of the foot is called the dorsal surface of the foot;
- The ball of the foot (chest area) is called the metatarsal pad;
- The sole of the foot is called the plantar surface of the foot.

This then is the purpose of the work: to challenge, propose possible answers and to question. I believe that Reflexology has discovered no more than a third of its potential, leaving at least two-thirds left to discover. We all have a long way to go.

Hopefully this book allows for a solid foundation upon which these uncharted territories and discoveries can rest.

Time will tell.

Welcome to my journey of discovery.

May it add some colour to your own journey.

SECTION 1
Reflexology Theory

FEET FIRST —
I touch. I feel. I think. I am.

CHAPTER 1
Introduction to Reflexology

The therapy known as Reflexology (or in some parts of the world: Reflex Zone Therapy) comes from the concept of medical reflexes. Basically the theory pertains to an external stimulus being transferred into nerve impulses which are then sent to the Central Nervous System (CNS) or the Spinal Column and Brain, where a response is generated, thus returning from the Brain and CNS to the peripheral. Or more simply put: Input going in and a response coming out.

It is worth noting that the word "reflex" in this context refers to reflection, as in mirror image, with the reflexes of the feet (also the hands) acting as miniature "mirrors", reflecting the entire organism (Anatomical Reflection Theory: see Chapter 7 for a detailed analysis).

The very basis of Reflexology is a communications system, which operates from external to internal and then generates a response action. By working the feet and/or hands, messages are sent to the body to help it correct imbalances.

Reflexology is a unique science and art for promoting balance and well-being. The basic techniques of Reflexology seem simple, yet once mastered, are profound. The major techniques are the use of the thumbs and fingers on areas of the feet, which correspond to all characteristics of the human being. The procedures used are relatively easy to learn.

The applications of Reflexology range from relaxation and

stress reduction, and improved circulation and nerve supply, to the treating of physical, emotional, mental and spiritual imbalances. Once mastered, Reflexology becomes a powerful form of therapy. Its scope and range of uses are limitless, bound only by our current understanding and interpretations.

MY JOURNEY TO REFLEXOLOGY

My Reflexology journey is an interesting one, an important background to this current work. When I first studied Reflexology, along with many other therapies, I dismissed Reflexology as extremely inconsistent. My teacher could not answer what I thought were simple yet important questions. These inconsistencies arose as a result of the basic premise upon which reflexology is based: the two feet (and two hands) reflect exactly the anatomical positions of all parts of the body (Anatomical Reflection Theory: See Chapter 7 for a detailed analysis). In short, where things are in the body, they are reflected proportionately and accurately in the feet.

This premise in practice is not followed with any consistency, with the location of many reflex areas in the feet not even close to anatomically accurate. Further, the sizes of many reflexes are proportionately unrealistic to say the least. It was these inconsistencies that caused me to initially dismiss Reflexology.

Even after qualifying in Reflexology, I preferred other therapeutic approaches, yet I found that I was increasingly being drawn to the feet and working them. It was then I decided I had to confront the inconsistencies that I had perceived while studying. Nowhere could I find an explanation that answered my questions. In fact all sources appeared to simply reiterate, with minor variations, the original, with little or no attempt to expound a consistent approach to the theory and practice of the science of Reflexology. Supposedly advanced Reflexology techniques simply accepted the basics and attempted to build upon these inconsistencies.

With growing global interest in Reflexology, it is time to look more closely at this powerful therapy with deeper knowledge and understanding. My own studies, including TCM (Traditional Chinese Medicine), and my experiences began a journey which has led me to this current work of re-examining the basics of Reflexology.

It is not about teaching a 'right' way – the only way, but of teaching an expanded viewpoint, which allows Reflexologists to think for themselves and continue to grow and expand.

ORIGINS

There is enough evidence to suggest that the feet were significant and sacred to many, if not all, of the most ancient cultures, including Egyptian, Chinese, Indian, the Americas (North and South) and the Aboriginal society. However, little survives of the original practices, and Reflexology as we have it today comes from what was rediscovered about 100 years ago by American medical practitioners.

Reflexology only began just over a hundred years ago and has spread very quickly internationally over the last forty years. Today, Reflexology can be found in nearly every country in the world and it is significant that Reflexology has spread in such a very short space of time as such clearly demonstrates its potency.

MOVING INTO THE FUTURE

This rapid expansion, however, has come at a price. Throughout the world, Reflexologists have concentrated on promoting Reflexology rather than on analysing the principles and premises upon which it is based, and thus forming a solid foundation upon which to expand and grow.

Until recently, there has been very little within Reflexology that is actually new. This book has been written to expand the foundations and premises upon which Reflexology is based: to question these and to begin the process of developing a sound basic understanding of the science of Reflexology theory and practice.

This is a process that needs to happen in Reflexology, all natural therapies and the medical health care system so that mechanics that do the same thing every time are not produced. If the therapist does not need to understand anything other than the techniques and to simply perform these as instructed verbatim, these questions may not matter. In fact, they are avoided by this approach. This may be one of the reasons for such an approach. However, it is apparent that this approach is not a wholistic one.

The best therapists are those who have a consistent perspective and a thorough grounding in the theoretical and practical skills of their modality. As free-thinking independent therapists, they are capable of making decisions by firstly choosing the appropriate techniques for a given situation with understanding and insight, knowledge and intuition. They are then capable of tailoring a treatment to the needs of the individual.

If you believe everyone is the same and you are treating a dis-ease, then perhaps this does not matter. But if you are helping a unique individual, it does matter. This is the choice all Reflexologists face.

"I do not wish to produce mechanics who do not understand what they are doing and why. The challenge for a therapist is to turn the science of Reflexology into their own unique art. To achieve this, anyone using Reflexology needs an excellent understanding of the basics."

CHAPTER 2
Why the Feet? A Sacred Art

The beauty of Reflexology is that everything you need to work is taken with you wherever you go: your knowledge and understanding, and your hands. I have worked feet in the strangest of places: the street, intermission at the theatre, buses, trains and airplanes, beaches, park benches: anywhere and everywhere. There is no other therapy so mobile and easily accessed as Reflexology.

A much neglected and yet profound insight is that Reflexology is the only body therapy that can work from the inside. This imbues Reflexology with a huge advantage over all other body therapies, as these have to work through the bulk of the body (layers of muscles) to access the inner or the deep structures. Reflexology does not. Why? This will be explained in more detail in Chapter 7: Anatomical Reflection Theory, but briefly, if the two feet reflect the whole body, and each foot is half the body (front, back, outside and inside), then the inside of the feet reflects the inner body, allowing Reflexology to work from the inside without having to work through the bulk. This is a huge advantage when treating a person with Reflexology.

WORKING THE HUMAN BEING THROUGH THE FEET

Reflexology does not work the feet, but the human being through the medium of the feet as the door. The key to unlocking that door is Reflexology. This is important as the purpose of Reflexology is to work with the human being to help the body achieve its aim, which is healing and balance. 'Foot problems' may be helped with Reflexology, but are not its primary focus which is to work with the entire human being.

This is another important aspect in which Reflexology differs from other therapies, and therefore nothing should be done to the feet that would not be appropriate for the body. (This will be explained further in Chapter 19, "Holding the Person, Holding the Feet")

WHY THE FEET?

Why use this medium: the Feet? There are a number of reasons for this that need to be clarified and explained. They are:

1. REFLEXOLOGY IS NON-THREATENING:
The most obvious reason for this is that, unlike other body therapies, you do not have to take your clothes off. Many people, especially the young and mature, are reluctant to do this. Taking your clothes off also brings up questions of propriety, decency, appropriateness, safety, etc in the mind of the receiver, which does not occur with Reflexology. Very few people, if anyone, feel in any way threatened by removed shoes ands socks.

2. EXTERNAL TO INTERNAL: THE FEET ARE ONE OF THE FOUR REFLECTIONS:
There are four parts of the body that reflect the whole, or four external structures which reflect internal structures.

These are the eyes, ears, feet and hands and the associated therapies that go with them are:

- Iridology, the diagnostic tool used to read the internal through the eyes
- Auricular therapy, performed on the ears
- Reflexology, practiced on the feet and/or the hands.

All these reflections are based on the same premise of the individual and external part of the body reflecting the whole, and further, each of these reflections is a mirror image of the body reflected anatomically accurately and in the foetal position.

3. NERVE ENDINGS IN THE HANDS AND FEET:

On a purely physical level, the hands and feet occupy a disproportionate share of the brain due to the fact that they together comprise our major sensory organ of touch. It is through the hands and feet that we interact with the outside world, and there are far more nerve ends in these structures which enable the body to sense what is happening in the outside world. In fact the hands and feet are covered with nerve endings or nerve receptors. This makes them the most sensitive of all structures of the body, much more so than the eyes and ears or anywhere else for that matter. This is part of the explanation of the Nervous System Theory of Reflexology, which will be discussed later (Chapter 8) in detail.

4. THE FEET AS OUR INSTRUMENT OF MOVEMENT:

The feet, unlike the hands, are our instrument of movement. It is through the action of the feet that we are able to move. The hands grasp and the feet walk. This is a minor but significant difference. The feet get us moving, keep us moving, and movement brings about change. So, on a physical and psychological level the feet are a very important factor in both external and internal movement and change. All ancient cultures (India, China, Egypt, Northern and Southern American Indians, Australian Aborigines and other native cultures) realised this and so placed significance on the feet.

For example, ancient artworks show bare feet, feet of religious figures, religious 'foot maps', foot binding, ritual dance, stamping, foot cleansing and foot baths. All the most ancient civilizations on earth have significant references to the feet, including religions such as Buddhism, Hinduism, Judaism and Christianity. Working the instrument of movement is in itself a significant aspect of change and therefore has an impact on the health, healing and wellbeing of the human being.

5. THE COMPUTER (BRAIN/MIND) AT WORK:

Another important aspect of the significance of the feet is that the brain/mind or computer of the human being has learnt to override the body. With the elevation of the brain/mind over the spirit and increased knowledge about the physical functioning of the body, the computer has learnt not only to ignore the body's messages, but also to over-ride them. Experience has demonstrated that the body is no longer as accurate as it should be.

This is evidenced by the fact that messages (e.g. pain) from the torso are not as reliable as they should be when it comes to reporting what is happening to and within the body. The computer has learnt, largely through experience and programming, to modify, alter, or switch off the messages/signals the body puts out. For example, on a purely physical level, the nerve impulses (messages) from the body go via the Central Nervous System and spinal chord to the brain where these impulses or messages are interpreted by the brain/mind (via previous knowledge and programming), and a response is generated. This same process happens not only on a physical level but also on an emotional, mental and spiritual level as well.

The computer or brain/mind has not yet learnt to override the messages of the feet. With the hands this is not the case: for example, hand/eye coordination links the brain/mind more consciously with the hands. The feet act as instruments of movement and change and as a reflection of the whole human being, and therefore are still reliable and accurate reflections of the whole. Experience over the years continues to confirm this.

Furthermore, the computer or brain/mind is not the human being. It is but the instrument of creation and destruction, depending on how it is used. Many argue that it is the human being, but it is not. So much actually happens within the human being independent of the computer/ brain/mind. For example, many vital processes, such as cellular communications, occur without computer involvement. This point is vital to understand why I talk about 'working with the body' rather than the computer, brain or mind. Experience has demonstrated repeatedly that the body understands so much more than the computer, which works via programming, just like your home computer. There is so much to this point and we have only just begun to scratch the surface of our understanding of the human being.

6. Reflexology is a Balanced Therapy (Yin and Yang):

When performing Reflexology, one works on the feet with the hands. This is significant as the hands are yang (active and doing) compared to the feet, which are yin (receptive). The reason for this is that the human being stands on the earth but reaches for the heavens, and so heaven energy, universal energy or God's energy, which is yang, enters the human being through the upraised hands and arms, and flows down into the earth through the human's feet. At the same time, Earth's energy, which is yin, flows upwards entering the body through the feet. This is the explanation of the Chinese energy flow system called Meridians. The Yin Meridians flow upwards from the feet and the Yang meridians flow downward from the hands.

Therefore the hands working on the feet complete the picture: Heaven's energy joining with Earth's energy; or to put it another way, the hands, a yang instrument, working upon the feet, which is yin. And so, by its very nature, working the feet (yin) with the hands (yang) is innately balancing.

7. THE FEET NURTURE AND CLEANSE ON AN ENERGY LEVEL:

The feet are the most yin structure compared to the rest of the body. Yin is the deeper and more powerful, while yang is more superficial. The feet are particularly important as the first destination of yin (Earth) energy. Yin energy, compared to yang, is nurturing, deep and powerful, feminine and gentle. The role of yin energy is to nurture, feed and cleanse. This is a very significant and vital role.

Expanding this theory further, it is not by accident that in the Chinese system there is only one acu-point on the sole of the foot, which is acu-point Kidney 1 (the beginning of the Kidney meridian). Its name is Bubbling Spring, signifying the beginning of the flow of water (yin energy) from the Earth upwards to nourish life. Thus it is through this acu-point that the Chinese theory explains how the human being is nurtured by yin energy. It is the root or foundation of each individual human being's on-going life. You can't get more important than this.

So, it is through the soles of the feet that yin energy enters the body and nurtures and feeds the whole structure. But the feet are also the instrument of cleansing via the Bladder (the partner of the Kidney) meridian. Its role is to connect to every structure, organ, cell and atom of the body and take used-up or waste energy and drain it down through the body into Mother Earth through the feet and especially, and specifically, via the fifth digit or little toe.

Therefore the feet are the entrance point of yin/Earth energy and the exit point of yang/Heaven's energy. This is why the feet are the most powerful and significant of the external areas of the body that reflect the whole.

8. MOTHER/CHILD RELATIONSHIP: A SACRED ART:

The feet are our connection to the earth, and the earth (yin) is our mother who nurtures and cleanses us through our feet. We, as human beings, connect to Mother energy through our feet. All of us therefore are the children of Mother Earth. The relationship between a mother and child is the first and most significant of all the relationships we human beings have. It is also the most powerful of all relationships, whether we realise that consciously or not. Our mother brings us into the world (ashes to ashes, dust to dust) making this a powerful and sacred relationship. A mother nurtures her child, takes care, feeds, and cleanses her child. This is the yin relationship of Mother Earth and her children, humanity. It is a yin, nurturing and extremely important, powerful and sacred relationship. Ask any mother and you will quickly see the deep bond that is formed. So the feet deserve a great deal of respect and when working the feet one is becoming a bridge between Mother Earth and one of her children. Thus one is entering this most primal, basic and sacred of all relationships. It is the foundation relationship upon which all others are based. Ancient native cultures understood this connection, but it has been forgotten over the eons. Reflexology, whether consciously or not, provides a reconnection.

Foot Reflexology is the only therapy where this is the case. When one practises Reflexology, one is not only working a powerful reflection of the whole human being, but also entering the most sacred and sanctified of all relationships, that of mother and child. The Reflexologist by virtue of working on a person's feet is being placed squarely between the child (the receiver) and his/her mother; The earth beneath thy feet. Therefore whether the receivers are conscious of this or not, the body knows they are entering into this most sacred of relationships. This is not an authoritarian, dictatorial, restricting, or abusive relationship, but rather a gentle, nurturing and loving one. Thus, when performing Reflexology the giver needs to demonstrate the deepest of respect and honour to the receiver and their mother the earth, by respecting this relationship, by promising to 'Do no harm' and by offering themselves to the receiver as a nurturing intermediary. The practitioner gives oneself over to the process of the receiver rather than working the feet.

This is a major reason that a standard stimulation-type approach is especially inappropriate when working the feet. Stimulation by its very nature is a yang approach and is not as appropriate for the feet. The feet are asking for nurturing, cleansing and helping. Once you realise this, and you show the feet the respect they deserve, you will find that the human being opens to you, allowing you access and letting you in.

If you ever experience this connection you will know of its power for good and the huge responsibility that comes with it. There is nothing like entering this relationship and the body opening to you. It is the most wonderful and extraordinary of experiences, but with it comes a huge responsibility, for once the body lets you in, its defences are down, and you are capable of anything. An awesome experience with an awesome responsibility, which is why it is extremely important to 'err on the side of caution' while performing Reflexology: 'If in doubt, don't!'

A significant aside is that the majority of Reflexologists around the world are women, approximately eighty to ninety per cent as a guess-stimate. Perhaps intuitively women are drawn to Reflexology as they innately understand this most powerful and primal of relationships, that of mother and child.

One last point worth reiterating is that you are not working the feet but the entire human being, including all aspects through the feet. The feet are the medium in to the human condition and so each section of the foot represents a part of the body.

One should do nothing to the feet that one would not do to the body. In this way you are demonstrating an extremely important expression of deep respect, responsibility, love and true consideration and value of the human being. This is another benefit that has evolved from the mother/child relationship and the sacred art of Foot Reflexology.

CHAPTER 3
What is Foot Reflexology and What is Not?

Anything that involves working the feet in any form has come to be considered as Reflexology. This is the broadest definition of Reflexology, and one that many would use. However, it is not correct. There are significant differences between Reflexology and other foot treatments including and especially foot massage.

WHAT IS NOT REFLEXOLOGY?

A foot (or hand) massage is not Reflexology. There are significant differences between massaging the feet and Reflexology. Many aromatherapy, massage and body therapy trainings have included a module of reflexology (broadest definition of the term), but very few of these trainings are actually Reflexology. Foot massage differs significantly from Reflexology. They are not the same therapy, nor do they have the same therapeutic basis, history, science, art and benefits. In fact they are significantly different.

ILLUSTRATION 1: Table: Reflexology vs. Massage (Foot Massage)

REFLEXOLOGY	MASSAGE (Foot Massage)
1. Reflexology uses no oils, creams, lotions and potions on the feet.	1. Massage usually uses a carrier oil other lubrication such as essential o
2. Reflexology uses significantly different and specific relaxers/openings and treatment techniques, such as thumb and finger walking	2. Massage uses massage techniques, s as effleurage, on the foot.
3. Reflexology works the human being through the feet, rather than working the feet, i.e. all physical, emotional, mental and spiritual aspects are worked through the feet.	3. Massage is massaging the feet and structures (e.g. muscles, tendons, l ment, fascia, nerves, etc.) of the feet
4. Reflexology works just the feet (and possibly the hands and ears), which are all reflections of the human being.	4. Massage works the whole body, inc ing the feet as a structure of the bod
5. Reflexology does not diagnose dis-ease through the feet	5. Massage may use the foot diagnostic *NOTE*: Some body therapists have b taught to use the feet diagnostically
6. Reflexology accesses individual reflexes in the feet that need treatment and Reflexologists understand where the reflexes are and how to treat them.	6. Massage works the whole foot, with emphasis on working the muscles tissues of the feet, and perhaps all reflexes as well.
7. Reflexology is a method of aiding the body to heal itself, working all the systems of the body through the feet.	7. Massage emphasises the muscular skeletal systems when working.
8. Reflexology does not use massage techniques	8. Massage uses massage techniques.
9. The benefits of Reflexology are not the same as those of massage, although they may include these. Reflexology is therapeutic in nature as the emphasis is on treating imbalances.	9. The benefits of massage are less spe and more general in their applicat with an emphasis on relaxation, working through the skeletal and r cular systems.
10. Reflexology has its own history and development separate from massage.	10. Massage has its own history and de opment separate from Reflexology.
11. Reflexology has never attempted to incorporate massage into its theoretical and practical approach.	11. Massage has attempted to inco rate Reflexology into its theoretical practical approach.
12. Specialist Reflexology training institutions are independent of massage trainings.	12. Massage trainings often incorpo foot massage (which is termed Refl ogy).
13. Relatively short historical development of Reflexology: a little over one hundred years. Reflexology does not have any significant historical tradition.	13. Massage has a longer and more an historical context than Reflexology.

It is obvious that Reflexology and foot massage are not the same thing and yet, as they both are body therapies, they have many similar characteristics which have made the independent development of the profession of Reflexology more difficult. It is a pity that Reflexology and Massage (and specifically foot massage) have tended to be combined, to the detriment of Reflexology as a legitimate and independent natural therapy profession. It is also a pity that this combination has resulted in a blending of the two and a blurring of the boundaries between them. For example, the contra-indications and/or safety precautions of Reflexology are actually those of massage (See Chapter 22 for more details), and in fact have been taken from massage.

The last point mentioned above (history) is significant and is one of the major reasons that Massage and Reflexology have been blended together, as is the fact that massage, having a longer historical tradition, has tended to incorporate Reflexology (and other body therapies) into its domain. Further, Reflexology, with a lack of a long historical tradition was initially linked with massage to gain acceptance. Often massage therapists have expanded their therapeutic approaches by learning Reflexology, further blurring the boundaries, and this is still currently the case.

There is another historical reason for this blurring. Reflexology, as we have it today, began in the USA and to this day Reflexology has had great difficulty in the US standing on its own two feet, although Reflexology has tried and is currently making in-roads. Nevertheless, many US States have legislated Reflexology under massage, and to perform Reflexology, one must be a registered massage therapist.

It is about time that Reflexology stood on its own two feet (excuse the pun) as a separate therapeutic approach. This is one of the major challenges that lie ahead. Reflexology is a natural therapy profession, with its own unique therapeutic science and art as well as history.

So, WHAT IS REFLEXOLOGY?

Reflexology is a unique science and art for promoting balance and wellbeing. It has its own evolution separate from other body therapies and is based on the Anatomical Reflection Theory. The basic techniques of Reflexology are the use of specific thumb and finger techniques on areas of the feet that correspond to all aspects of the human being.

Reflexology is both a science and an art. It is a unique therapy of working specifically with the feet (and hands) to activate the natural healing potential of the human being. It is based on the premise that there are four superficial structures of the human being that reflect the whole and that the feet (and hands) reflect the human being as they are, and anatomically accurately, which allows the feet (and hands) to be used to access all aspects of the human condition. It is a therapy and a treatment designed to activate the healing potential within each human being.

As a science, Reflexology requires medical and scientific knowledge, including an understanding of the body's anatomy and physiology, as well as a sound and practical knowledge of the theory and practice of Reflexology. Unique practical skills need to be learnt, developed and practiced until the Reflexologist is competent in their implications and application to the human being.

As an art, the Reflexologists, armed with the science, use their dedication, patience, intention and intuitive abilities to shape the tool of Reflexology into their own hand for the benefit of others. The art therefore is the unique quality brought to the therapy of Reflexology by each individual Reflexologist working through knowledge, understanding and compassion. So, Reflexology brings to the therapeutic situation unique skills for accessing the healing potential of the individual, which is best achieved through the foundation of knowledge and the practical application of this knowledge through the incorporation of each individual Reflexologist's uniqueness: the production of artists rather than mechanics.

Reflexology as a medical science, and as an art form, is expanding both in its theoretical and practical applications. It is past time for Reflexology to step out of the shadows and into its rightful position as a legitimate and professional therapy, with professional qualified Reflexologists recognised by a professional Reflexology association or natural therapies association, and not a massage organisation.

When looking for a Reflexologist, one should look for either:

a) A qualified Reflexologist (with a Reflexology qualification) that is recognised by a national Reflexology professional organisation in your country,

OR SECONDLY

b) A qualified Reflexologist (with a Reflexology qualification) that is recognised by a national natural therapies professional organisation,

OR THIRDLY

c) A qualified Reflexologist (with a Reflexology qualification) that is recognised preferably by the national health system professional organisation.

Even once you find a Reflexologist ask them some simple questions about their qualifications and experience, such as:

1. Explain Reflexology?
2. What Reflexology qualification do you hold?
3. Where did you train?
4. Are you a member (eligible for membership) of a professional Reflexology organisation?
5. What professional associations are you a member of?
6. Do you have current professional and public liability insurance?

These questions should be a good guide to the professional standing of the Reflexologist. For example, if they are in a professional association and it is a massage one, follow this up with: Are you eligible for membership of the national professional Reflexology Association? Also question the Reflexologists about Reflexology to gain an insight into the level of their understanding.

> **NOTE** – The general standard of training for professional membership varies from country to country, and it would be worth finding out what the minimum standard for professional recognition is in your country, state or area before searching for a Reflexologist.

CHAPTER 4
Why Reflexology? What can it do?

Reflexology, like other body therapies, has had difficulty defining the purpose of its therapy. This had led to confusion among the health care system and the general public, and thus Reflexology has done itself a disservice. Ask any Reflexologist the question: What can Reflexology do? and they will answer vaguely about the general benefits, ranging from relaxation and stress reduction to treating all types of imbalances. That is,

Reflexology is anything and everything. Whatever you want.

OR

Anything and everything for anyone and everyone.

One can begin to see the connection to massage and other body therapies, and the vagueness that this engenders firstly in the Reflexologist and secondly in the eyes of the health care system as well as those of the general public. This is another dilemma Reflexology needs to confront.

Is Reflexology a therapy? What type of therapy is it? These questions so far have been largely ignored. Reflexology can be used as a beauty therapy, and/or as relaxation and feel good therapy. By this approach Reflexology, by working all the reflexes, is very similar to a general massage: work everything and help people feel better. Another dilemma. This is, however, a valid and useful therapeutic approach. Many argue that this type of approach is therapeutic, but it is not treating anything specifically.

At the other end of the scale, Reflexology as a therapy is an approach designed to assist the body to heal itself via the treating of specific reflexes for specific purposes. And so, at this end of the spectrum, Reflexology is a therapy that can help the body to deal with all forms and types of imbalances superficially (externally) and within the human being.

The profession of Reflexology needs to decide what is done and why. This will then lead to how to work. The choices are:

1. **Reflexology as Beauty and Relaxation Therapy:** Work all the feet (human being) and cover everything; OR
2. **Reflexology as a Therapy:** Work the reflexes in the feet that are relevant to specific imbalances, and then balance the human being to encourage healing to occur.

Reflexology, therefore, can be (and I would argue should be) divided into at least two distinct professional groups:

1. Relaxation or Salon Reflexology, and
2. Professional Therapeutic Reflexology or Clinical Reflexology.

RELAXATION or SALON REFLEXOLOGY

This is the older approach to Reflexology and has evolved from massage, or perhaps due to its link to massage. This approach involves ALWAYS working all the reflexes of the feet in a specific order every time, i.e. all the reflexes of one foot (preferably the left) and then work all the reflexes of the other foot.

> **NOTE** – This approach of working all the reflexes of one foot and then the other, is slowly evolving towards working both feet together as it is more therapeutic to work the complete reflexes (both halves as it were) together.

Then either:

a) Spend more time and effort on sore/tender (out of balance) reflexes as they arise, OR

b) Work both feet and all reflexes completely and then go back over the sore/tender (out of balance) reflexes after finishing each or both feet.

Such is based on the belief that by stimulating ALL the reflexes one is activating the healing potential of the human being, and so it emphasises the benefits of stress reduction and relaxation. It is a valid and useful general tool of wellbeing and health maintenance, and so the other aspect of this approach, which is emphasised, is the feel good aspect and preventative health care.

Further, as a result of this stimulation approach which stimulates everything, there are more dangers involved (Contraindications and/or Safety Precautions), and so the Reflexologist is advised not to work on receivers who have dis-eases. They can however, work on receivers who have everyday, run-of-the-mill problems.

As Reflexologists are only aiming to relax and decrease stress, any other outcomes are the result of simply, through relaxation and stress reduction, the human being's own healing potential. So the tendency here is for the Reflexologist to lay claim to the positive results and the negative ones are the result of the healing crisis.

Under this approach, the Reflexologist needs only a general knowledge of the theory upon which Reflexology is based, including only a generalised understanding of the Anatomical Reflection Theory. Accuracy is not necessary as everything is worked. There is little need for a thorough and detailed theoretical understanding of Reflexology, including and especially where the reflexes are in the feet. All that is necessary is to learn the sequence and skills necessary to perform the sequence, and then use it every time.

It produces mechanic-type Reflexologists who always do the same thing every time. This is the preferred module as it is easier to justify and more likely to gain recognition and acceptance. It also makes very few claims that may be considered controversial. It is designed to be appealing to everyone, and therefore safe and non-threatening. Further this approach emphasises promotion and recognition as its first and foremost aim.

PROFESSIONAL THERAPUETIC REFLEXOLOGY or CLINICAL REFLEXOLOGY

The other approach is the professional therapeutic Reflexology or Clinical Reflexology method, which includes all the benefits mentioned above, but with the emphasis on a consultation and treatment of imbalances, and on helping the receiver more specifically. So, relaxation and stress reduction does not have to be emphasised and in fact are a result of the treatment rather than the aim.

This approach, which has evolved more recently (and is still evolving), rather than working all the reflexes, involves learning how to work all the reflexes and then tailoring the treatment to the needs of the receiver. It also involves working the reflexes (across the feet) together and at the same time. This is more therapeutic as, for example, the head and neck (toes) are worked together, which is more therapeutic than working half the head (toes) and then approximately thirty minutes later, working the other half. This allows the Reflexologist to target the specific reflexes of the imbalance and to concentrate on these. As a result, in practice, it becomes increasingly more difficult to work all the reflexes. This working of all the reflexes actually does not therapeutically make a great deal of sense when you consider that not everything is involved in specific imbalances. Does everything need stimulating? Why stimulate everything?

Under this approach a greater range of practical tools are learnt, from which the Reflexologist can draw: Not only thumb and finger walking techniques but also stimulating and sedating as well as balancing techniques. So the Reflexologist has at his or her disposal a greater range of options, which is part of the reason that it is more therapeutic. Further, it is not simply a one-dimensional stimulation approach.

Under this approach, the Reflexologist needs a thorough theoretical understanding of the principles and applications of Reflexology as a health care and therapeutic modality, including Anatomy and Physiology (A & P) and especially the Anatomical Reflection Theory. This should also include an examination of the professional, ethical and moral aspects of the healing process.

Reflexologists as professional therapists need to understand their role in the healing process and the inherent dangers to be able to make an informed decision about what to do, when and how. The Hippocratic Oath should be paramount here: '*I shall do no harm.*' Working physically has risks involved, but the more wholistically one works, the greater responsibility there is involved. Knowledge is the key here: To work consciously rather than unconsciously, and to work from the premise of

- **If in doubt, don't** and/or
- **If in doubt, balance, and assist the body to do what it needs to do**.

This approach develops free-thinking, conscious and sensitive Reflexologists who have at their fingertips a variety of tools from which to choose. This also means that each treatment on a single receiver is unique. It is the more therapeutic approach, but also the more challenging one.

The benefits of this approach, is that it is designed to treat imbalances and to help the receivers, and therefore the aim is more specific and tailored to the needs of the individual. These benefits are that the Reflexologist works with the body, aiming to help assist the body to achieve its aims. It increases, as a Reflexologist works more consciously, the possibility of healing occurring.

This approach, however, brings with it different and a greater range of risks and responsibilities. Clinical Reflexology is more therapeutic and therefore more profound, in both a positive and negative sense of the word. The answer lies in knowledge and understanding, and being professional and responsible for the role one plays in the healing process.

These two distinct types of Reflexology so far have been mixed, linked and blurred together to promote the benefits of Reflexology. Both of these approaches have their advantages and disadvantages, and it is firstly the choice of each and every Reflexologist to decide these issues, and then to present themselves and their therapy clearly: another issue the Reflexology community needs to confront.

CHAPTER 5
The Don'ts of Reflexology

There are three DON'Ts of Reflexology and they are:
- No. 1: **NEVER DIAGNOSE**
- No. 2: **NEVER NAME A DISEASE**
- No. 3: **NEVER TREAT ONLY SPECIFIC CONDITIONS**.
  Rather ALWAYS treat the WHOLE PERSON by work-
  ing BOTH FEET and all reflexes, **but you can either**:
  a) Spend more time and effort on sore/tender reflexes as
     they arise, OR
  b) Work both feet completely and then go back over sore/
     tender reflexes after finishing each or both feet.

Let's look at each of these individually.

1. NEVER DIAGNOSE

This is the standard line taken by Reflexology, but the truth
of the matter is that all Reflexologists do diagnose. Diagnosing
will be looked at in greater detail in Chapter 26. But briefly,
how do Reflexologists diagnose?
  a) KNOWLEDGE: Initially a Reflexologist diagnoses by tak-
     ing a detailed medical and life history of the receiver before
     beginning to work on them, and the Reflexologist transfers
     the imbalances from the body to the reflexes of the feet. For
     example, take a person with a knee problem: the Reflexolo-
     gist notes down to work the knee reflex on both feet. This is

diagnosis.

b) LOOK & SEE & TRANSFER: Secondly, by looking at the reflexes of the feet, the Reflexologist gathers information on the imbalances found in the feet and then, via the Anatomical Reflection Theory (See Chapter 17), transfers the seen imbalance to the region of the body. Again, this is diagnosis.

c) TOUCH & FEEL & TRANSFER: Thirdly, while working the feet the Reflexologist often picks up imbalances in the reflexes of the feet and once more via the Anatomical Reflection Theory transfers the felt imbalance/s to the region of the body. Once more, this is diagnosis.

These forms of diagnosis are for the Reflexologist and not the receiver. The whole purpose of this form of diagnostics is to make the treatment as specific and accurate for the receiver as possible. Telling the receiver is a mistake that some Reflexologists make and it is an important error in judgment as there are always options rather than answers. All a Reflexologists can be sure about is the fact that an imbalance in a particular part of the foot is reflecting an imbalance in the related part of the body, and as there are so many different structures in any particular part of the body (such as skin, bones, muscles, tendons, ligaments, fascia, organs etc) and the fact that the body is three-dimensional and therefore the imbalance may be front, inside or even back, it is extremely difficult to be certain as to what is actually being reflected. The Reflexologist should note down what he/she thinks it is, but it is a mistake to inform the receiver of this, as it may not be correct. As well the Reflexologist is assuming that an imbalance noted is a physical one and this is not necessarily the case (and in fact often it isn't). An imbalance can manifest on a physical level, but it is also just as likely to manifest on an emotional, mental and/or spiritual level, and so the Reflexologist is on very shaky ground here.

Simply take not of what is seen and felt and work accordingly, but do not inform the receiver as you may do harm.

Better to diagnose imbalance rather than dis-ease.

2. NEVER NAME A DIS-EASE

Reflexologists should never name a dis-ease, or even a particular organ. Why?

Firstly because some argue that only a medically qualified health care provider has the legal and moral right to diagnose. This may in fact be correct, but there is a more important reason for not diagnosing dis-ease: such could lead to the Reflexologist treating a dis-ease and thus a label rather than helping a human being.

The other question here that needs mentioning is that Reflexologists have been known to tell receivers what they have found and plant the seed of disharmony, which may or may not be correct, and the Reflexologist relies on the chart they have been taught from. Furthermore, the Reflexologist risks their professional credibility. If incorrect, they have done harm to the receiver, to themselves and to the profession of Reflexology.

However, if one is absolutely certain that there is a major physical problem manifesting in the feet, then one has a moral obligation to inform the receiver of this. But what is important here is how this is done rather than actually doing it. In this scenario, which is extremely rare, the Reflexologist needs to inform the receiver that:

1. First and foremost, the Reflexologist is ONLY passing this information on as a concerned person and a professional, ethical Reflexologist.
2. The Reflexologist may be completely wrong.
3. It may just be an imbalance and nothing more (in other words, down play the situation).
4. From the Reflexologist's experience and knowledge, it may be a physical problem in this area of your body. Do not name a specific organ, dis-ease or label as there are always options.

This is one of the major problems with so many of the charts, which by nature are one dimensional and give the impression that the major organ in that area of the foot/body is the only thing that it could be. For example, in the upper abdomen it could be the organs in this area of the body, but it is just as possible that it could be skin, muscles, tendon/ligaments, fascia, bones, etc in the upper abdomen, and as the feet and body are three dimensional, it could even be the mid-back and all the structures found there.

5. The Reflexologist recommends that the receiver get a second opinion by visiting their health care provider and if necessary provides a referral for this purpose.

Following on from this, Reflexologists are often asked when something is tender: *'What's that?'*

Initially while learning, and in the early stages of becoming a professional Reflexologist, the tendency is to tell the receiver. This is partly for learning purposes so as to gain a better understanding of the feet and the Anatomical Reflection Theory, as well as to convince the giver that Reflexology actually works. This is understandable but it is not a valid reason.

What would be better is to simply ask a question. Something like: *'Do you have a problem in this or that area of the body, front and/or back?'*

Often this question alone triggers the receiver's memory and they will explain what you have picked up and what they have felt themselves. This is as far as one needs to go, but do make a note of this on your consultation sheets for present and future reference, i.e. what needs to be done.

However, the best option here is to downplay the whole process by:

1. Initially, if possible, giving the receiver back information they have already given the Reflexologist (from the medical and personal history taken before working). However, the Reflexologist should take note of this as it could be this but

could also be something else. It is the body's way of giving the Reflexologist a message and that message should be listened to. It does not have to be interpreted, just listened to and followed.

2. If this is not possible, the next best option is to state, 'It is just an imbalance. Nothing to worry about. It is no major problem and easy to rectify.' That is what the Chinese call psychological healing: the planting of no negatives.

3. If the receiver does not accept this explanation, the next best option is simply to give a region of the body. For example, if it is something in the head/neck region (toes), simply state that it is an imbalance in that area of the body, probably once again something simple, e.g. neck tension.

This is the most that should be conveyed to the receiver as again it is actually a message to the Reflexologist from the body that it needs help and should always be followed. Listen to the body, interpret the message and then obey the message. It is as simple as that.

All Reflexologist should do is diagnose an 'imbalance', which by its very nature is relative neutral, fairly simple to correct and of no major significance. This phrase is extremely general and neutral and therefore plants no seeds of destructive thought, action or emotion. It is the best option.

3. NEVER TREAT ONLY SPECIFIC CONDITIONS Rather ALWAYS treat the WHOLE PERSON by working BOTH FEET

This is once again the standard response from Reflexology and if the Reflexologist is working as a mechanic then it may be possible. For relaxation, general tone up, feel good response, and stress reduction this can probably be done, but if Reflexology is more than this, then experience demonstrates that this approach is increasingly more difficult to follow. As one begins to treat specific imbalances and their related helper areas (See Chapter 12 for an explanation of helper areas) and one begins to follow the messages of the body, it becomes increasingly more difficult to work the whole person by working both feet and all reflexes.

There is another problem with this approach. If a receiver is paying a Reflexologist to treat a specific problem then it is irresponsible and unprofessional of the Reflexologist not to do what they are being paid to do. So as a professional Reflexologist the number one priority should be what the receiver has asked for.

And what if this takes the whole time period? Again, experience is that in practice if one is treating and helping the body, one cannot always treat all the reflexes. There are so many restraints on a treatment that this is just not always possible, which is why another method of treating everything is needed to give the Reflexologist more flexibility: a sequence to balance the whole body in a few minutes. This way a Reflexologist can concentrate on what they are being asked to do and they can also listen and follow the messages of the body as they arise.

So a basic sequence of treatment would be:

1. Openings/Relaxers;
2. What the receiver has asked for;
3. Related reflexes/areas of the body (e.g. the system in which the imbalance is located and the related helper areas); and finally,
4. Balancing the whole system at the end.

NEVER TREAT ONLY SPECIFIC CONDITIONS. Rather ALWAYS treat the WHOLE PERSON by working BOTH FEET,

BUT YOU CAN: A) SPEND MORE TIME AND EFFORT ON SORE/TENDER REFLEXES AS THEY ARISE.

If one is going to work this way that is, working all the reflexes and the whole person by working both feet, this option

the Australian aborigines have incidences of foot use: in some tribes or clans women when menstruating were isolated from the group and tied stones to their heels. This is interesting but is not a complete therapeutic approach to the feet. So far this is the type of piece-meal evidence that has surfaced. It is interesting and lends support to the belief that Reflexology is an ancient therapy, but does not prove that this is in fact the case. All it does prove is that ancient cultures knew the feet were significant in many different ways, including for health purposes. Perhaps the reason that there is so little evidence is that most of these ancient cultures that appear to have used the feet therapeutically tended to be cultures that did not have a tradition of a written language and therefore did not keep detailed records.

So it can be argued fairly confidently that all ancient cultures saw the feet as more than just the instruments of movement, also seeing them as spiritual, cultural and perhaps therapeutic instruments.

There are currently no detailed records of the feet being used as a therapy in ancient cultures. There are plenty of ancient foot maps that may in fact be therapeutic maps of the feet, but the understanding of what these mean and their relevance to the therapy of Reflexology as we have it today is questionable.

Ancient maps and illustrations relating to the feet that are currently available do indicate the importance that so many ancient cultures placed on the feet, but do they indicate that foot therapy (Reflexology) was part of their cultures? The simple answer is no. As to the maps, we have lost the means to understand and interpret them. We are unable to translate them, especially into anything that can be significantly related to the therapy of Reflexology. The maps are more than likely not physical ones, but rather religious and/or spirituals ones, for many are representations of Buddha's feet, or the god, Vishnu's feet. When one compares these illustrations to

Reflexology Foot maps little or no correlations can be found. Our current understanding of both the ancient foot maps and Reflexology is such that we are unable to put them together in any meaningful therapeutic way.

A particular piece of evidence that needs discussing is the relief found on the tomb wall of the ancient Egyptian doctor Ankhmahor from about 2,500BC. This relief is of Ankhmahor working the hands and feet. The hieroglyphs above the scene reads: "Do not let it be painful" and the attendants reply: "I do as you please." This is extremely encouraging evidence to prove that Reflexology is an ancient therapy. But let's look at this in more detail.

Firstly, let's assume for the moment that this relief actually is showing the feet being used therapeutically. If this assumption is correct, we can then say that one Egyptian physician used the feet (and hands) therapeutically, but there are no other records (written or visual) to explain what this doctor did, when, why and how. Does it relate to Reflexology as we have it today? No one can say with any degree of certainty. Further, does it demonstrate that all Egyptian physicians used the feet therapeutically, and that Reflexology (hand and foot therapy) was used extensively in ancient Egypt? Currently, no other evidence has been found to support this assertion.

Next, an ancient Egyptian physician was much more a doctor and surgeon as we know them today. An ancient Egyptian doctor was everything from a make-up artist, aroma therapist and beautician through to doctor and surgeon. So, for example, this relief could be using the feet therapeutically, but it could also just as likely be manicure and pedicure, and anything and everything in between. There is not enough evidence to be sure. This physician could have been especially famous for taking care of hands and feet. The truth is that we cannot tell. It is an interesting piece of evidence for sure, but it is but a piece, and to draw the conclusion that Reflexology, as we have it today, is an ancient therapy from this is a large leap of faith.

An interesting aside is that all the evidence so far discovered (except the Egyptian physician's tomb relief) is in the cultures around the Pacific Ocean: China, Australia, the Americas (North and South), and to a lesser extent Indian. This is interesting in the light of an historical theory that the first major civilisation on earth was located in the Pacific Ocean and that they colonised the world outward from the Pacific. The most ancient sites on earth are located around the Pacific Ocean, which supports this theory. And if this is in fact the case, then perhaps Reflexology was one of the original therapeutic arts that these people discovered and developed and took with them on their journey of colonisation. If so, then perhaps Reflexology is an extremely ancient therapy and one of the original therapies on earth.

A desire rather than a fact, I think.

One last point: Assume that all the evidence listed above and sighted by so many Reflexologists, is in fact foot therapy. Does it support modern Reflexology of today? There is no evidence at all to indicate the therapeutic approaches of ancient cultures.

MODERN HISTORY

Reflexology's history as we have it today is quite modern. The history of Reflexology (Reflex Zone Therapy) begins in the late 1800s in Germany where there is evidence of Zone Theory, pressure points theory and practice on the body being investigated and developed.

The origins of Reflexology are a little over one hundred years old, dating back to the turn of the 19th century. It began within the medical profession in the USA. This is significant as Reflex Zone Therapy, as it was originally called, began and was accepted by the medical fraternity initially. It began with the work of Dr Fitzgerald (1872–1942), a nose, ear and throat specialist and surgeon, who later came to be known as the 'Father of Reflexology'.

Dr Fitzgerald was initially at Boston Hospital but then worked in London for two years where it is believed he visited Germany. It is strongly suspected that he came across the concept of Zone Theory and Zone Therapy while there. This, however, is pure conjecture as Dr Fitzgerald argued he invented Reflex Zone Theory, and never gave any other explanation of its origins.

After his return from London, in around 1909 he discovered Zone Therapy. Dr Fitzgerald, as a surgeon, discovered that he could use implements such as surgical clamps, rubber bands, wooden pegs etc. on parts of the hands and as a result he could numb parts of the body, which resulted in less anaesthetics being needed, less bleeding during surgery and better recovery for his patients. He published his findings in a book, which included his Reflex Zone Theory as the explanation for how this could be accomplished. Dr Fitzgerald postulated that there were ten longitudinal lines of zones dividing the body (five each side of the mid-sagittal plane or longitudinal midline of the body). See illustration below. (SEE also Chapter 8, Part A for a detailed analysis of Zone Theory, as well as Chapter 9, Zone Theory Revised: Energy Flow through the body).

Dr Edwin Bowers worked with Fitzgerald and they co-wrote *Zone Therapy or Relieving Pain in the Home* in 1917, and then published *Zone Therapy or Curing Pain and Disease* in 1919. From here, Fitzgerald began sharing his discovery and Reflex Zone Therapy with other medical practitioners. From 1915 to the 1930s, Reflex Zone Theory was controversial but did meet a degree of success with some doctors and dentists.

Dr Fitzgerald taught Zone Therapy to Dr D. C. Riley, who also published a book called *Zone Therapy Simplified*, which included the ears. In the early 1930s Eunice Ingham, who we would today call a physiotherapist or body therapist, worked with Dr Riley in Florida. Dr Riley encouraged Eunice to ex-

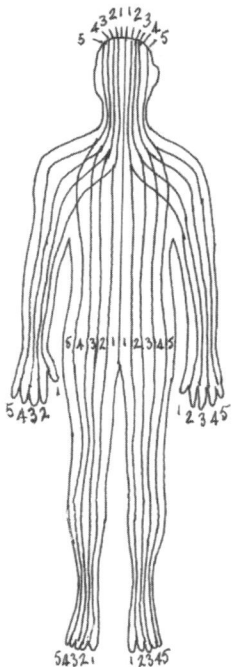

ILLUSTRATION 2: Zone Theory

periment with Zone Therapy. Eunice Ingham, who is considered the 'Mother of Reflexology' or more recently 'Grandmother of Reflexology', made three major contributions to the development of Reflexology or Reflex Zone Therapy. She transferred Reflex Zone Theory and therapy to the feet, developed the practical techniques that are the basis of Reflexology as we have it today, and was the one who took Reflexology to the non-medical community.

Eunice wrote a total of three books: *The Stories the Feet can Tell* published in 1938, *Zone Therapy and Gland Reflexes* in 1945, and *Stories the Feet have Told* in 1951. Unlike the doctors before her, she did not use implements or gadgets on the feet and only worked the feet with her hands. She began teaching her techniques within the medical profession, but as you can image, being a woman and a non-medical practitioner (not a doctor) she was banned by the American Medical Association. This is the point at which Reflexology (Reflex Zone Therapy) and the medical profession parted company. Eunice could no longer share her approach within the medical profession and so she took it to a wider community. From here onwards she spent her summer holidays traveling around North America, teaching anyone interested in learning. These were mainly such professions are physiotherapists, chiropractors and other body therapists that at this time were not medically recognised.

By 1949, this had grown to the point that she enlisted the help of her nephew Dwight Byers to help her teach Reflexology. Dwight Byers formed the International Institute of Reflexology and wrote his own book *Better Health with Foot Reflexology* in 1960, as well as putting together the Institute of Reflexology's foot chart. Eunice Ingham retired from teaching in 1970 and died in 1974. Dwight continued her work and it was he who took Reflexology to the world, lecturing for the first time outside of North America, even presenting in Australia in the early 1980s. So, with a few exceptions, Reflexology only left North America very recently and it has spread the world in a short space of time, an important and significant fact.

So Reflexology or Reflex Zone Therapy can be traced back to one person, Eunice Ingham, and was spread around the world by her and her nephew Dwight Byers.

From this beginning, Reflexology has, within some two to three generations, spread around the world to the point that Reflexology can be found in just about every country on earth. This is an amazing and rapid expansion for such a modern therapy. Dwight Byers' emphasis for Reflexology has been its propagation, and the control of the purity of his aunt's achievement. He will be remembered for the spread of Reflexology into a globally recognised natural therapy. This, however, has had a number of significant consequences:

1. Firstly, the rapid global spread of Reflexology
2. The existence of a variety of Reflexology charts and books as Dwight has attempted to maintain control of Reflexology teaching and products. Therefore, those who wanted to go into print on Reflexology had to make sure they did not break the copyright laws, resulting in literally thousands of Reflexology chart variations. These are, once recognised, not significantly different from the original.
3. The price of this expansion and control has been the lack of critical analysis of Reflexology as a science, art and therapy. Reflexology has concentrated on promotions, recognition and expansion with little time for critical analysis, and detailed understanding of Reflexology until extremely recently.

As a result, there have been little or no significant developments in Reflexology from the Eunice's & Dwight's original approach from the 1930s to the 1990s. However, in the 1990s the process of development and expansion of the theory and practice of Reflexology began. Christine Stormer, a nurse and Reflexologist from South Africa, was the first to question the original approach and thus initiate this process. Chris developed the first significantly different Reflexology foot chart and published a number of books, including her specialty *The Language of the Feet* (1995) and *Reflexology: The Definitive Guide*. The Reflexology community owes a great debt to Chris, and I acknowledge here the significant contribution she has made to the profession of Reflexology. Her love, her inner beauty and quest for knowledge are also acknowledged.

Others have continued the process Chris began, and Chi-Reflexology is one result, as is this current work. Others who have expanded both the theory and practice of Reflexology include Inge Dougans, the first to combine Reflexology with Meridians; Susanne Enzer with Maternity Reflexology; Lyn Booth with Vertical Reflexology; and Pauline Wills with Colour Reflexology, to mention just a few. However, one of the problems with new and advanced approaches is that all have based their approach upon the foundations laid by the original without a critical analysis of these foundations.

Something that is worth mentioning here is that the most exciting developments in the science of Reflexology have actually come from those drawn to an 'energy' or non-physical approach, and this includes Lyn Hatfield from the Western Australian School of Reflexology, is a metamorphosis or metamorphic technique (another energy approach) specialist, who has developed the best physical chart I have so far seen.

Currently Reflexology can be found in most, if not all, countries of the world, yet it is largely alternative or complimentary rather than part of the standard health care system. However, it is medically recognised in China, Denmark and South Africa, and is being taught in some universities in the United Kingdom. As well, much medical research into Reflexology has been completed, mainly in Denmark, but also in the United Kingdom and the United States, and more recently here in Australia. The Maternity Department of the Gosford Hospital on the central coast of New South Wales completed medical research into Reflexology in Midwifery and childbirth. Maternity is one area, both in Australia and around the world, where Reflexology is making major inroads in the health care system. The other area where Reflexology is making great strides is in Palliative care, where the advantages of Reflexology are being increasingly recognised.

CHAPTER 7
Anatomical Reflection Theory: Perspective of the Feet

The basic premise of Reflexology is that the two feet reflect the body, and that the two feet reflect the body anatomically accurately in what is called 'The Anatomical Reflection Theory'. Either this theory is accurate or it is not. It cannot be fifty percent accurate, or seventy, or even ninety nine percent. It is either valid or it isn't. Either the feet do reflect one hundred percent anatomically accurately or they do not.

When studying, I dismissed Reflexology as a valid science and therapy as there was no consistency based on this premise. These inconsistencies will be explained below. I could find no attempt to even look at these inconsistencies in the Reflexology community. Both Reflexology books and foot maps, although cosmetically changed, are copies that have perpetuated the inconsistencies of the original. All that occurred was a brief statement that the two feet reflect the body anatomically accurately and then they went on from there, perpetuating the inconsistencies.

Further, these publications have paid lip service to this important basic premise, with little or no detailed explanation of the perspective, such as:

1. Is the sole of the feet the front or the back of the body?
2. Is the back/top of the feet the front or the back of the body?
3. Is the inside of the feet, inside or outside of the body?

4. Is the outside of the feet, inside or outside of the body?

How can one use a tool without understanding its basics? I certainly could not. As a result, I dismissed standard Reflexology and went in search of energies through the feet, and I did not care where I found them. Ironically this search led me back to the basic theory of Reflexology and to the Anatomical Reflection Theory: that the two feet do reflect absolutely anatomically and proportionately accurately.

First, one needs to discover these inconsistencies. To this end, following is a simple representation of these basic standard foot maps as a point of reference, so that these inconsistencies can be pointed out and discussed.

Reflexology indicates, although it does not usually state this, that:

1. The TOES are the HEAD/NECK region of the body,
2. The BALL OF THE FOOT is the CHEST of the body,
3. The ARCH OF THE FOOT is the ABDOMEN region, and
4. The HEEL area is the PELVIC REGION.

SOLE (Plantar) REFLEXES

Looking at Illustration 3 below (page XX), and working down from head (toes) to buttocks (bottom of the heel), the inconsistencies and explanation are as follows:

1. Pituitary Gland Reflex:

The Pituitary Gland is located at the base of the brain between the two hemispheres in the mid-line of the body. Therefore, if you cut the body in two equal halves, you would slice through the Pituitary gland. As the two Big toes together are the whole head and therefore each Big toe is half the head, the location of the Pituitary gland in the diagram below is in the centre of each half your face. This is not the physical location of this gland, but in fact the major feature of half the face is the eye and the eye socket. This makes much more sense when you realise that this reflex on literally everyone is tender, and would indicate that every body has an imbalance in the Pituitary gland. Does this make sense? NO. However, when you realise that this reflex is actually the eye reflex, and the eye is a very tender instrument as it is designed to take in light rays or vibrations and transmit these to the brain/mind, it makes sense that it is sensitive as it is designed to be. Try pressing into your own eye socket: it is tender, as is its reflex on the Big toe.

Another aspect needs to be brought in here, and that is the proportions of a reflex to the body. If the feet reflect anatomically accurately, then the size of the structure in the body MUST be much smaller in the feet, that is, the structures must be proportionate to the size in the body compared to the size of the feet. Therefore, the Pituitary gland reflex on the illustration above is simply way too large. The Pituitary gland in the body is a very small structure and on the feet it would actually be smaller than the tip of a pin.

This is another major aspect of the Anatomical Reflection Theory: if the feet are an accurate reflection of the body, they must not only be anatomically accurate in location, but also proportionately in size.

2. Heart Reflex:

This reflex, on the left side of the body/foot, is absolutely amazing. The Heart Reflex is so large that it takes up over three-fifths (Zones 1, 2, 3 and part of Zone 4) of the left side of the chest cavity. Where is the left lung? There are two lungs, one either side of the body (feet), and the left lung has only two lobes (the right has three), to accommodate the majority of the heart, which is on the left side. The Heart in the chest cavity is midsagittal, i.e. in the middle of the body, with the majority of the heart on the left side of the body (feet). Further out from the heart is the smaller left lung, but on the map below there is very little room for the left lung at all.

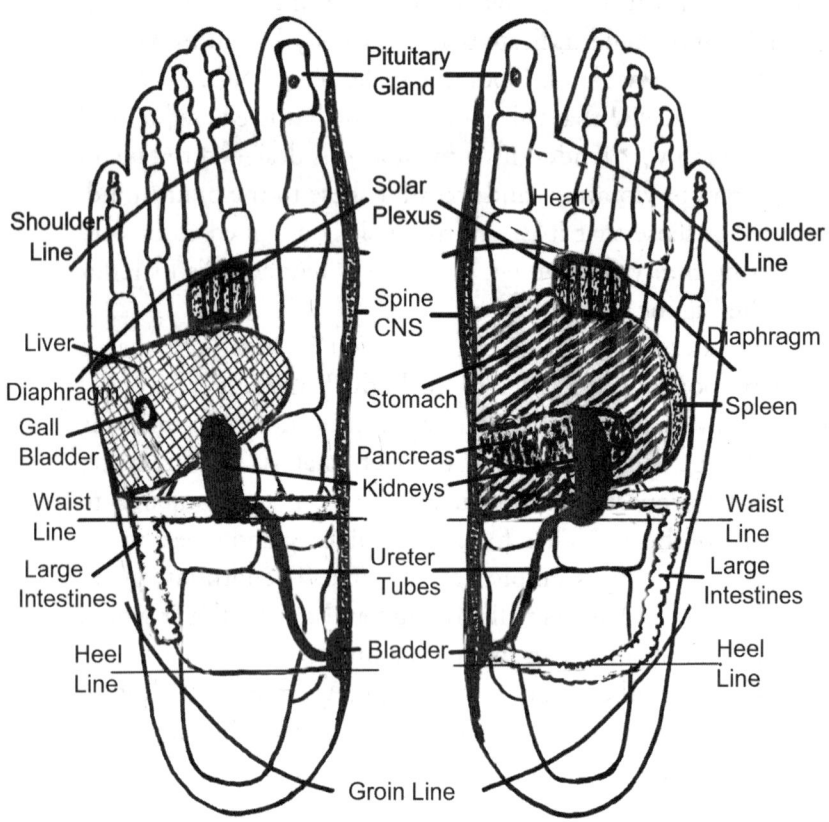

**ILLUSTRATION 3: Basic Standard Reflexology Chart
– Sole View**

3. SOLAR PLEXUS REFLEX: (SEE CHAPTER 10 FOR A DETAILED ANALYSIS)
  Solar Plexus is an energy vortex or chakra from the Indian
Chakra (energy) system and its location, as shown on the map
above, is between the second and third toes, under the ball
of the foot (chest area), and there are two, one each side of
the body. Is it anatomically accurate? NO. The Solar Plexus
Chakra, like most of the Chakras of the body, is located in the
midsagittal plane (middle or mid-line of the body) in the hol-

low below the sternum or breastbone, and there is just one.

So if the feet reflect anatomically accurately, then this reflex cannot be Solar Plexus.

4. PANCREAS AND LIVER REFLEXES:

Although predominantly on one side of the body, both these organs are actually on both sides of the body as they transverse or cross the body, and if you cut the body through the mid-line you will cut through both these organs. The Liver, which is predominantly on the right side of the body (right foot), does have a significant tail-type structure on the left side (left foot). The Pancreas, although largely on the left side of the body (feet), actually sits in the duodenum, which is on the right side of the body (right foot). So the pancreas should also appear on the right foot, but does it?

5. BLADDER REFLEX:

Note: This relates to some extent to point 7 below.

The Urinary bladder is very frontal (towards the front of the body), just behind and slightly above the front pelvic bone (symphysis pubis), and again in the mid-line of the body. In the sitting position the bladder is just off the seat of the chair. It is very low in the torso, much lower than illustrated above, which places the bladder approximately half way between the Waist Line and the buttocks. This cannot, if the feet reflect anatomically accurately, be the Bladder.

6. NO REPRODUCTIVE REFLEXES:

If the sole of the feet is the front of the body, then there must be reproductive (both male and female) reflexes on the sole of the feet, but there are not. And the male and female reproductive system is not located in the same physical place, so there should be two sets of reproductive reflexes on the sole of the feet, one for male feet and the other for female feet. Again there is not even one.

7.THE HEEL AREA (PELVIC REGION)

is basically empty: (Also Point 5 above.)

Look at the map above: nearly the whole heel area is empty, that is approximately one-fifth of the feet (and therefore one-fifth on the torso) is empty. That means there is nothing much below the navel, which is approximately one-fifth up from the pelvic floor, or one-fifth of the whole torso.

What part of the human body is empty? None of it. There is no part of the human body that is empty. Therefore, if the feet reflex anatomically accurately, then all reflexes need to be taken down, much lower than illustrated above. So much of the Small and Large Intestines, as well as the Urinary Bladder and Reproductive (male and female) reflexes are located in the heel area, which is the reflection of the pelvic region.

8. SPINE REFLEX:

The spine is commonly called the back as it is located towards the back of the body. It is definitely not at the front of the body. Therefore, placing this reflex towards the sole of the feet indicates that this is actually the back of the body. But as we will see from the back, inside and outside of the feet reflexes, the front and the back of the body (and the feet) are intermixed, with both the sole and back of the feet being both the front and the back of the body (feet). Confused? Me too.

Again, if the feet reflect anatomically accurately this is just not possible. Something is definitely out of place. And it is the spine here, which is located inside towards the back of the feet (back of the body), which is where it should be if the feet reflect anatomically accurately.

When one realizes this and moves the spine towards the back of the foot, the amazing result is that the bones of the feet (which are located inside and towards the back of the feet) reflect proportionately accurately the bones of the spine. Thus:

- The inside aspect of the 1st bone (distal phalanx) of the Big toe reflects the skull;
- The inside aspect of the 2nd bone (proximal phalanx) of the Big toe reflects the seven cervical bones of the neck;
- The inside aspect of the 1st metatarsal bone, reflects the twelve thoracic bones of the mid-back;
- The inside aspects of the cuneiform, navicular and part of the talus bones reflect the five lumbar bones of the lower back; and finally
- The joint between the inside aspects of the talus and calcaneus (heel) bones reflect the sacrum and coccyx.

9. Shoulder Line, Diaphragm Line, Waist Line and Heel Line:

These are the divisions commonly used in Reflexology. Three of these, the Shoulder Line, the Diaphragm Line and the Waist Line, are divisions of the body and are all located at the front of the body, with the Shoulder Line and the Waist Line being both at the front and back of the torso, and the Diaphragm being inside the body. But where is the Heel Line? It is on the feet. It is not a division of the body. This is another problem that arises. Three of the four are body divisions and one is not. Further there is one division of the torso that is missing: the Groin Line. This is commonly located on the back of the feet (back of the torso), which will be discussed in more detail below. If the feet reflect anatomically accurately, there is a problem here and something is wrong.

What about the location of the Waist Line on the illustration above? It is once more extremely high, making the upper abdomen quite small and cramped. But what is the Waist Line? It is an imaginary line found by drawing a line around the whole body (front and back) below the elbow with the arm in a relaxed position at the side of the body (foot). It is quite low and runs through the lumbar vertebra of the spine or back. Amazingly, the Elbow reflex is found on the outside of the feet at the 'bump' (proximal head of the 5th metatarsal bone) of the outside metatarsal bone. On most feet this 'bump' is quite prominent. Once the 'bump' is located the Waist Line is drawn across and around the feet below this bump (sole, inside, outside and back of the feet), just as it is around the torso.

The fact is the Groin Line is located on the sole (front of the body), but it cannot be seen unless one removes the tissues of the feet as the groin is created by the bones of the pelvis and the leg (femur), and so it can also be found on the feet in the calcaneus or heel bone. Therefore, the sole of the feet is in fact the front of the torso, with all the divisions of the body located anatomically accurately here.

Let's now look at the illustration of the back of the feet below, which is the back of the body (and feet), or is it?

BACK (Dorsal) REFLEXES:

1. BACK OF HEAD/NECK, UPPER BACK/BACK OF THE CHEST & MID-BACK REFLEXES:

The back of the toes reflects the back of the head and neck. This is anatomically correct, as is the upper and mid-back reflexes, yet on the same surface (back of the body, which all these reflexes indicate) there is the groin, lymph and fallopian tube, which are on the front of the body, not the back. So three of the reflexes above indicate that the top or back (dorsal surface) of the foot is the back of the body, and there are three that indicate it is the front of the body. If the feet reflex anatomically accurately, either the three back reflexes are incorrect or the groin, lymph, fallopian tube reflexes are incorrect. Both cannot be right.

2. GROIN/LYMPH/FALLOPIAN TUBE REFLEXES:

This is particularly significant reflex and so let's look at each individually.

a) *Groin:* The groin is located on the front of the body. As

physically in different places. (See Illustration 6: Outside Foot for the testes) the male testes are inside and frontal, and below the groin and front pelvic bone and therefore in the torso, much lower than the female reproductive organs. NOTE: the testes are inside, not outside. So the male and female reproductive organs are just not in the same place on the body but they are on the feet.

c) The next problem with this reflex is the fact that it is much too high, and is nearly out of the pelvic (heel) region completely. The ovary/testes are very low, as is the whole reproductive system of both men and women. It is all just too high. Why?

d) It is ironic that most Reflexologists actually work Kidney energy (acu-point K.5) for the reproductive reflex rather than the reflex itself. The location of most reproductive reflexes on the inside of the foot is actually working a Kidney acu-point. Why does this have an effect on the reproductive system? Because Kidney energy 'rules' reproduction. But it is not the reflex.

e) Lastly, below the uterus is the vagina which is between the uterus and the outside world. Where is the vagina on the above illustration? How long on the above illustration would the vagina be? How long is the vagina in the pelvic region? Another problem with proportional reflection.

OUTSIDE (Lateral) REFLEXES:

1. Shoulder/Arm Reflex:

The outer tip of the shoulder (the acromion process) is on the outside of the body and the upper arm (humerus bone) goes from there to the elbow joint, which is just above the waistline. This reflex is far too small to cover the tip of the shoulder to the elbow. In fact, the humerus bone is proportionately equal to the Fifth Metatarsal bone, and the proximal head (towards the heel) of the Fifth Metatarsal (the 'bump') is the elbow. Finally the waistline is found by drawing an imaginary line across the body just below the elbow. The same applies to the feet.

2. Upper Back/Back of Chest Reflex & Mid-Back Reflexes:
This again has been discussed above.

3. Knee/Leg Reflex:
This is a particularly important reflex for the Anatomical Reflection Theory, which will be discussed later in this chapter. Suffice to say here, this reflex is again rather small when compared to the actual thigh, leg and knee. The leg attaches to the torso at the hip, which is very much lower in the pelvic (heel) region, but this reflex does not go anywhere near the hip, heel or pelvic region.

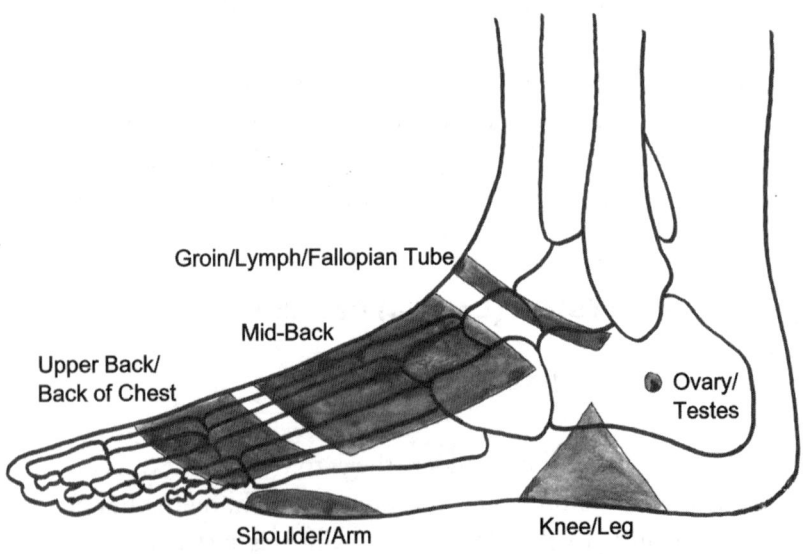

Groin/Lymph/Fallopian Tube

Mid-Back

Upper Back/
Back of Chest

Ovary/
Testes

Shoulder/Arm

Knee/Leg

**ILLUSTRATION 6: Basic Standard Reflexology Chart
– Outside View**

4. REPRODUCTIVE REFLEX AND PELVIC AREA REFLEX:

Again this has been discussed above, other than the label that is placed upon it by standard Reflexology. It is particularly interesting that the outside of the foot and body is labelled the "Ovary/Testes", as these are significant aspects of the system and yet are placed on the outside of the body. If this is the outside of the body (feet), then men have their testicles hanging out and women have their ovaries hanging out too. So how can this reflex be the Ovary and Testes?

A possible explanation again comes from energy (chi) as this is actually a Bladder acu-point which as mentioned earlier, has a relationship with and impact on reproduction.

5. LYMPH/FALLOPIAN TUBE/GROIN REFLEX:

This has been covered earlier.

You can now begin to understand, from the above discussion, the many contradictions found in Reflexology charts and the reason why you can identify them as copies. Either the feet do not reflect anatomically accurately, or most of the reflexes currently considered correct in the feet are not in their right locations and are not anywhere near proportionally accurate to the physical structures of the body, but not both.

The way around this dilemma, is either:

1. That the whole question of the Anatomical Reflection Theory does not matter as a Reflexologist always work all the reflexes of both feet in every treatment, therefore one does not need to be accurate (which is what most argue),

OR

2. To discover a consistent perspective of the feet so that one can accurately locate anything or everything: thus the Anatomical Reflection Theory.

As I do not work all the reflexes (and have not for a long time) and the fact that I access an imbalance very specifically and accurately, has led to the necessity to understand how the feet actually reflect. To be able to work this way, one must have a thorough understanding of the feet and how the feet work: Anatomical Reflection Theory. Decisions have to be made, and accuracy becomes an important and significant issue.

I had to understand the reflection of the feet to the body to be able to do this. This led to a re-examination of the basic premise of Reflexology (that the feet reflect the body anatomically accurately), and the development of the Anatomical Reflection Theory.

ANATOMICAL REFLECTION THEORY EXPLAINED

This Theory has evolved as my understanding of the theoretical and practical components of Reflexology have evolved, and it is still evolving. It is a process of understanding and development whereby, the more you understand the more accurate you become, and the more accurate you become the more you understand.

So the major theory upon which Reflexology is based is the Anatomical Reflection Theory. The first aspect of this interpretation is fairly consistent across the science and art of Reflexology, which is summarized in the following Table.

ILLUSTRATION 7: TABLE:
Anatomical Reflection of the Body to the Feet

ANATOMICAL Area of the Body	ANATOMICAL REFLECTION in feet	DIVISIONS of the body and Feet
Head and Neck	Toes	Shoulder Line
Chest	Metatarsal Pad or Ball of the foot	Shoulder and Diaphragm Lines
Upper Abdomen	Upper Arch	Diaphragm and Waist Lines
Lower Abdomen and Pelvis	Lower arch and Heel	Waist Line and Groin Line

Note that some schools of Reflexology have a Heel Line rather than a Groin Line, as mentioned earlier. The Heel Line is placed at the colour change between the arch of the foot and the heel area. The problem with this is that all the other divisions of the feet are body divisions, except for the Heel Line. You do not have a Heel Line on your torso, yet you do have a Groin Line, which is a curved arch rather than a straight line. The Groin Line is located in the body at the bottom of the torso, and so on the feet it is located below the colour change of the arch and the heel area. It is actually created by the bones of the lower pelvis and the thigh (Femur) bone. So it is not a tissue structure but rather is formed by the bones. This is also reflected in the feet where you need to remove the tissue of the feet to see the Groin Line in the structure of the calcaneus bone. It is a curved arch just as it is on the body, which takes the reflexes of the lower abdomen downwards into the heel area. This is consistent both anatomically and reflectively.

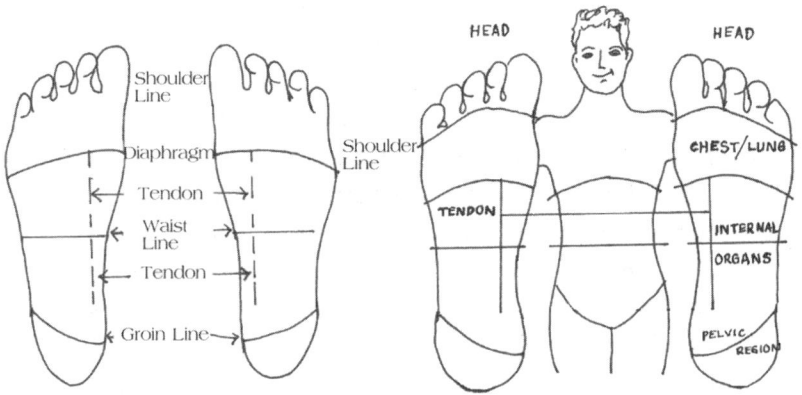

ILLUSTRATION 8:
Anatomical Reflection of the Body to the Feet

With the above in mind, if the Anatomical Reflection Theory is correct then it must be consistent. The above table is a step along the way. The other aspect of this reflection theory is that the four surfaces of the body (front, back, inside and outside) reflect consistently the four surfaces of the feet. I am yet to find a clearly stated and detailed outline of this perspective, and one of the reasons for this is that the Ingham method of Reflexology is accepted as 'the bible' of Reflexology. Most seem to have accepted the original and worked from there, leading to inconsistencies and an un-stated stance on the perspective used in Reflexology. Pick up any Reflexology book and the one glaring omission is a clearly stated and explained perspective of the feet.

The following is my perspective and it is consistently followed throughout this work. It may in fact be incorrect, but at least there is consistency.

My perspective is that:

- The sole of the feet REFLECTS the front of the body.
- The back of the feet REFLECTS the back of the body.
- The inside of the feet REFLECTS the inside of the body.
- The outside of the feet REFLECTS the outside of the body.

There are many reasons for these assumptions. There is the fact that the soft tissues of the sole of the feet reflect the soft tissues of the front of the body, just as the harder tissues of the back reflect the harder surface of the top of the feet; as does the relative softness of the face reflects the softness of the toe pads. The bones of the feet proportionately reflect the bones of the body, especially the pelvic structures when viewed from the above perspective. The spine and spinal cord are located toward the back of the body, and again reflect the bones and curves of the spine through the bones of the feet. There are so many pieces of supporting evidence that could be cited.

Finally, there are significant correlations between the yin and yang surfaces of the body and the yin and yang surfaces of the feet.

- The front of the body is yin compared to the back, which is yang. This reflects with the sole of the feet as yin, compared to the back of the feet, which is yang.
- The outside of the body is yang compared to inside of the

body, which is yin. This reflects perfectly with the inside of the feet being yin compared to the outside of the feet being yang.

And so, this perspective is also consistent with the Chinese perspective of the body and the feet.

ILLUSTRATION 9:
The Anatomical Perspective of the Feet

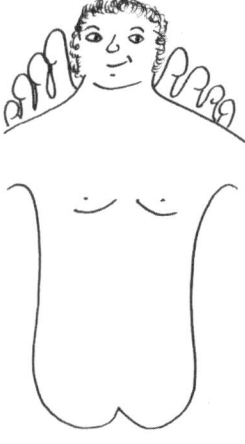

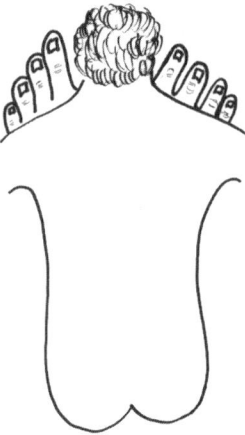

**Front of the body
= Inside Feet**

**Back of the body
= Outside Feet**

**Inside of the body
= Inside Foot**

**Outside of the body
= Outside Foot**

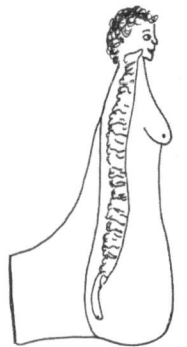

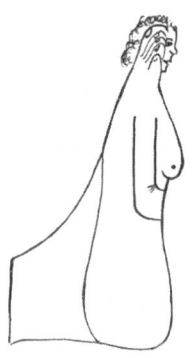

One important and often-neglected aspect of Reflexology and particularly this perspective is that many Reflexologists don't even realise that Reflexology is the only body therapy that can work from the inside. As each foot reflects half the body, the inside of the feet (and hands as well) is actually inside the body. Remember, the human being is three-dimensional, so when working the inside of the feet a Reflexologist is working 'from the inside'. This is hugely significant as there is much more than just the spine and spinal cord here. The inside of the feet is actually inside the muscles, tendon, ligaments, fascia, tissues and most significantly the majority of the organs of the body, particularly those organs and structures that are bi-lateral (the majority of the major organs and glands), that is they are located on both sides of the body and transverse or cross the mid-line of the body. This includes most glands including the Pituitary, Thyroid/Parathyroid and Thymus, as well as the Heart, the Liver, the Pancreas, the Intestines (Small and Large), the Bladder, and most of the Reproductive system. So, unlike other body therapies, Reflexology can access many of the body's structures from the inside.

Another unrealised and neglected aspect of Reflexology is that the lateral and medial aspects of the second, third and forth toes are actually inside the head and neck. (SEE Chapter 8 for a detailed explanation of this.) Again Reflexology has a huge advantage over all other body therapies as Reflexologists can access aspects of the head and neck from the inside.

The following table summarises this perspective.

ILLUSTRATION 10:
TABLE: Surfaces of the Body Reflected in the Feet

BODY SURFACE		FEET SURFACE
Front of the Body	**Yin**	Sole of the Feet
Back of the Body	**Yang**	Back of the Feet
Inside of Body	**Yin**	Inside of the Feet
Outside of Body	**Yang**	Outside of the Feet

WHY IS THIS THE CASE?

The Anatomical Reflection Theory overcomes all the inconsistencies outlined above, and so the reflexes are as follows:

1. The Pituitary gland is no longer located in the Eye reflex (centre of each Big toe) but is cut in half on the inside of both Big toes.
2. The Solar Plexus Chakra is not located under the second and third toes, below the diaphragm, but is located anatomically accurately on both sides of the inner aspect just below the chest (ball of the foot).
3. The Liver Reflex is mainly on the right foot, but is also on the left, and the Pancreas is mainly on the left foot, but is also on the right.
4. The Bladder Reflex is in the lower pelvic (heel) region, and is on both feet as it is in the centre of the body.
5. The Reproductive system can be accessed from the sole of both feet in the pelvic (heel) region, and on the inside (medial) lower pelvis (heel).
6. The Heel area (pelvic region) is no longer empty.
7. The Spinal reflex is located towards the back surface of the inner aspect of both feet, and actually reflects in the bones of the feet.
8. The back reflexes are located on the back of both feet.

All that follows (and proceeds) in this work is based on the Anatomical Reflection Theory perspective of Reflexology, and is consistent with this perspective.

However, there is more. This *reflection* in each individual human being is in the foetal position, which is in his or her mother's womb. There are a number of reasons why this is the case.

The first and perhaps most striking reason for this foetal position for the Anatomical Reflection Theory is that, as stated earlier, there are four external parts of the body that reflect the whole body: the eyes; the ears, and the hands and feet.

The ears are definitely in the foetal position, as are the eyes. It would follow then that the hands and feet are as well.

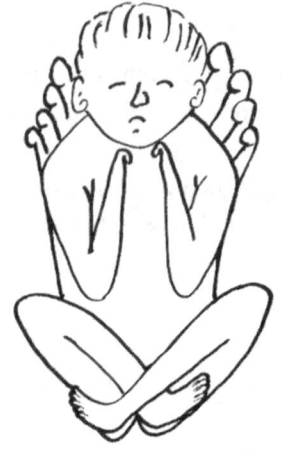

ILLUSTRATION 11:
The Foetal Position
Reflected in the Feet

Further aspects that led to this conclusion are the following:

1. The Reproductive reflexes, especially the testes in the male and the ovaries in the female can be accessed together in the up position (both the testes and the ovaries are located in the same place on the sole of the feet).

2. The reflexes of the shoulders/arms and knees/legs.

The most significant evidence for this proposition is that the testes and ovaries are located in the same position. How? We know that this is not physically the case, for the female reproductive organs (ovaries, fallopian tube, uterus and vagina) are located in the lower abdomen while the penis and testes are physically lower. Yet, they began in the same position while in the womb, and as the male foetus develops during the gestation period, the testes moved downward, finally residing in the scrotum. Yet they can be accessed in the up position as reflected through the feet. The logical conclusion is that the reflex or imprint must have happened prior to the testes downward movement, and therefore must have occurred early while in the womb.

So the male reproductive reflexes are actually in two places of reflection in the feet. They can be accessed in the up position (in the same location as the ovaries), as in the early stages of foetal development when the reflection of the developing foetus was 'mapped', but they can also be accessed in their current location, in the down position. So the male reproductive reflexes (testes and penis) are also located on the medial corner of the lower inner pelvis (heel) below the bladder reflex, which is physically where you will find them.

This leads into the next point and that is that the Anatomical Reflection is not static. The foetal reflection is the blueprint and underlying patterning of the feet (and hand, eyes and ears), but as we grow, evolve and change so do the reflections. This is an extremely important point to realise. The first and major 'map' of the feet occurs in our mother's womb, at a particular time and space during the gestation period, but it is not the last. As we grow and develop, evolve and change, learn and experience, as well as age, so do the feet and the Anatomical Reflection of the feet. Nothing is ever static. Change is the basis of life, including the reflections.

The limbs (arms and legs) also provide evidence of foetal positioning. The arms (humerus bones) are located on the outside of the feet, following precisely the fifth metatarsal bone which accurately *reflects* the humerus. But, where are the forearms, wrists and hands? Located on the sole of the feet, from the waistline (elbow) up through the abdomen and chest between the fourth and fifth toes (longitudinal Zones 4 and 5). Again, this is in a foetal position. (See Illustration 11 above.)

And where are the legs reflected on the feet? The leg reflex is located on the outside of the feet, below the proximal head of the fifth metatarsal. It is in the folded foetal positioning, with the femur moving up from the base of the outer heel (pelvis/outer hip/outer buttocks) to the knee (patella) and the tibia and fibula returning back down. The femur connects to the pelvic bones at the base of the outer heel. The legs, knees and feet are reflected in the outer view of the foetal position.

This leads to the next question: Where are the feet reflected on the feet? The answer lies in two places as a result of an outside and frontal view of the foetal position:

- Viewed from the outside, the feet are reflected at the base of the outer heel/pelvic area, while at the same time,
- Viewed frontally, the feet are reflected on the sole surface at the base of the heel/pelvis.

And as the legs and feet are crossed in the womb,

- The Left Foot reflects on the sole at the base of the right heel (pelvis) and secondly at the base of the outer right heel (outer hip/pelvis).
- The Right foot reflects on the base of the left heel both on the sole and outside.

Therefore, one can access the Right Foot Reflex in two places:

1. On the outside of the left foot, right at the very bottom of the outer heel (outer pelvis), towards the sole surface, and this reflection is largely accessing the toes;
2. On the sole of the left foot, at the very bottom of the heel/pelvis, where you can access mainly the back (dorsal) or top of the feet.

Conversely, the Left Foot reflexes are in the same position as described above, except they are located on the Right foot.

The next logical question is that, if the feet reflect the human being in the foetal position, just when does this 'imprint' occur? Obviously before the testes begin their downward journey but exactly when is open to debate. Could it be at the point when the soul of the developing human being makes the conscious choice to 'go through with it'? That point, in time and space, when the soul commits to this journey of life?

When does this happen: over nine months while in the womb? I theorise that it happens at a particular point during the gestation period, and is not exactly the same for each human being, as such depends on what was where at that point in time. For the majority of souls it occurs around the 20 week gestation period, roughly up to the point that the foetus can naturally abort or miscarriage. However, some souls are quick committers while others are rather slower. Supporting evidence for this hypothesis is that the knees are located on the outside of the feet, but are in slightly different positions for each person, depending on where his/her knees were at the time of imprinting the feet.

For those who are slow committers, the reflexes of especially the limbs (arms and legs) could be found just about anywhere. The foetus tends to be rather still in the first half of the gestation period, but begins increasingly to move around, including their limbs, in the later stages in the gestation period. Therefore, late committers are more likely to have their arms and legs in another position other than the foetal one.

As a result of the foetal positioning of the Anatomical Reflection Theory, much can be said about the person, not just whether they are fast or slow committers, but also such things as small baby in a large mother; a large baby in a small mother; left or right sided babies; positioning of twins (and reflective personality characteristics), etc. The confirmation of the foetal reflection is amazing and tells a great deal about each individual human being, not just physically.

This is just another example of each human being unique. And no map can be one hundred percent accurate. By its very nature, the uniqueness of human beings precludes this. However, this does not mean that one cannot find consistency in the Anatomical Reflection Theory perspective. All Reflexologists must keep this in mind: that all Reflexology theory is by its very nature generalised and for the majority of people it will be accurate, but there will always be exceptions. Once you know and understand the Anatomical Reflection Theory, one does not need any charts, maps or books to guide you. The knowledge will be the framework within which the intuition works.

ANATOMICAL REFLECTION THEORY
A Summary

There is a lot of explanation and information provided in this chapter. It is difficult to avoid detailed analysis of Standard Reflexology initially and then the Anatomical Reflection Theory. It is the only way to explain it.

So to summarise the basic premises on which Reflexology and this work are based, the reflection of the human body to the feet is:

- The anatomical divisions of the body are reflected in the anatomical divisions of the feet perfectly;
- Front, back, inside and out of the body and feet correlate.
- The reflexes in the feet reflect proportionally accurately with the anatomical structures of the body;
- The reflection of the feet to the body occurred at a particular point is space and time while the human being was in the foetal position in the womb, and therefore before birth.

All that follows is based on these premises of the anatomical reflections. For me, these perspectives have been remarkably verified. The Anatomical Reflection Theory deals with the physical reflection of the human being from the body to the feet and vice versa, but there is more here than just a physical reflection. The physical is just the beginning: where the actions of the other levels of existence are played out.

Although the Anatomical Reflection Theory is about the physical reflexes and their logical location, this reflection is not just a physical one. There is the emotional reflection, the mental reflection and the spiritual reflection (the Four Level of Existence), as well as reflective evolution of the individual over time.

It is also a reflection of the energies of the body (whether this is prana or chi), which also reflect anatomically accurately. It is all there, waiting to be accessed for the good (or ill) of each and every human being. Knowledge is power and sharing and spreading the knowledge is the best way to keep it alive and growing (and expanding and developing), allowing each to more consciously choose their way of performing Reflexology.

It is ironic that my journey of discovery, searching for the energies (chi) of the feet, has led me back to the basic premise of Reflexology and its absolute accuracy on all levels and in all ways.

as can be seen, this is just not the case in Reflexology, and all Reflexologists use foot charts to learn the location of reflexes and whether consciously or not, actually diagnose through the feet (to be discussed in detail in Chapter 16.)

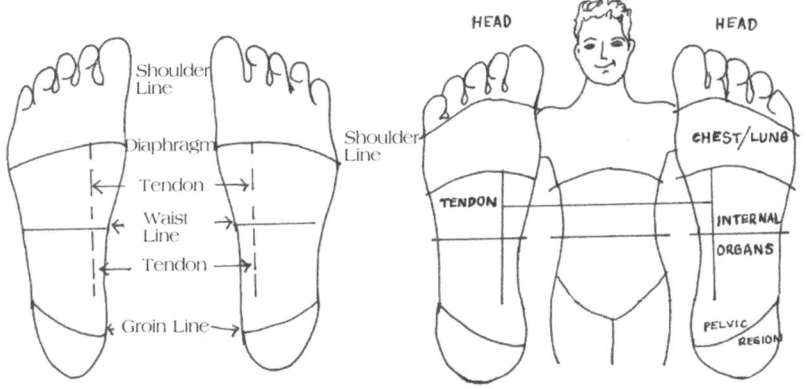

ILLUSTRATION 14: Divisions of the Body

As can be seen in the illustration above, when Reflex Zone Theory (i.e. the ten longitudinal zones, five each side of the body as applied to the feet/hands) is combined with the divisions of the body, that is the top of the shoulder or Shoulder line, the Diaphragm line, the Waist line and Groin, one gets a grid-like structuring of the body and the feet. This is the major use of Reflex Zone Theory as it allows Reflexologists to transfer from the body to the feet and from the feet to the body. It is ironic that Reflex Zone Theory, which proposes not to diagnose, is actually used by Reflexologists to diagnose.

Thus, for example, if a person has a problem with a frontal rib, then the Reflexologist can locate the area where it will reflect in the feet, via the zone/s the rib imbalance/injury falls into and the fact that it is below the shoulder and above the diaphragm. Again, a problem that arises from Reflex Zone Theory, for experience has demonstrated to Reflexologists that they can in fact transfer from the body to the feet and vice versa. If this is in fact the case, then the above-mentioned point (anything within a Zone can show up anywhere within said Zone) in Reflex Zone Theory does not hold water.

Zone Theory was used as the basis through which the reflexes in the feet were charted. Thus, it is via Reflex Zone Theory that Reflexology charts were developed, and yet it is contrary to the Theory.

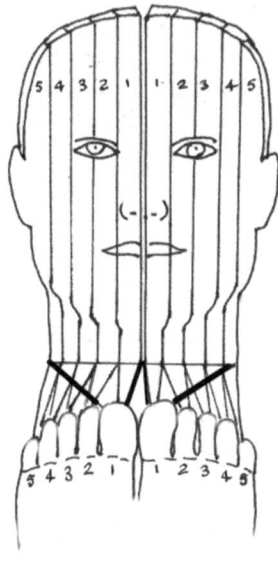

ILLUSTRATION 15:
Reflex Zone Theory
& the Head & Neck

Another important aspect of Reflex Zone Theory, as illustrated above, is that of explaining the Head reflex, which is reflected in the toes (or fingers) of the feet (or hand). One has five digits (toes or fingers) and yet one has but one head. So how does this work? There are two aspects of Reflex Zone Theory that explains this. The first part is that the two Big toes are in fact half your head (left and right half). When you cut the head through the mid-line, one gets two halves, and so each Big toe is half of the head, with the right Big toe the right half of the head and the left Big toe is the left half of the head.

Also, there are ten zones (five each side of the body) and

ten digits (five on each foot/hand). Therefore each toe (finger) from inside to out is actually each of the zones of the head, that is:

- The Big toe (thumb), is both the whole half of the head as well as Zone 1 of the head;
- The second toe (index finger) is Zone 2 of the head;
- The third toe (middle finger) is Zone 3 of the head;
- The fourth toe (ring finger) is Zone 4 of the head;
- The fifth or little toe (little finger) is Zone 5 of the head.

The explanation for this is that, with the brain and major components of the Central Nervous system (CNS) located in the head, and with the Big toe as half the head, one cannot access anything accurately and therefore the other toes reflect Zones 2 to 5 (i.e. different slices of the head), so that detailed aspects of the head can be accessed more accurately. This is where the significance of the 2nd to 4th toes as slices of the head and therefore the inside and outside of these toes is actually inside the head and neck. So Reflexology, other than surgery, is the only therapy that can access aspects of the head and neck from the inside. To reiterate these significant and neglected aspects of Reflexology Zone Theory: the inside and outside of each of the 2nd through 4th toes is actually inside a slice of the head and neck.

2. The Brain and Nervous System Theory

This theory is the next major theory and the one most commonly used, either with or instead of Reflex Zone Theory and the Anatomical Reflection Theory to explain how Reflexology works.

Briefly, the theory is that all the nerve endings are in the feet (and hands) and therefore by working the feet (hands) and all areas and reflexes of the feet with stimulatory techniques, one is stimulating each and every individual nerve and thus the whole nervous system that goes to every part, gland and organ of the body. Therefore Reflexology is working through the nervous system by improving nerve supply to the whole body, although it is not clear how this is achieved.

This is the nice neat little package that can be presented to both the general public and the health care professionals to give an acceptable explanation of how Reflexology works. It also supports the assumption that Reflexologists do not have to understand how the feet work. As all the reflexes and all nerves are worked, Reflexologists therefore do not have to understand their own therapy, as one simply stimulates everything, thus stimulating all the nerves, and improving nerve supply to the parts of the body that are out of balance (and those that are not).

A bonus of this theory is that it has been designed to justify Reflexology theory and practice, rather than an attempt to actually explain how Reflexology works. In this sense then, it has many similarities with Reflex Zone Theory in that they both were designed after the event to attempt to justify, validate and promote what is.

There are a number of other problems with this theory and briefly they are:

1. Why stimulate everything?
2. Does everything need stimulating?
3. Why work every nerve and the whole nervous system?
4. Under this theory, Reflexology would be of no benefit to those that have no nerve supply to their feet, as it is only working through the nervous system.
5. Again Reflexologists cannot, and it is not desirable under this theory to, attempt to work out what is where and why. Therefore, it is again a nice, neat package that avoids many of the issues presented in this book, especially the assumption that by working everything, what needs to be done, is done. And of course the whole attempt to map the body on the feet. Once more there is no need to understand, or to have Foot Charts, and yet Reflexology does.

3. Nervous System: Crystal Deposits Theory

This is actually not a separate theory but is an extension of the Nervous System Theory. It is based on the same assumptions as above, with the added dimension that: human beings are very toxic and toxins, due to gravity, are drawn down to the feet and over time build up around the nerve endings as crystalline deposits, thus interfering with the normal functioning of the nerves of the feet and therefore the body. So, during a Reflexology session, these crystal deposits are broken down, thus improving nerve supply to the feet and the body.

Firstly, the discussion above concerning the Nervous System Theory also applies here. Secondly, is the question of gravity pulling toxins down to the feet. As most people are quite toxic for one reason or another, if this theory is valid, then most people's feet would be quite toxic, perhaps even quite discoloured. Is this the case?

If this theory is valid, then all the feet would be very toxic and Reflexologists would regularly find these deposits all over the feet and in every treatment. Is this the case? Reflexologists regularly and consistently find these crystalline deposits all over the feet: sole, back, inside and outside. Is this the case? These deposits are not always found and definitely not over the whole foot (body) and yet toxins are in every cell of the body to varying degrees. Logically there is a problem here. These crystalline deposits are not always found in the feet and when they are they tend to be most commonly and often found in the ball of the foot area: the Chest.

4. External Reflecting Internal: Theory of Reflection

There is one other major theory worth expounding that tends not to be included, but is implied by Reflexology and

yet is ignored and so far has not been dealt with, is there are four external parts of the body that reflect the whole and they are:

1. The eyes
2. The ears
3. The feet
4. The hands

Under this theory, the two feet (and hands) are a reflection of the human being, not only physically (Anatomical Reflection Theory) but on all levels: emotionally, mentally and spiritually as well. This imprint (not only on the feet, but the hands, eyes and ears) occurs in the foetal position while in your mother's womb, at the point in time and space when the soul, spirit or essence chooses to go through with this journey. Further, this reflection changes over time: it evolves and grows as we do.

So the two feet reflect not only the foetal position but also:

1. **The present** (and possibly the future) through the sole of both feet (palms of both hands);
2. **The past** through the back of the feet (back of the palms of both hands);
3. **Deep inner aspects**, through the inner aspect of the feet (and hands);
4. **Superficial, everyday aspects**, through the outside of the feet (hands).

Also, the left foot (hand) reflects the yin aspects of these perspectives, while the right foot (hand) reflects the yang aspects. Lastly, the feet are the most powerful of all, due to the fact that they are our connection to Mother Earth, which is the first and most primal of all our relationships and is a nurturing and cleansing one. This then is the theory of Reflection (and on an energy level, reflexion). The simple fact that the two feet do reflect the human being.

5. Other Theories

There are many other theories that are increasingly being proposed for how Reflexology works, and many are in fact from body therapies generally, rather than Reflexology specifically. They are generally combined with the major theories of how Reflexology works outlined above rather than as stand alone Reflexology theories. They include such aspects as stress and deep relaxation, Body Chemistry, Meridian Theory, Vibrational Healing/Medicine Theory, Energy Theories, Intention, Relationship of giver and receiver, Love, Spiritual energy/healing, environment in which Reflexology is conducted, Wholistic approach, etc.

Note: many of these are also part of the story, but are not an explanation in themselves. Some are worth mentioning here.

A. DEEP RELAXATION (SEE CHAPTER 4 FOR A MORE DETAILS)

This theory is used by all body therapies and is based on the assumption that stress is the cause of all our major imbalances and problems, and best countered by deep relaxation. With deep relaxation there is a decrease in brain activity and an increase in alpha brain waves, which allows the natural healing potential of the body the opportunity to heal.

This has become a trend that has spawned a complete industry, especially and including many of the body therapies, in particular massage. This is the feel good explanation. Basically by having Reflexology (or any of a range of body therapies) regularly one decreases stress levels and increases deep relaxation, which allows the body to function better.

There are many things that could be mentioned here. There is, no question about the value of deep relaxation and, assuming Reflexology brings about deep relaxation, it is a valid explanation. But is this it? Is that all Reflexology is? Is this all Reflexology does?

If this is it, then all people have to do is find their own way of attaining deep relaxation. There is no need for therapies, including Reflexology, except for the justification that people would not do it for themselves. That is possible.

However, is deep relaxation a difficult thing to achieve during a Reflexology session? Does it take an hour to achieve? Is it that hard a thing to do? Deep relaxation is actually easy to attain. It is not difficult. It is a consequence of the treatment rather than an end in itself. It happens quickly, easily and naturally, if the Reflexologist is working with the body. So deep relaxation is a consequence rather than an end it itself.

One other point worth mentioning here is that this theory is based on the assumption that stress is the cause, and if we can only get rid of stress then life would be wonderful. A little simplistic, don't you think? Again a nice, neat package to present to the general public to sell our wares. Perhaps it would be better to consider the level of stress rather than stress itself. Human beings need stress to achieve. A level of stress is good for us all.

B. BODY CHEMISTRY

This theory is a theory explaining all forms of touch: the simple act of two human beings touching anywhere, and is one of the theories for all body therapies, including but not exclusively Reflexology. There is now evidence that touch brings about chemical changes within the body, and specifically such chemicals as encephalins and endorphins. Although this theory is definitely part of the explanation, if this was the complete story, then no matter how, when or where one touches, the results would be the same. All body therapies would be the same and should gain the same results, irrespective of the approach and techniques. Is this the case? Clearly it is not.

C. MERIDIANS AND ENERGY PATHWAYS

The Meridian system is the theory of how energy moves

about the body. There are six of the twelve energies flowing through the legs, the Liver/Gall Bladder, Spleen/Stomach and Kidney/Bladder. Along these pathways there are acu-points, which along with the pathways, may be accessed during a Reflexology treatment, and so some of the benefits of Reflexology may be due to the meridians and acu-points. The meridians that do not run through the legs and arms are Heart/Small Intestines, Pericardium (Heart's Protector)/Triple Burner, and Lung/Large Intestines. Theoretically these energies are not accessed through the meridians and acu-points that run through the legs and feet. This is also the case for the arms and hands. So, the meridians and acu-points do not explain Reflexology, as there are only half the meridians running through the legs and feet, yet Reflexology accesses all the energies of the body through the feet.

Theoretically the meridians are one long interconnected pathway, which has no beginning or end, and so by accessing one pathway you are in fact accessing them all. This is another possibility, but again it does not explain how Reflexology works. In fact, the original Chinese approach was a point approach, and the meridians or energy pathways developed later. It is the acu-points that have their own unique name and are powerful. The meridians are the theoretical way energy moves around the body to every cell, every atom and every structure, and are where the pathway is closest to the surface and therefore can be accessed. Finally, the meridians are also simply connecting the acu-points (which are far more therapeutically significant), that is linkage of acu-points with similar characteristics, and so it is not the pathways that are important but the acu-points. Reflexology rarely, if ever, actually accesses the acu-points themselves as the techniques are significantly different.

So the Chinese meridian and acu-point system do not fully explain Reflexology. It again adds to the overall therapeutic qualities and potential of Reflexology, but it does not explain how Reflexology works.

D. VIBRATIONAL HEALING/MEDICINE THEORY

This theory is that everything, including the human being, is a form of vibration. It is a theory of change: a theory purporting that everything is in a state of flux and so everything is moving. Every cell and atom of the human being and everything else in the universe is vibrating. Therefore, the vibration oscillates between a balanced state and an imbalanced state and so changes with imbalances and this imbalance can be influenced: to correct, adjust, modify and improve the vibration of the human being and therefore bring about a more harmonious vibration for the individual. This is actually an energy theory, without using the word energy.

Once again this theory is designed to explain working with and on the whole body rather than specifically Reflexology, and yet may have a role to play in how Reflexology works. However, everything that is done to the human being (and therefore the feet and hands), has an impact on the vibration at the microcosmic and macrocosmic level of human existence. So again, although this may have a role to play, it does not explain Reflexology.

E. ENERGY (CHI/QI OR PRANA) THEORIES

There are many energy theories and the most popular ones are the Chinese Chi or more accurately Qi and the Indian prana and Chakra theories. The basic theory here is that energy blockages result in stagnation of energy and this brings about imbalance, illness and dis-ease, if the blockages can be removed wellness will result. However, as science teaches energy never ceases to exist, it only changes form. Energy flows and moves. It cannot be stopped, nor can it be blocked. Energy flows like a river from the source to the stream into the river and on to the sea. It will always find a way to flow.

Energy is everywhere in everything. Nothing in the universe exists without energy. And so this general theory of life is interesting and adds to our understanding of the human being and the universe, but it unfortunately does not explain Reflexology.

This is another of those nice, neat packages to explain Reflexology in a generalized, non-specific way: "I am working with energy." And I myself fall under this category.

MY THEORY: So, How does Reflexology Work?

The theories that hold the greatest appeal for me are a combination of:

1. External Reflecting the Internal: Theory of Reflection;
2. Anatomical Reflection Theory;
3. The Feet: A Sacred Art;
4. Energy.

With the 'External Reflecting the Internal: Theory of Reflection' incorporating both the Anatomical Reflection Theory and Energy Theories as well, as aspects of the other theories mentioned above, plus providing a philosophical framework within which Reflexology can be placed, this then is my explanation of how Reflexology works. Is it complete?

• Yes.
• No.
• Closer.
• Hopefully getting there.

Perhaps any and all theories are based on the beliefs of the person or group proposing the theory. Interesting. Yet the truth is we do not know. In fact, there is more we do not know than we do.

Reflexology is a therapy used through the feet (and hands). Why the feet? (or hands?) Are they different from working anywhere else in the body? What makes them different? Special?

But what is the theory upon which this is based? At this

stage of our understanding we are grappling with the unknown, attempting to explain something that at this point in time we cannot. The above discussion indicates that all the theories of how Reflexology works, to varying degrees, fall short of explaining a simple truth: Foot Reflexology works.

The beginning of wisdom is the statement: I do not know!

CHAPTER 9
Reflex Zone Theory Revisited: Energy Flow through the Body

Reflex Zone Theory proposes that there are ten longitudinal lines or zones dividing the body (five each side of the midsagittal plane or longitudinal mid-line of the body) creating a slice of the person so that all the organs and parts of the body lie along one or more of these zones or slices.

The theory also proposes that anything within any particular zone could manifest anywhere in that zone. Therefore, as this is the theory, one cannot diagnose. This is what Dr Fitzgerald proposed. However, if this is in fact the case, there would be no foot charts or diagnoses at all, as anything could show up anywhere within said zone. One cannot find the location of anything in the feet in relation to the body under Reflex Zone Theory and it is contrary to the Anatomical Reflection Theory. This is another of the problems with this theory. It is used as the basis of the practice of Reflexology and yet is not followed with any consistency whatsoever.

There are two significant points worth mentioning here. Firstly, Dr Fitzgerald, as a western medical practitioner, should have described Reflex Zone Theory in the anatomical position, but he did not. This is rather amazing when one realises that the anatomical position is the very first thing all medical students learn and the stance through which the body is described by all medical practitioners. This anatomical position is a person standing, legs apart facing forward with their palms forward (See illustration below).

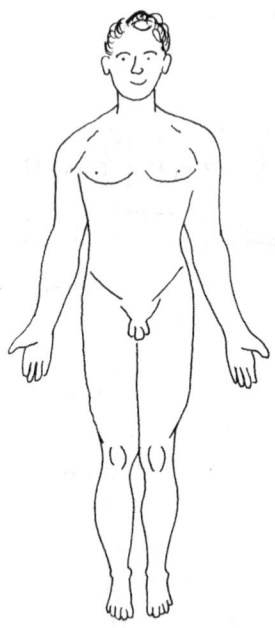

ILLUSTRATION 16: Anatomical Position

The anatomical position was changed for Reflex Zone Theory as the thumb related to Zone 1 had to be close to the body, but in the anatomical position the thumb is on the outside. So Dr Fitzgerald himself actually changed the anatomical position. Why? Because he knew that the thumb related to the centre of the body and therefore had to be Zone 1. Did Dr Fitzgerald himself actually realise that there was a problem with Reflex Zone Theory from the very beginning? Did he use this theory simply because he was unable to explain his discovery any other way? Or, as some have suggested, did Dr Fitzgerald actually know about the Chinese energy flow (meridians) and used Zone Theory to explain energy flow so as to avoid the issue of energy?

Dr Fitzgerald as a medical practitioner and surgeon, would have explained his discovery via the nervous system if that was possible, as this was one explanation that would have easily been accessible to doctors at this time, yet Dr Fitzgerald did not even attempt to do this but rather invented Reflex Zone Theory. This indicates that Dr Fitzgerald knew that his discovery was not working through the nervous system. This is significant because the most popular and generally promoted theories of how Reflexology works, is that it works through the nervous system. Interesting that the inventor or re-discoverer himself never used this explanation.

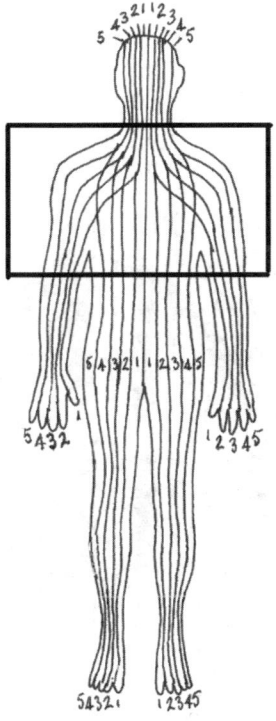

ILLUSTRATION 17: Zone Theory

The other major problem with Reflex Zone Theory can be seen on the illustration above. The shoulder area is a problem due to the fact that if you follow each zone from head to foot, they are clearly in a particular zone and there is no doubling up effect. However, the problem arises when one follows the zones from the fingers up the body. In the shoulder area the zones overlap, and which zone are they in? And where do they reflect in the hands and the feet? Remember, Dr Fitzgerald proposed Reflex Zone Theory as an explanation for the hands, not the feet, and yet it is these very zones that cause the problem. See Illustration below, which is a larger representation of this area.

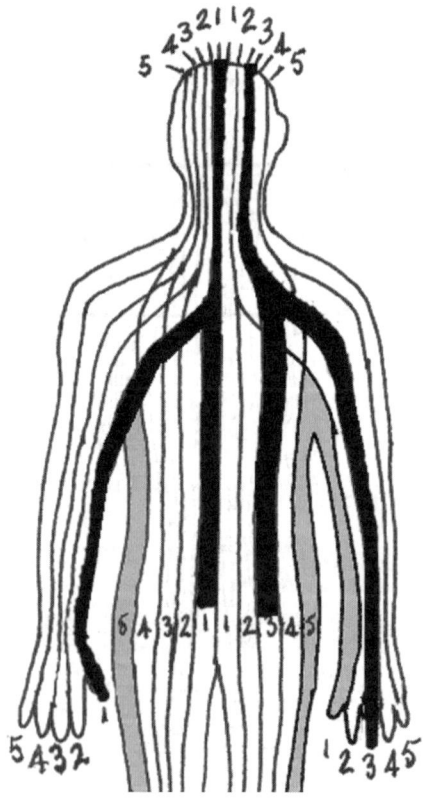

ILLUSTRATION 18: Zones Through the Shoulders

As illustrated above, Zone 3, which flows from the Middle finger upwards in the shoulder area crosses Zones 5 and 4 so that it can join with Zone 3 running head to toe. Another example, following Zone 1 from the thumb upwards, one can easily see that Zone 1 from the thumb crosses Zones 5, 4, 3, 2 to enter Zone 1 flowing from the head to toes. Also, you might notice that Zone 1 actually ceases to exist in the Chest/Upper Back area and re-emerges in Zone 1 inside. This problem in the shoulder area, is the case with all the Zones from the fingers:

- Zone 2, crosses Zones 5, 4 and 3;
- Zone 4, crosses Zone 5;
- Zone 5 is a particular problem, especially if you follow the illustration above from the toes upwards as it disappears completely in the outer chest/shoulder area. (See grey area on above illustration) Furthermore it actually joins Zone 1 that runs to the thumb. Interesting.

The questions that arise in the Chest/Shoulder/Upper Back region are:

1. What happens to the Zones here?
2. What Zone is where?
3. How does one know, in this region, what Zone one is dealing with?

What is the solution to this problem?

One proposal is that Reflex Zone Theory has no limbs, especially arms, and so the Zones (and therefore the reflection in the feet and hands) are only of the torso and head rather than the whole body: an interesting way around the problem, but Dr Fitzgerald himself was interested in the hands. And this is his explanation of how the zones work through the hands. So this solution seems to simply be a means to avoid the problem. Is there a better alternative?

Yes, there is, and it lies in the Anatomical position. In the anatomical position the thumb is on the outside and the little finger is on the inside, but in Reflex Zone Theory's illustration it has been reversed. The Zones are actually in the anatomical position with the thumb on the outside. But how?

SIMPLE: in the anatomical position, raise the arms above the head!

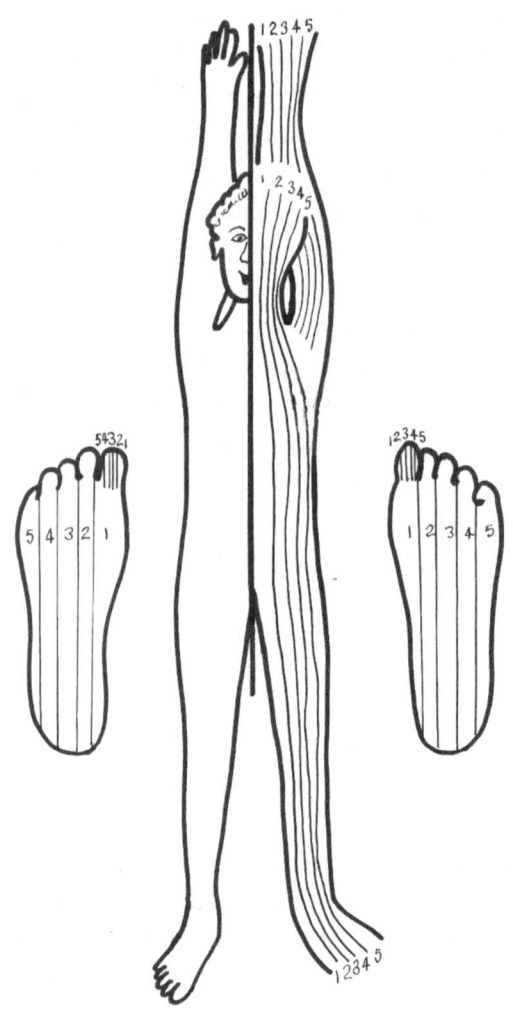

ILLUSTRATION 19:
Zones through the Body, Fingers to Toes

By doing this the contradictions of the Shoulder/Chest/ Upper Back Zones eliminated Having done this, all longitudinal zones can run not from head to toe, but rather from fingers to toes.

Keep in mind that Reflex Zone Theory states that the zones followed the contour of the body so that where the body is wider, so are the zones; and where the body is narrower, so are the zones. Therefore, the zones are proportionate to the dimension of the body (and feet or hands) and are of equal proportions in a particular part of the body (and feet or hands) but are not of equal proportion throughout the whole body. Further the head ten Zones (Zones 1 to 5, each half of the head) run from the head to the toes.

But why raise the arms above the head, as illustrated above? Is there any justification for this solution? Yes, there is.

Firstly, structurally and biomechanically the shoulder joint is designed for upward action that is above the height of the shoulder. The explanation for this is that when human beings were apes swinging through the trees the arms were in the upward position. Biomechanically the shoulder joint is designed for these upwards actions rather than all the downward actions people use their shoulder joint for. So why do we have so many shoulder problems? Simple, we do not use the joint as it was originally designed.

Secondly, a more poetic and flowing explanation, comes from the Chinese philosophy. The Chinese say that we stand on earth, but we reach for the heavens. In this position (as illustrated below) heaven's energy, universal energy, cosmic energy, God's energy or Yang energy flows down through the human being into the earth, and at the same time, earth energy, Mother energy or Yin energy flows upward back to the heavens. This is the explanation of the meridians or energy pathways and how they flow through the human being.

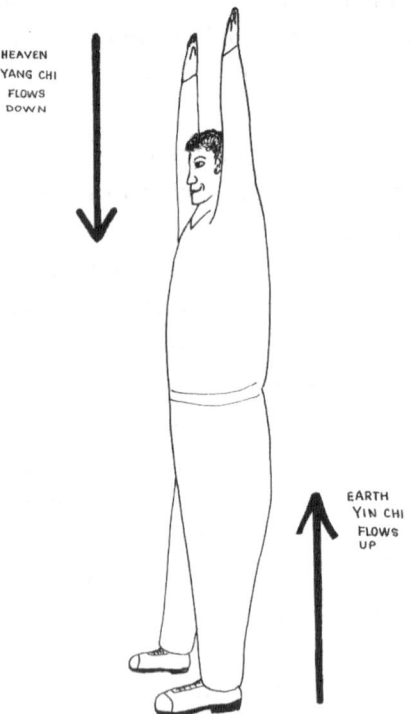

HEAVEN
YANG CHI
FLOWS
DOWN

EARTH
YIN CHI
FLOWS
UP

ILLUSTRATION 20: Energy/Chi Flow through the Body

So Dr Fitzgerald tapped into the natural energy flow through the human being and yet had no framework within which to understand, least of all explain, this phenomenon. So, as he had come across Zone Theory while he was in Germany, he used this to explain his discoveries. Dr Fitzgerald, as a western medical practitioner, had no understanding of the Chinese philosophy and specifically Traditional Chinese Medicine (TCM) and energy flow through the body. (Or did he?) If he had, he would have explained his discoveries in a completely different way, and Reflex Zone Theory would never have been proposed. Reflex Zone theory, therefore, was a doctor's attempt at explaining energy flow without the realisation that that was what he was tapping into.

With this, the contradictions within Reflex Zone Theory are overcome, but at the same time it decreases, if not the historical significance of Dr Fitzgerald and Reflex Zone Theory, Reflex Zone Theory as an explanation of Hand and Foot Reflexology. It's major contribution, other than historically, is:

1. The establishment of the grid framework of the body and the feet for students to learn what is where and where is what;
2. The transfer from the body to the feet and vice versa, i.e. for diagnosing purposes (See Chapter 16);
3. Its explanation of the head.

Other than this, Reflex Zone Theory is but an attempt to explain energy flow without an understanding of energy flow, which the Chinese understood and explained thousands of years ago.

CHAPTER 10
Solar Plexus Explained

Reflexologists all around the world recognise the Solar Plexus reflex in the feet, which is located under the second and third toes (longitudinal zones 2 and 3), just below diaphragm and chest or ball of the feet. All acknowledge its significance and usefulness as a powerful reflex for most, if not all, imbalances. It is arguably the most powerful point on the feet and is called Solar Plexus in nearly every Foot Chart. But is it in fact Solar Plexus? Let's examine this assumption a little closer.

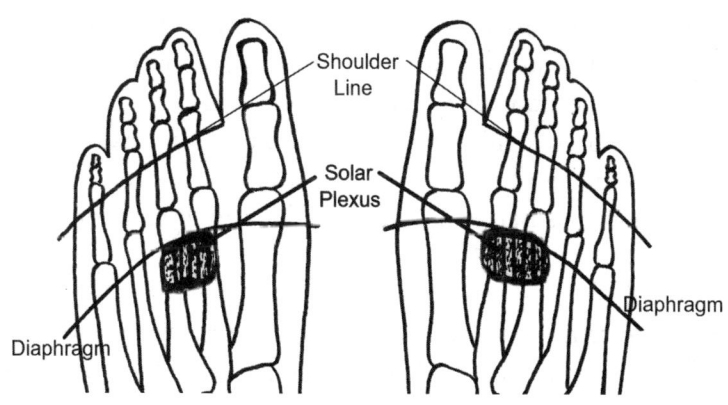

ILLUSTRATION 21: Solar Plexus Reflex in Reflexology

This location indicates that there are two such reflexes on the feet. You do not have two Solar Plexi (plural of plexus), one on each side of the body. You have one located on mid-line of the body below the diaphragm. So this cannot be Solar Plexus. This was one of the first things I questioned when I initially studied Reflexology, and no one could give me an adequate response.

But what is the Solar Plexus? Correctly labelled it is the Coeliac Plexus, but in Reflexology and common usage it is known as the Solar Plexus. The Coeliac Plexus is a collection or network of nerves found in the upper part of the abdomen, behind the stomach and in front of the aorta, where nerves come into the plexus, mix and then travel outward to various parts of the body. It is in a sense a nerve junction box, just like an electrical sub-station, where the major heavy-duty electrical wires come into the sub-station from the power station and are redistributed to every dwelling within the sub-station's jurisdiction. It is not the only plexus in the body. Is it the largest, or most important?

Any plexus in the body is a nerve centre where nerves are redistributed to a particular region of the body: the abdomen in the case of the Solar or Coeliac Plexus. Is the Solar Plexus a particularly significant and especially powerful plexus of the body? No. It is just a sub-station or junction box as are all the plexus of the nervous system. Important and necessary, but not particularly significant as such, and no more anatomically and physiologically powerful than any other plexus. Yet it is the only plexus that appears on nearly every Reflexology foot chart.

Why?

If Western medicine does not provide an answer we will have to look elsewhere. The Solar (Coeliac) Plexus is commonly considered to be located in the mid-line just below the sternum due to the fact that a blow to this area can have a detrimental effect on the Coeliac Plexus. This relationship provides a connection between the physical Coeliac Plexus and its common location on the body. It also links with the Indian energy system, known as Chakras. I do not want to delve too deeply into the Chakra system. Suffice to say that the Solar Plexus Chakra, or energy vortex, is located just below the sternum in the centre or middle of the body. Most Reflexologists believe that this is the explanation for the Solar Plexus reflex on the feet, and this explains its significance. But does it?

What about the Anatomical Reflection Theory and Solar Plexus? (See Chapter 7, Anatomical Reflection Theory) Under this theory, the Solar Plexus, which is located in the centre of the body on the midline would have to be located on the medial aspect of the feet. Is this where it is located on the feet? Again the simple answer is no. See the Illustration below, which shows the front of the body correct location of Solar Plexus chakra.

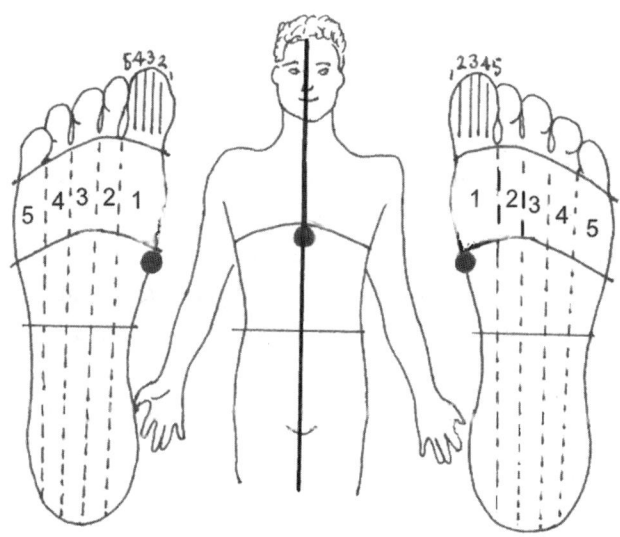

ILLUSTRATION 22:
Solar Plexus Chakra through the Feet

As illustrated above, anatomically the Solar (Coeliac) Plexus is located toward the sole on the inner aspect of the foot.

The front of the Solar Plexus Chakra would be located in the same place. As the Chakras actually passes through the body, ending (and beginning) in the spine, it would be more accurate to locate the Solar Plexus Chakra in the thoracic region of the spinal reflex toward the back of the foot, along the first metatarsal bone on the inside aspect of the foot. What is known as the Solar Plexus in Reflexology circles is not the location of the Solar Plexus Chakra. So, it is not the Coeliac Plexus, anatomically accurate, nor is it accurate within the Indian energy system.

The hollow is significant in explaining why originally it was thought to be Solar Plexus, and that if you come down your chest in the mid-line, at the end of the sternum, one falls into the hollow which is known as the Solar Plexus Chakra. At the same time, when you come down both halves of the chest (ball of the feet) of the feet in Zones 2 and 3, one falls into a hollow beneath the diaphragm. So both are a hollow structure, which is why they were put together; the hollow in the feet reflects the hollow in the body.

A further explanation is that when Reflexology was being initially developed and understood, they could not find any physical, medical or anatomical explanation for this reflex and its potency, and so looked for non-physical explanations that might justify its significance and power. The result was the Indian Chakras system and specifically Solar Plexus, as there was no other possible explanation at the time that appeared to suit.

NOTE: it is the only Chakra that appears on literally every Foot Chart.

It seems surprising that so few Reflexologists have critically analysed Reflexology theory and practice since its inception.

If it is not a physical reflex and it is not Solar Plexus Chakra, then what are we dealing with in the hollow below the second and third toes (zones 2 and 3) and the diaphragm on each foot? It cannot be the Solar Plexus physically or anatomically, or even in the Indian Chakra energy system, when transferred to the feet.

The answer lies in the Chinese energy system and in the life-force creation process as illustrated below. In Traditional Chinese Medicine (TCM), the Solar Plexus reflex on the feet is actually the first point of the Kidney meridian, that is, acu-point Kidney 1 called Bubbling Spring: the reflection of the beginning of the Kidney energy (which is the Root of Life) and the starting point (and possibly more significantly, completion point) of the chi or life force creation process.

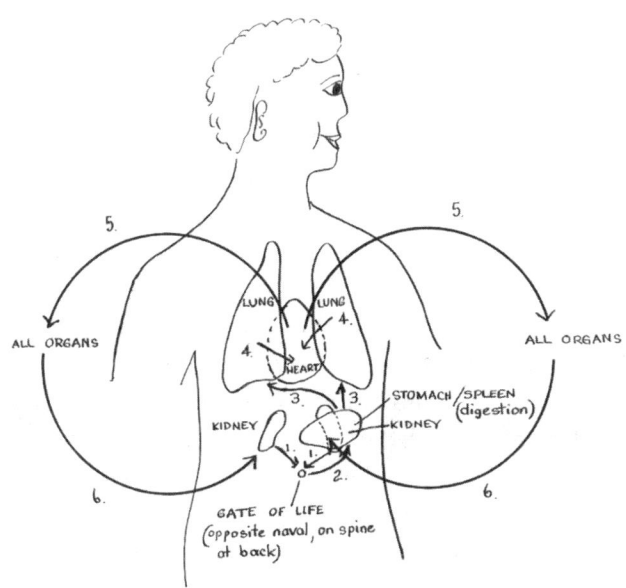

ILLUSTRATION 23:
Chi (Life-force) Creation and Distribution Process

At the very centre of this reflex is located the Kidney chi or energy, composed of Original Chi (Pre and Post-natal Chi). Kidney chi, which flows up from the earth into the human being via acu-point Kidney 1: the Bubbling Spring or beginning of a river: a poetic image for the beginning of life. This is our connection to Mother Earth who nourishes and nurtures us all. In TCM, this is the only acu-point located on the sole of the feet, and the only acu-point they wanted philosophically on the sole of the feet and is one of the reasons for its potency. The conclusion that arises from this is that this point reflects Kidney chi, as it does. But it is more than this. It is the beginning, as well as the completion, of the process of life-force creation within the human being. To explain, it is the beginning: the Bubbling Spring but its reflection in the Anatomical Reflection Theory is on both sides of the body, at the base of both lungs: the completion point of life-force creation process within the human being.

The above illustration of the chi creation process shows that all the components needed for this process finally come together at the base of both lungs. Where is this reflex located on the sole of the feet? Below the diaphragm, at the base of each lung, below the second and third toes (in zones 2 and 3), as reflected on the feet. The correlation is clear. This reflex is reflecting not only Kidney chi, but also the point at which all the necessary components for chi-creation (Kidney {pre- and post-natal} chi, Spleen or Grain chi, and Lung or Air chi) come together in the individual, which is at the base of both lungs, reflected on the feet.

This reflex then is actually two reflexes in one (See illustration below). The beginning of the process, at the very centre, is Kidney chi, and around this lies the end of the process, the place where all the components come together, the base of both lungs. This pure chi essence point lies around the outside of the acu-point Kidney 1. Therefore, there are two very powerful energies in the same location. No wonder this reflex is the only acu-point on the sole of the feet.

In other words, the original definition of the Triple Burner, which is the life-force creation and distribution of chi throughout the whole being. It is how we create chi and how we distribute that chi through the meridians to the organs and to every cell and atom of the human being. All this is reflected perfectly in the Kidney 1/Triple Burner acu-point reflex in the feet. This is actually what this point reflects and why it is so powerful and significant. Use it for everything, as it deals with Bubbling Spring, the beginning of life and the root of life, as well as the life-force creation process, or creating your own unique chi.

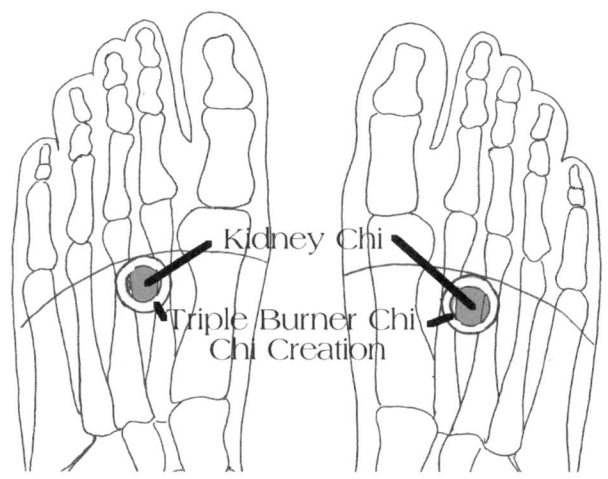

ILLUSTRATION 24: Kidney 1/Triple Burner Reflex

The Triple Burner is what is reflected at the base of both lungs on both feet. Around acu-point Kidney 1 you will be able to locate the Triple Burner process. These energies are quite distinct so it is important to locate them correctly. You will notice on yourself that if you use the tip of your thumb and press into acu-point Kidney 1, you will access Kidney chi. If you then work around the edge of this point you will discover the Triple Burner chi, a distinctly different feel altogether. Two powerful energies in the one reflex. One of these powerful energies is Kidney chi, the Root of Life, and the other is the Triple Burner, which is the whole process of chi-creation. No wonder this is such a powerful and useful reflex. Use it with renewed respect, for just about everything.

CHAPTER 11
Divisions of the Foot and Landmarks

An important aspect that is added to the Anatomical Reflection Theory and Reflex Zones (Zones 1 to 5 each side of the body) is the Division of the Feet and Body, and Landmarks. With these three combined, one can grid the feet as illustrated below.

DIVISIONS OF THE FEET and LANDMARKS

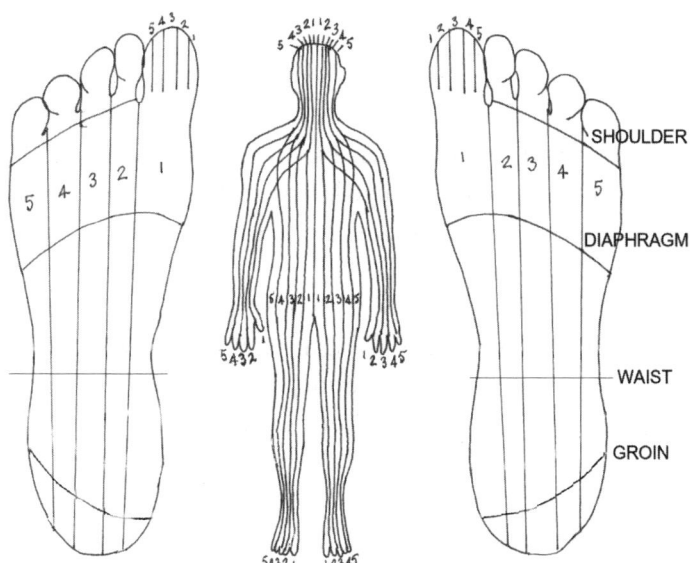

ILLUSTRATION 25: Zones & Divisions of the Body Through the Feet

The natural divisions of the body are:

1. **The Shoulder**, or the top of the shoulder, which is the division between the head and neck and the chest area;
2. **The Diaphragm**, which is above the bottom of the ribs, which is the division between the upper cavity or the chest and the middle cavity or the upper abdomen;
3. **The Waist**, which is an imaginary line of the body that separates the middle cavity or upper abdomen, from the lower cavity or the lower abdomen;
4. **The Groin**, which is the bottom of the lower cavity or lower abdomen, or the end of the torso created by the pelvic bones and the heads of the femurs (leg bones)

As illustrated above, these divisions can also be found in the feet. The feet reflect the body anatomically accurately.

The Shoulder Line or top of the shoulder is reflected at the base of the toes (neck) and is sometimes called the shoulder pad in Reflexology. It is the division between the toes and the ball of the feet and therefore reflects the top of the shoulder, which is the division between the head and neck and the chest.

The Diaphragm, or Diaphragm Line, as in the body is found up under the ribs and is the muscle of breathing (respiration). It is a line, much like the muscle is in the body, located by the colour change between the ball of the feet (the chest or upper cavity) and the beginning of the arch of the feet (upper abdomen).

The Waist Line of the feet cannot be seen, just as the waist cannot be seen on the body. On the body the waist is found with the arm (or humerus bone) in the relaxed position by the side of the torso, it is a line drawn across (transverse) the torso below the distal head of the humerus (arm) bone, that is below the elbow.

As illustrated below, the Fifth Metatarsal bone (Little toe long bone) reflects the arm (humerus) bone, and the distal head of the humerus bone is the proximal head of 5th metatarsal bone. Therefore the distal head of the 5th metatarsal bone is the reflection of the elbow. So, to locate the Waist Line on the feet, just as it is found on the body, find the proximal head of the 5th metatarsal bone, which on most people sticks out the side of the feet, and directly below this 'bump' draw a line straight across the sole and around to the back of the feet, which is the Waist Line on the feet.

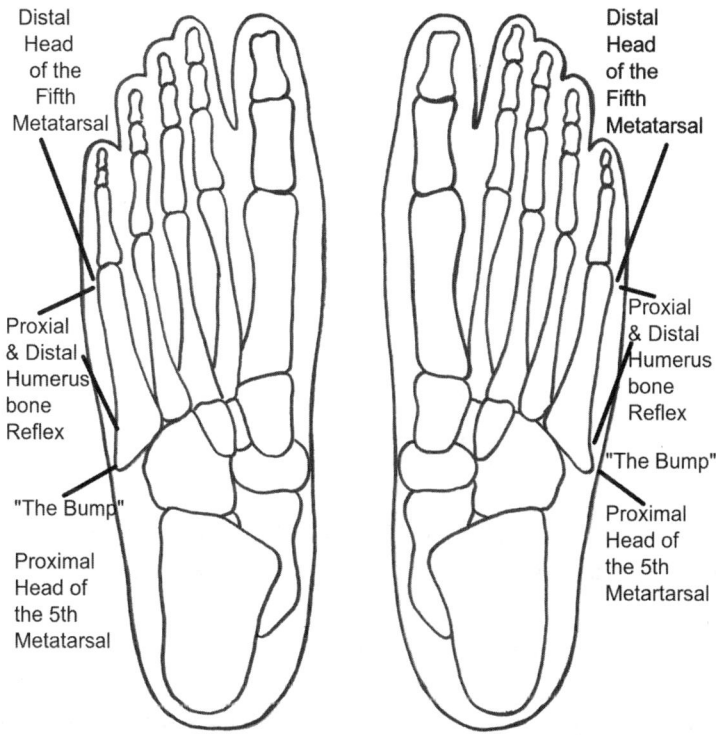

Distal Head of the Fifth Metatarsal

Proxial & Distal Humerus bone Reflex

"The Bump"

Proximal Head of the 5th Metatarsal

Distal Head of the Fifth Metatarsal

Proxial & Distal Humerus bone Reflex

"The Bump"

Proximal Head of the 5th Metartarsal

ILLUSTRATION 26:
Heads of the Fifth Metatarsal bone or Elbow

NOTE: The proximal head of the 5th metatarsal bone: "the bump', therefore, is one of the important landmarks on the feet as it reflects the Elbow and therefore allows for the location of the Waist Line on the feet, as it does on the body.

NOTE: Another important reflection is the distal head of the 5th metatarsal bone which is the proximal head of the humerus bone, and therefore is the shoulder joint.

The Groin on the body or Groin Line on the feet is created by the bones of the pelvic region and the femurs (upper leg bones) of the leg, and thus the Groin Line can only be viewed once the tissues have been removed down to the bone structures of the feet. The Groin Line then becomes visible. It is an arc (just as it is on the body) moving downward from outside to inside across the sole of the feet. It is formed by the shape of the calcaneus or heel bone and is the attachment point across the sole of the feet of the fascia of the feet.

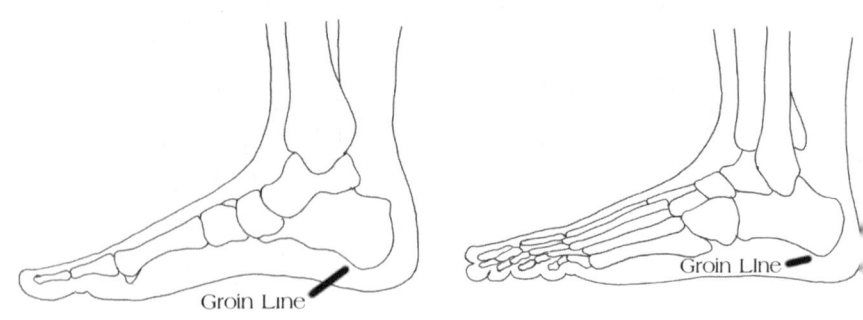

ILLUSTRATION 27: Groin Line on the Feet
Medial View   **Lateral View**

These then are the Divisions of the body located on the feet, and one of the two important landmarks of the feet. The other important landmark is related to the fascia of the feet mentioned above.

This fascia runs across the arch of the feet or instep, from the calcaneus or heel bone to the distal (toe end) heads of the five metatarsal bones, and there is a thick band of this fascia that runs between the Big and Second toes (longitudinal zones 1 and 2) from the distal heads of the 1st and 2nd metatarsal bones to the heel bone, when the toes are pulled back (See Illustration below), this think band of fascia stands out. On

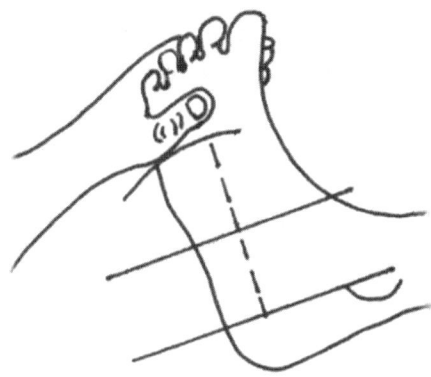

**ILLUSTRATION 28: Finding the Tendon Line
(or Thick band of fascia)**

some individuals this fascia is quite tight while on others it is relatively less tight. It is this fascia as well as other structures of the feet that help to create what is commonly called the arch of the foot (high or low arches), which is called the Medial (inside) Longitudinal (length) arch (See Chapter 25 for more details).

Historically, in Reflexology's formative years, the medical profession thought that the thick band of fascia of the feet was actually a tendon, which is a connective tissue of the body that connects bone/s to muscle/s but this is not the case here in the foot. Yet in Reflexology this thick band of fascia was originally called the Tendon Line and this has remained as Reflexology jargon. Well trained Reflexologists will know that it is not actually a tendon at all, but is in fact fascia. So, in Reflexology terminology it is known as the Tendon Line, while at the same time, medically it is fascia.

The importance of the division of the feet and the landmarks are that when combined with the Anatomical Reflection Theory and the Zones of the feet, the feet and body both are formed into a grid so that Reflexologists, and especially Reflexology students, can learn where the reflexes are and can also transfer imbalances from the body to the feet and from the feet to the body. The feet reflect the body, anatomically accurately and once one understands this perspective and the zones and divisions, then one can find anything and everything either in the feet or in the body (as imbalances reported by the receiver, or seen or felt in the feet).

For example, if a receiver has a headache, the Reflexologist will know to concentrate on the toes, and conversely (diagnostically: to be discussed in detail in Chapter 16) if the Reflexologist either sees or feels (touch) imbalances in the toes then they can be transferred to the head, and more specifically perhaps the zone of the head and neck, e.g. 2nd toe is Zone 2.

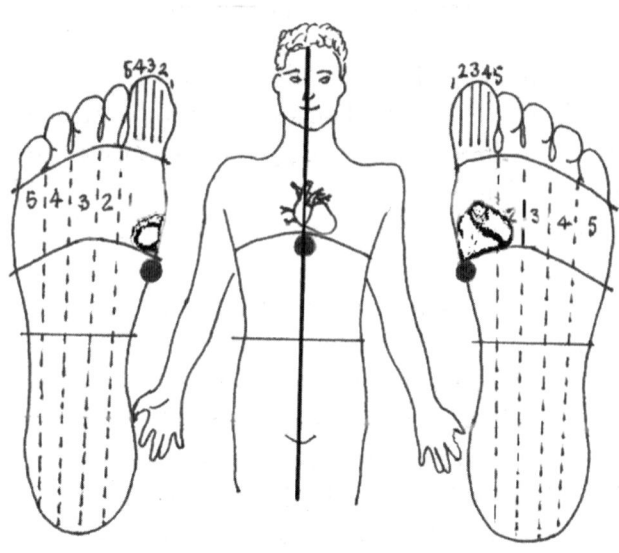

ILLUSTRATION 29: Mapping the Feet

As the illustration above demonstrates, the location of the heart in the body can be found in the feet quite easily. The heart is bi-lateral, that is on both sides of the body, and in Zone 1 as well as a little in Zone 2 of the left side of the body, and therefore the left foot as well.

A further example from the above illustration is of particular interest as it is the actual location of the Solar Plexus Chakra (See Chapter 10). The Solar Plexus Chakra or nerve plexus is in the mid-line of the body (Zone 1) and just below the end of the sternum and diaphragm. Therefore, on the feet it is located inside on both feet, just below the Diaphragm line.

With this knowledge then, Reflexologists can easily, accurately and effortlessly locate anything and everything from the body to the feet and from the feet to the body. Knowledge is power, and when combined with the necessary practical skills, makes Reflexology an even more powerful therapy.

CHAPTER 12
Referral and Helper Areas

Referral and Helper Areas are an important aspect of Reflexology as they add a significant dimension to the treatment. Together they aid in being able to work under varying circumstances as well as helping to put the body back together as a wholistic human being.

REFERRAL AREAS

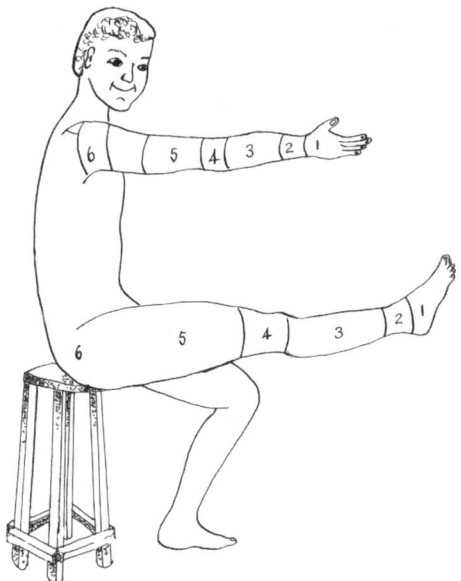

ILLUSTRATION 30: Referral Areas

A Referral area is an anatomically related area, which can be worked instead of, or in addition to, the area of imbalance. This is true for all referral areas. The basic reason these areas are called *referrals* is simply because of the anatomical relationship existing between them.

To understand Referral Areas you have to think of the human being on all fours like an animal. The explanation for this is when we were animals and we did not have two arms and two legs, but four limbs or legs, and we were running around on all fours. Then it is easy to see the parallels that exist, for example, the movement of the ankle corresponds to that of the wrist.

Another explanation of Referral Areas comes from Reflex Zone Theory. The five (Zones 1 to 5) Reflex Zones run up from the toes to the head and vice versa, as do the same five Reflex Zones run up from the fingers to the head and vice versa.

Referral Areas are areas of the foot and leg that reflect parallel areas of the hand and arm. They are used when:

- The Reflexologist cannot work the feet due to injury, inflammation and swelling or due to the feet being too sensitive for any reason;
- The receiver for either self-help or for between Reflexology session self-help, for any reason cannot use the reflexes in the feet, or as additional areas to work with the reflexes of the feet.
- Reflexologists and receivers can use the Referral Area of an imbalance located in the hand and arm as well as or instead of the feet.

For between treatment work, allow the receiver to find the point of pain in the appropriate Referral Area him or herself and that way they will remember where it is as well as find the correct location. If it is acute, I recommend working regularly and as often as the person can, but if it is chronic, I recommend two or three times a day, such as morning and evening, or after meals.

The Table below outlines the referral areas that exist between the lower and upper limbs, that is, the legs and feet to the arms and hand and vice versa.

ILLUSTRATION 31: TABLE: Referral Areas

LOWER LIMB – LEG/FOOT	UPPER LIMB – ARM/HAND
FOOT:	*HAND:*
Right Foot	Right Hand
Left Foot	Left Hand
SOLE of foot:	*PALM:*
Right Sole	Right Palm
Left Sole	Left Palm
BACK/TOP of foot:	*BACK of palm:*
Right back of foot	Right back of palm
Left back of foot	Left back of palm
TOES:	*FINGERS:*
Right toes	Right fingers
Left toes	Left fingers
Big toe	Thumb
2nd toe	Index finger
3rd toe	Middle finger
4th toe	Ring finger
5th (or little) toe	Little finger
SOLE of toes:	*FRONT (PALM SIDE) of fingers:*
Right plantar toes	Right front of fingers
Left plantar toes	Left front of fingers
BACK/TOP of toes:	*TOP/BACK of fingers:*
Right back of Toes	Right top/back of fingers
Left back of Toes	Left top/back of fingers

ANKLE:	WRIST:
Right ankle	Right wrist
Left ankle	Left wrist
Inner ankle	Inner (Thumb side) wrist
Outer ankle	Outer (Little finger side) wrist
Dorsal ankle	Back of wrist

LOWER LEG:	FOREARM:
Right lower leg	Right forearm
Left lower leg	Left forearm
Inner lower leg	Inner forearm (soft surface)
Outer lower leg	Outer forearm (hard surface)

KNEE:	ELBOW:
Right knee	Right elbow
Left knee	Left elbow
Front of knee	Outer elbow
Back of knee	Inner elbow

FEMUR/THIGH:	UPPER ARM:
Right femur/Thigh	Right upper Arms
Left femur/Thigh	Left upper Arm
Inner thigh	Inner upper Arm
Outer thigh	Outer upper Arm

HIP:	SHOULDER:
Right hip	Right shoulder
Left hip	Left shoulder
Outer hip	Back of shoulder

HELPER AREAS

Helper Areas are far more important as they are Reflexology's way of putting the body back together. Anatomy and Physiology, the medical explanation of the systems of the body, divides the body up into separate systems, and the problem with this method of understanding the human body is that it does not deal with the human being wholistically. So, Helper Areas are Reflexology's attempt at putting the systems of the body back together and dealing with any imbalance or problem wholistically.

For example, a reproductive imbalance by the Systematic approach to the human body would work the Reproductive System, but the glands (or Endocrine System) are an integral part of the process of reproduction, and yet are not included in the Reproductive System. Therefore, the Helper Areas are a method of looking for other aspects of the human being that may help a particular imbalance, which lies outside the direct reflexes and the system in which the imbalance is placed.

Helper Areas are additional areas worked to aid a specific imbalance. They are the reinforcement you send to aid the specific imbalance. So they are reflexes in the feet which, when worked in conjunction with the direct reflexes, help in relieving the imbalance. They are reflexes that have a direct effect on the afflicted area and are the reinforcement needed to make sure you reach the desired result of a more balanced state of existence. Helper Areas involve looking at body systems and lateral thinking and include the interrelationships of the human being and the human body as a whole.

So the concept of Helper Areas is Reflexology's attempt to help Reflexologists think laterally and wholistically. They are extremely important, if not vital, if the Reflexologist's approach is based on a systematic approach to the body, which deals with the bits in isolation from the rest, and the body cut up into separate systems, which have become arbitrarily locked in and are now 'tradition'.

To Be A HELPER AREA THE REFLEX MUST :

1. Not be the direct Reflex/es of the imbalance in the feet but other reflex/es, and
2. Lie outside the system in which the imbalance is placed.

And the question Reflexologists need to constantly ask is: *"What might help this imbalance, other than the obvious?"*

So, for a menstruation imbalance, the direct reflexes are

the Reproductive reflexes in the feet, and the system in which menstruation would fall is the Reproductive system. Therefore, the Endocrine system or the glands, and specifically the Pituitary and Thyroid/Parathyroid glands would be Helper Areas for these are not the direct reflex/es and they are outside the Reproductive system in the Endocrine System.

Helper Areas then are extremely important to wholistically help the human being and the particular imbalance. There are a number of general Helper Areas for any imbalance, although please keep in mind that they are generally helpful for any imbalance, but not necessarily helpful for every imbalance. These are listed in the table below.

GENERAL HELPER AREAS
ILLUSTRATION 32: Table

CENTRAL NERVOUS SYSTEM (CNS), ESPECIALLY THE SPINE
As this is one of the two major communication systems of the body, and as it is the faster of the two systems, this is often useful, especially specific spinal nerves that relate to a specific imbalance.

DIGESTIVE SYSTEM
There are those that argue the Digestive system is a good Helper Area for many imbalances and this has some merit. However, as the digestive system contains nearly every major organ of the body and runs from the mouth to the anus and covers nearly everything in between, most imbalances are either part of this system and therefore fall under the Digestive system, or are related in some way to this system. It is one of the problems of a systematic approach to the body that will discussed in Chapter 27.

ENDOCRINE SYSTEM
As this is the second of the two major 'communication'

systems of the body (glands excrete hormones through the blood) it also is often a good Helper Area for many imbalances, especially digestive, growth and development, and reproductive imbalances.

IMMUNE SYSTEM

Strictly speaking there is no system called Immune System. However many speak about it as if there is, and further, literally everything in the body is part of the immune system, so literally every imbalance falls under the Immune System. So it cannot be a Helper Area. Nice little vicious circle.

KIDNEYS

The kidneys filter the blood, often a good Helper Area for many imbalances, as better blood and less toxins in the system, helps.

LIVER

As the Liver works through the blood, it is a generally good Helper Area for just about any imbalance, as better blood is just about always of assistance.

LYMPHATIC SYSTEM

This is a good system as it helps to break down and dispose of complex molecules from the blood, and therefore helps to clean the blood. Once again better blood is always a good thing.

SOLAR PLEXUS OR K.1/TRIPLE BURNER

'**Solar Plexus**': Some would argue that this reflex is good for many imbalances as it strengthens the personality. As it is actually **K.1/Triple Burner**: This reflex is good for just about anything and everything as it deals with the 'roots' of the person and the process of Chi (energy) creation.

CHAPTER 13
FOOT MAP: *Physical Anatomical Location of the Reflexes*

As a prelude to the chart that follows, a discussion of the foot maps that are currently available and their consistency is necessary.

There are hundreds, if not thousands, of foot charts available. Why are there so many? The reason for this is twofold:

1. To go into print, Reflexologist must make sure their chart is significantly (or at least cosmetically) different enough from the original so that he/she would not be sued, as the original chart is copyrighted and a breach of copyright, without authority and compensation, may result in legal action.

2. As a minor point, Reflexologists have added detail to the understanding of the feet, based upon the original. These developments have been added to the original, but are based upon the original. They are still essentially the same chart with minor information added. They are, when you compare them, not significantly different from the original.

Most charts are not significantly different from the original. Therefore, one must conclude that the major reason for these minor changes is related more to point 1 above than actual developments. Cosmetically, so many of these foot charts appear to be different, but once one begins comparing them to the original it becomes increasingly clear that they are simply copies.

Look at the Foot Chart Illustrations from Chapter 7 and compare these illustrations (and the evaluation from this chapter), as well as the Anatomical Reflection Theory, with other charts and it becomes quite obvious that these charts are but copies. They all have basically everything in the same place, and have perpetuated the same flaws as the original.

There are two exceptions I know of to this, (There may be others that I have not seen.) the foot chart of Chris Stormer (the oldest that I know of) and the Western Australian School of Reflexology foot chart. These two charts are significantly different from others as they have begun analysing the premises and basics of Reflexology. These two foot charts are important for the development of all Reflexologists and Reflexology itself for they have questioned the original and attempted or begun to understand Reflexology theory and present some sort of consistency. Ironically, both of these foot charts have evolved from a non-physical and energy-type approaches.

To these two charts I acknowledge a debt as they aided me in my attempt to understand Reflexology better with the result being this current work. As mentioned elsewhere, Chris Stormer's approach is emotionally based, and Lyn Hatfield, from the Western Australian School of Reflexology, is Metamorphosis or Metamorphic Technique approach, which is also an energy and non-physical type approach.

There are two comments that need to be made here before moving to the actual chart. Two facts arise as a result of the Anatomical Reflection Theory which few Reflexologists appear to understand and that is that:

1. **The inner aspect of the feet is actually inside the body**;
2. **The inner aspects of the Big, 2nd, 3rd, 4th and 5th toes and the outer aspect of the 2nd, 3rd and 4th toes are actually inside the head and neck.**

The first of these two points most Reflexologists appear to vaguely know, but it is left at that: simply a statement.

Generally, however, these two facts appear to have been

either missed or glossed over by most Reflexologists, despite being hugely significant, as Reflexology is the only body therapy that can actually access the organs and structures inside the head/neck and body. This is simply stated as one of the basic premises upon which Reflexology is based and then left aside.

The deep inner physical, as well as the other three levels, can be accessed where it resides: within. So, Reflexology has a huge advantage over all other body therapies, as the inner aspect of both feet is down the mid-line of the body, which cuts through all the major organs, except the lungs, spleen and kidneys, as well as most of the glands and many other structures of the body, including the deep muscles that cannot be accessed any other way.

So, Reflexology, through the inner aspect of the two feet, is working inside the body, and there are actually four lines or planes that can be worked here. They are, from back to front of the body (feet):

1. The superficial structures and the superficial and deep muscles of the back;
2. Inside the spine and sacrum and central nervous system (cut in half with half on each foot);
3. Inside most of the organs and structures of the body;
4. The front tissues and superficial and deep muscles of the front of the torso.

Also the inside and outside (as mentioned above) of most of the toes are actually inside the head and neck. This is hugely significant as again Reflexology is the only therapy (other than surgery) that can access slices of the head and neck from the inside. To explain, one must return to the Reflex Zone Theory of the Head/Neck (toes).

With the previous explanation (See Chapter 8) in mind, it is obvious that:

1. The Big toe is both the whole half the head, and therefore the inner aspect of the Big toe is along the midsagittal plane

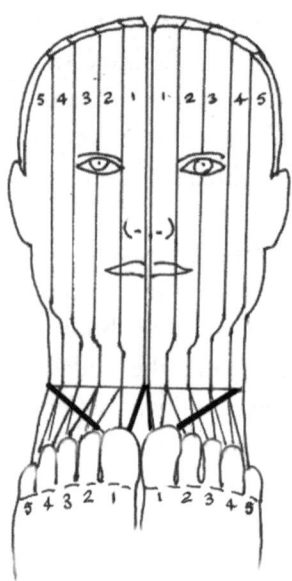

ILLUSTRATION 33: Reflex Zone Theory and the Head

or mid-line of the head and neck and therefore is inside the body, and it is also Zone 1 of the head/neck and therefore again inside the head and neck, closest to the mid-line of the body.

2. The inner and outer aspects of the 2nd, 3rd, and 4th toes are slices of the head, that is Zones 2, 3, and 4, and therefore the inner and outer aspects of these toes are in fact inside the head and neck.

3. The inner aspect of the 5th toe is also inside the head and neck with the outer aspect being the outer head and neck.

One other point before proceeding to the physical anatomical location of the reflexes in the feet is that, on the sole view of the feet the Reflexologist is looking at the sole from the bottom and therefore the Reflexologist's:

• Right hand is on the Left foot, and

• Left hand is on the Right foot.

It is important to keep this in mind; otherwise you may get confused as to right and left.

One last point before illustrating the systems of the body and their reflexes through the feet; as the Sole view of the systems of the body is quite complicated, it has been broken into two divisions based generally on the depth of the system from deep to superficial. As the body is three dimensional and is not a flat one dimensional object, no one location of the feet (body) is any one thing.

ILLUSTRATION 34: PHYSICAL FOOT CHART

a) SOLE (PLANTAR) VIEW:

I. CARDIOVASCULAR, ENDOCRINE, REPRODUCTIVE, SENSE ORGANS AND URINARY SYSTEMS:

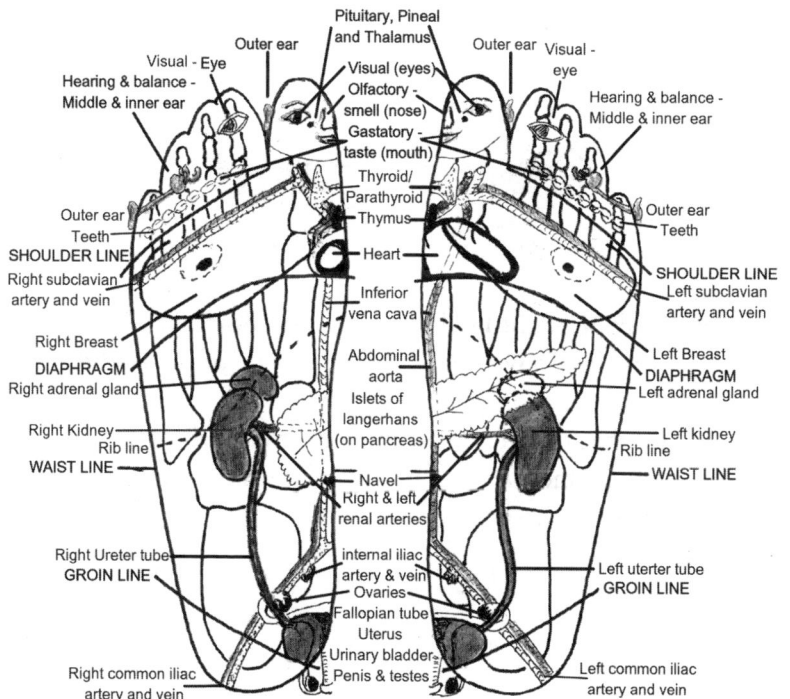

Right Foot/Right Half of the Body

Left Foot/Left Half of the Body

NOTE that the Muscular and Integumentary (skin) systems have been left off the above Foot Chart.

129

2. DIGESTIVE, LYMPHATIC, NERVOUS AND SKELETAL SYSTEMS:

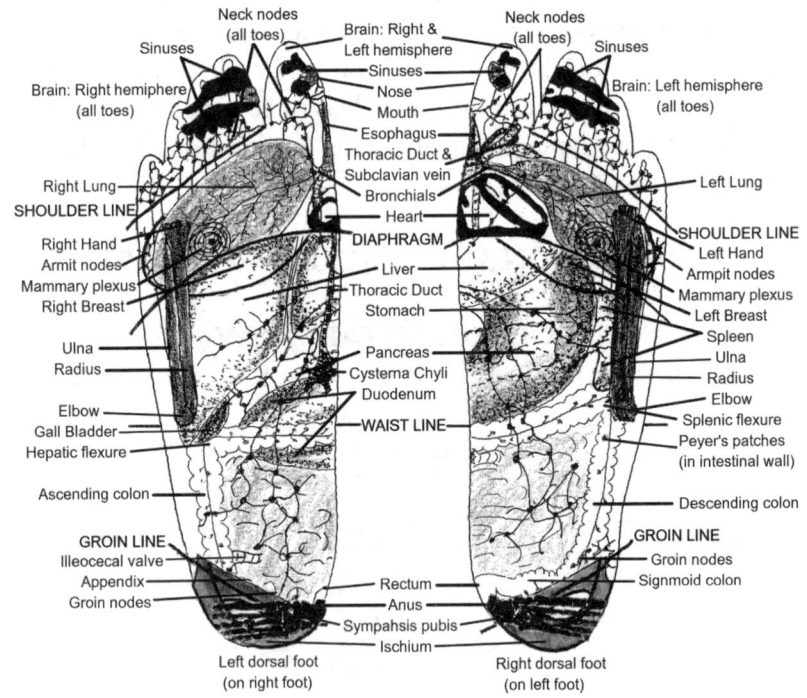

**Right Foot/Right Half
of the Body**

**Left Foot/Left Half
of the Body**

NOTE that the Muscular, Integumentary (skin) and most of the Skeletal and Nervous (brain) systems have been left off the above Foot Chart.

b) TOP/BACK OF THE FOOT/BACK OF THE BODY (DORSAL) VIEW:

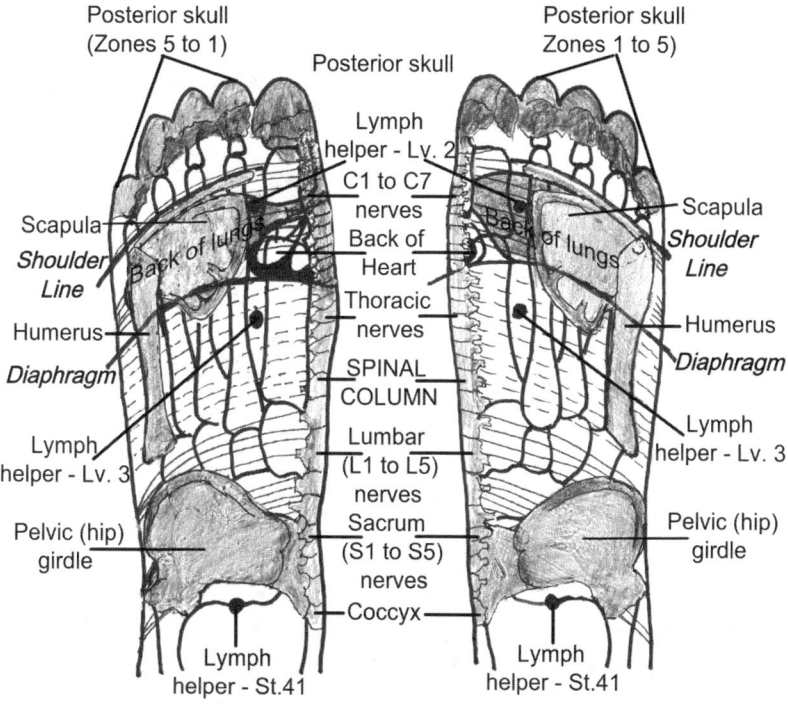

Posterior skull
(Zones 5 to 1)

Posterior skull

Posterior skull
Zones 1 to 5)

Lymph
helper - Lv. 2
C1 to C7
nerves
Back of
Heart
Thoracic
nerves
SPINAL
COLUMN
Lumbar
(L1 to L5)
nerves
Sacrum
(S1 to S5)
nerves
Coccyx

Scapula
Shoulder Line
Back of lungs
Humerus
Diaphragm
Lymph
helper - Lv. 3
Pelvic (hip)
girdle
Lymph
helper - St.41

Back of lungs

Scapula
Shoulder Line
Humerus
Diaphragm
Lymph
helper - Lv. 3
Pelvic (hip)
girdle
Lymph
helper - St.41

131

c) INSIDE OF THE FOOT/INSIDE THE BODY (MEDIAL) VIEW:

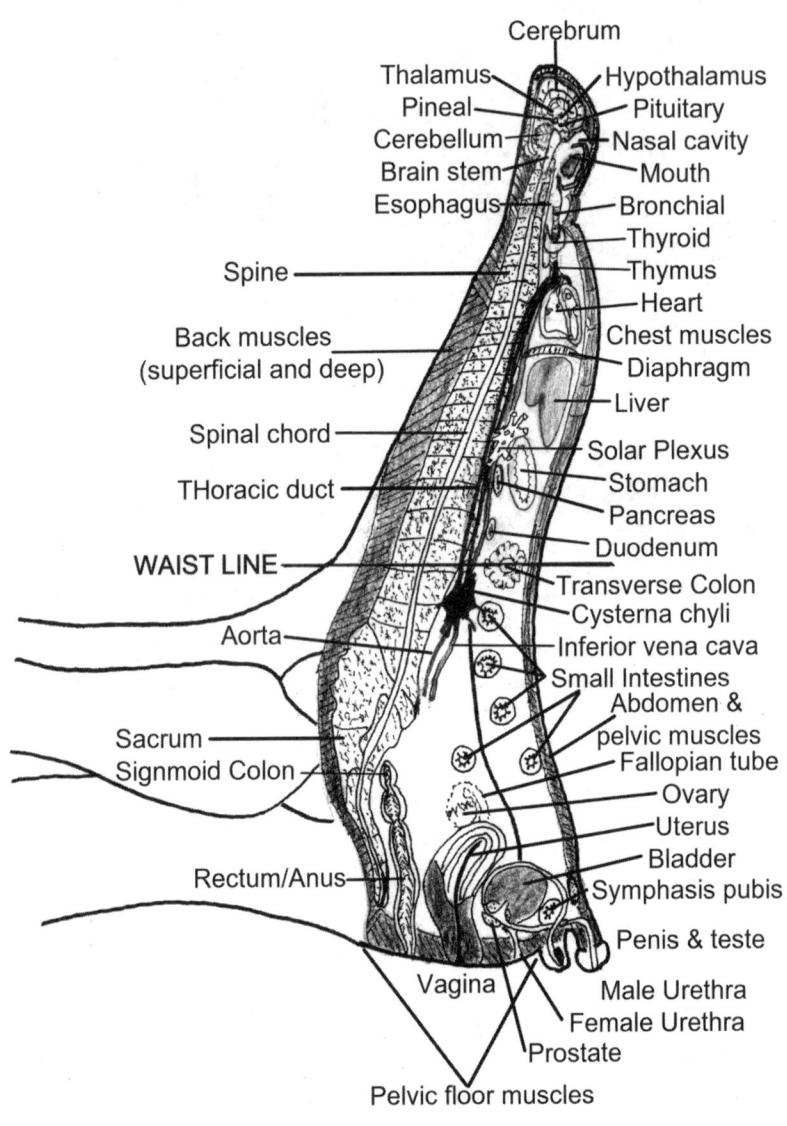

Cerebrum
Thalamus
Hypothalamus
Pineal
Pituitary
Cerebellum
Nasal cavity
Brain stem
Mouth
Esophagus
Bronchial
Thyroid
Spine
Thymus
Heart
Back muscles (superficial and deep)
Chest muscles
Diaphragm
Liver
Spinal chord
Solar Plexus
THoracic duct
Stomach
Pancreas
Duodenum
WAIST LINE
Transverse Colon
Cysterna chyli
Aorta
Inferior vena cava
Small Intestines
Abdomen & pelvic muscles
Sacrum
Fallopian tube
Signmoid Colon
Ovary
Uterus
Bladder
Rectum/Anus
Symphasis pubis
Penis & teste
Vagina
Male Urethra
Female Urethra
Prostate
Pelvic floor muscles

d) OUTSIDE OF THE FOOT/OUTSIDE THE BODY (LATERAL) VIEW:

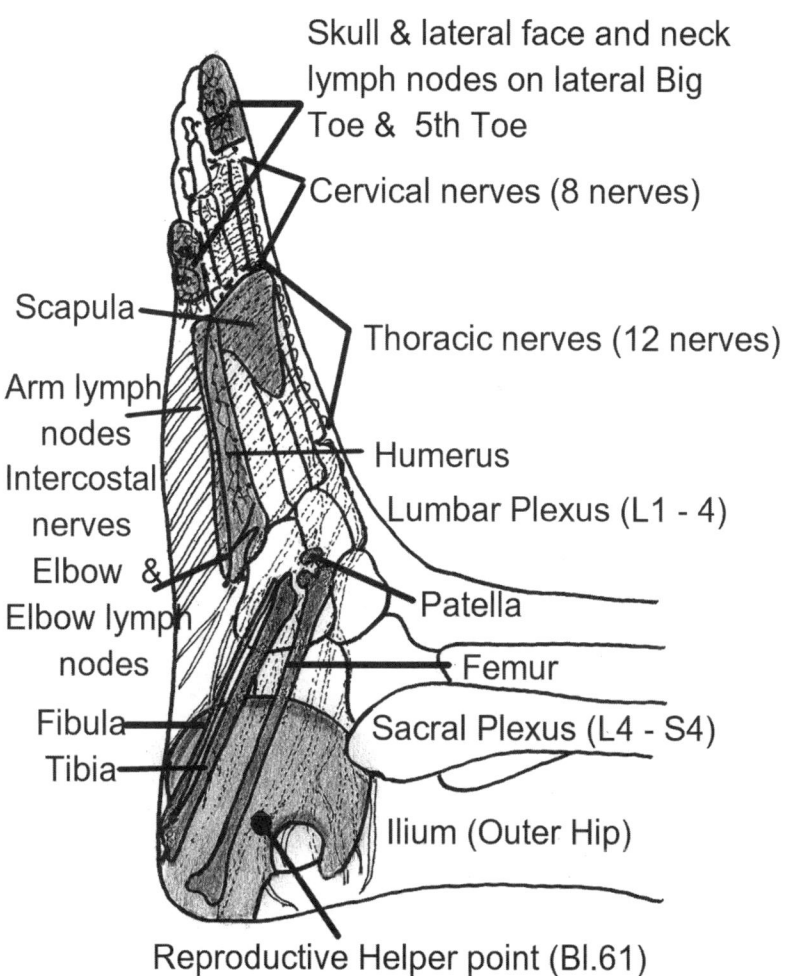

Skull & lateral face and neck lymph nodes on lateral Big Toe & 5th Toe

Cervical nerves (8 nerves)

Scapula

Thoracic nerves (12 nerves)

Arm lymph nodes

Intercostal nerves

Humerus

Lumbar Plexus (L1 - 4)

Elbow & Elbow lymph nodes

Patella

Femur

Fibula

Sacral Plexus (L4 - S4)

Tibia

Ilium (Outer Hip)

Reproductive Helper point (Bl.61)

SECTION 2
Reflexology
Practical Techniques

"Your eyes deceive you —
let your thumb and fingers
become your eyes,
and see anew."

CHAPTER 14
Visual Assessment of the Feet:
Introduction to Foot Reading

There are three methods of simple diagnosis through the feet and they are:

1. Medical history and transfer to the feet;
2. Look and see in the feet, and transfer to the body;
3. Touch and feel in the feet, and transfer to the body.

And of course, vice versa, that is transfer from the body to the feet. (For a detailed analysis of diagnosing, see Chapter 16). The first of these two points will be briefly covered here, and the second point will be discussed in the following chapter.

As an introduction to Foot Reading, one can simply look at a pair of feet, take note of what one sees, and then via the Anatomical Reflection Theory, the zones of the feet and the divisions of the body, transfer to the body.

Further useful information includes:

- The sole of the foot, reflects the front of the body and therefore the present (and possibly future);
- The back of the foot, reflects the back of the body and what is behind, and therefore the past;
- The inside of the foot, reflects inside the body and therefore the deep inner stuff;
- The outside of the foot, reflects the outside and superficial, everyday matters.

And still more details of:

- The right foot reflects the yang, active, doing, masculine aspects of the human being;
- The left foot reflects the yin, passive, intuitive, feminine aspects.

Just with this information alone, one can begin to see and interpret information gleaned from the feet. A visual assessment of the feet, therefore, is a worthwhile beginning as much is revealed on a physical level as well as on emotional, mental and spiritual levels.

The two leading Reflexologists of foot reading are Avi Grinburg of Israel and Christine Stormer of South Africa. If interested in foot reading, the writings of these two would be a good beginning, but recently there have been others who have delved into 'palmistry of the feet'.

BUT WHAT CAN ONE SEE IN THE FEET?

The list is endless, but includes:

- Variations in Temperature (Hot/Cold)
- Overall colour: Pink, Red, Yellow, Grey, Black, Blue, etc.
- Changes in colour
- Moisture: Clammy, wet/moist; perspiration
- Distinguishing marks, areas and reflexes
- Injuries and scars (Recent bone fracture/breaks) and operations
- Dry, rough and scaly skin
- Corns, bunions, calluses, plantar warts and spurs
- Freckles, beauty spots, moles and hair concentration
- Ulcers, wounds, wrinkles, creases and skin folds
- Changes in skin texture and shape and bone structure
- Prominent veins and nail condition
- Shape of the toes and their position
- Enlarged toes joints; hammer toes
- Swelling and oedema (Fluid retention)
- Eczema and tinea (any skin condition)

- Odour and weight distribution
- Shape of the feet compared to the shape of the body
- Angle of each foot in relation to each other
- Arches: high, low or normal
- Connective tissue appearance and muscle tone: Good, moderate, poor
- Ankle flexibility

There is so much to be observed and interpreted. As one can now easily see, by looking and seeing and then interpreting, one is actually diagnosing an imbalance, perhaps physical but not necessarily, in the part or region of the body. The more one does this, the more one sees.

As an exercise, get a blank pair of feet: sole, back, inside and outside and with a pair of feet in front of you, take a good look at both feet and record down what you see. Then choose one of these things that you have recorded down and attempt to interpret it. As a suggestion, simply accept the first thought that comes into your mind. It is usually the most accurate. Now discuss this, being very conscious of the fact that you are talking about this person, and see what happens. Both of you will be amazed at how accurate this often is and how much it reveals.

There are so many different interpretations of foot reading, but do not let this discourage you. Learn them all. They are all worthwhile. The key is to find one that you relate to the most and use this as your basis, and what will happen is that, especially if you learn to follow your first thought, your intuition will choose from your knowledge the most appropriate meaning for each individual. This is an excellent way of developing your intuition and training your mind to accept your intuition. Realise that it is knowledge that frames and structures the intuition. Without knowledge, intuition is like water or sand; it flows through your fingers without being of much use. But on the other hand, knowledge without intuition is dead, and lacks vitality, accuracy and creativity. You need both.

CHAPTER 15
Touch as an Evaluative Tool:
Thumb and Fingers become the Eyes

As mentioned in the previous chapter, there are three methods of simple diagnostic through the feet. As with Foot Reading of the previous chapter, with touch one can simply feel what is happening in the body through the feet, and take note of what one feels, and then via the Anatomical Reflection Theory, the zones of the feet and the divisions of the body, transfer to the body.

Like looking and seeing, the sense of touch is extremely worthwhile as it reveals information on a physical level, as well as on an emotional, mental and spiritual level.

Touch is an important consideration, and is one of the Reflexology Theories (see Chapter 8 for more details). Not only is touch important, but also the type of touch is of particular concern. How one handles the feet sends a clear message to the body about your attitudes to the feet, to the body and the receiver. Remember, when working the feet, you are working the body and the human being through the feet. These matters will be discussed in detail in Chapter 19 and in Chapter 20.

The eyes see what is on the surface of the feet, but cannot see beneath the surface. The eyes are not as reliable an instrument as most think they are. This is because the impulses which the eyes pick up are transferred to the brain/mind, and it is actually here in the brain/mind that the impulses are translated into meaningful information. So the ability to take in light and vibrations is the major function of the eyes, but the ability to translate and understand those vibrations actually occur in the brain/mind, and this is based on previous experiences, knowledge and programming of the computer.

For this reason alone I would recommend not using your eyes when performing Reflexology. As a suggestion, use your eyes to get to the general area where you are going, and then either:

- Work with your eyes closed, which is what I did for many years, OR
- Work with your eyes turned away, not watching what you are doing, which is what I tend to do now.

This way you will train your working thumb and fingers to be your eyes. Over time and with practice, your thumb and fingers will become sensitive to the reflexes and you will increasingly feel what is going on within. You must always be under the skin, and initially to develop this feel, you need to have medium pressure, but with experience and increased sensitivity your pressure will lighten. You will always need to be under the skin, but it is all there just under the skin, to be felt. Too strong a pressure actually decreases one's sensitivity and masks the messages under the skin. In fact, over time, it will actually cause imbalance in the system. Therefore, medium pressure at the most is all that is necessary.

Pressure should be varied from reflex to reflex and throughout different parts of the body (feet). There is no one pressure, and as you develop your ability to feel what the body needs in different locations, you will actually increase and decrease your pressure as you work, much like a musician playing an instrument where the vibrations or notes increase and decrease, creating an harmonious whole: a song. So Reflexologists should vary their pressure, from very light to medium, from:

- Reflex to reflex;

- Treatment to treatment on the same person;
- From one receiver to another.

This is one of the keys to listening to the body and following the body's messages. Where there is softness, the body is asking for stronger pressure and where there is hardness the body is asking for less. It is as simple as that. Why? Because what the body (feet) puts out as a message is it is asking for its opposite.

Let me explain. If the body is hot, what is it asking for? More heat? No. Coolness. If the body is cold, what is it asking for? Coldness? NO. Heat. So where there is hardness in a reflex or area of the foot (body), the body is asking for softness or sedation techniques. Where there is softness, the foot (body) is asking for hardness or stimulation. This is one of the fundamental aspects of working with the body, not against it. It is so simple and obvious that many have not seen what is there before their eyes (and their thumb and fingers).

So whenever there is any form of hardness, heat, inflammation, bumps, crunch, pop, crinkle, etc. the body, through the feet and reflexes, is asking for sedation. Something worth remembering is that whenever the body is in trouble the one thing that alwaysss occurs is inflammation (heat), whether it be superficially, for example skin and muscles, or whether it be deep inner organs. So what is the body asking for? Sedation.

Take the analogy of an old fashioned steam train running along a flat and level track (the balanced state of existence), let's say the train uses 10 tonnes of wood per hour to maintain a speed of 60 kilometres per hour (miles if you like). If you incline the track to 45 degrees (which is what stimulation does: it makes it harder for the body to do what it is trying to do), to maintain the 60 kilometres per hour speed, the train would use probably three times the amount of wood per hour, say 30 tonnes per hour. If the train began going up hill, say a 75 degree slope, then to maintain the 60 kilometres per hour speed the train would need say 60 tonnes per hour.

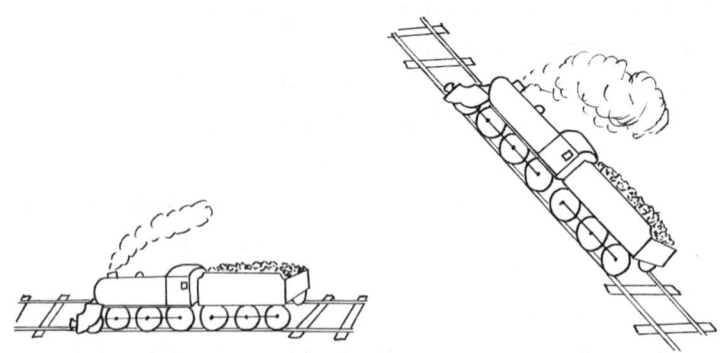

ILLUSTRATION 35: The Steam Train (Stimulation)

So when the body is in trouble and puts out a message of inflammation or hardness, it is not asking for stimulation but its opposite. This is why there are so many safety precautions and contraindications with a stimulatory approach. It is disobeying the body's messages and taking risks with the body and the human being, and making it harder for the body to do what it is already trying to do. Not a very wise course of action.

Taking the analogy further, when the body is in trouble, it is already on a 45-degree slope. What is needed is not making it harder for the body, by stimulating and increasing the workload, but the opposite, sedating, or decreasing the workload, so rather than the train needing 30 tonnes of wood (fuel or energy) to maintain the 60 kilometres per hour it will only need 10 tonnes, which frees up 20 tonnes of wood (fuel or energy) for the job at hand. Much more sensible and safer.

One further point here is that when there is dis-ease the tendency is as mentioned in the previous chapter, that is extreme inflammation and the body is working four or five (or even ten) times harder to maintain itself, and so the body is asking for sedation, or to make it easier for the body to maintain itself, so that it has a better chance to work on the dis-ease and to heal itself.

Conversely, where there is emptiness, hollow, cool, holes, etc. the body is asking for stimulation. Note that if this is actually the case, there will be little or no pain, especially no sharp pain, but only a dull ache or a good pain if anything.

So touch is extremely important, but the type of touch is far more important. Learn to listen to the body through your touch and you will know what the body, through the feet, is asking for and you can begin the journey of listening to the body and following the body's messages. It is all there; it just takes experience, knowledge and sensitivity. It is not hard, but easy.

> "HEALING IS NATURAL AND EASY.
> IT CAN HAPPEN IN THE BLINK OF AN EYE."

AND

> "MIRACLES CAN HAPPEN.
> OPEN THE DOOR FOR MIRACLES TO HAPPEN."

OR

> "HEALING IS HARD. LIFE IS HARD.
> AND ONE MUST STRUGGLE AND SUFFER TO HEAL."

Which is the better belief system? Which is a better premise from which to work?

CHAPTER 16
Diagnosing through the Feet

Much has been written in various other chapters of this work concerning diagnosis. So let's reiterate and pull all this information together here.

One of the two DON'Ts of Reflexology is: **NEVER** diagnose or **name a disease**.

Reflexology argues quite clearly that Reflexologists should never diagnose, and yet uses the diagnosis of others to treat. Interesting. Why? Are others more qualified to diagnose? Does this say something about the profession of Reflexology or perhaps about the desire to be accepted by the health care system and so there is a desire to present a sanitized, non-threatening Reflexology in a way that is acceptable to a specific group: the health care system and perhaps the general public. This then is the standard line taken by Reflexology, but the truth of the matter is that all Reflexologists do diagnose, and there is nothing wrong with this.

HOW DO REFLEXOLOGISTS DIAGNOSE?

a) **Transfer from the body to the feet**: Initially a Reflexologist diagnoses by taking a detailed medical and life history of the receiver before beginning to work on them, and the Reflexologist transfers these imbalances to the reflexes of the feet. For example, with a person with a knee problem, the

Reflexologist notes down to work the Knee reflex in both feet. This is diagnosis.

b) **Look and see**: Secondly, by looking at the reflexes of the feet, the Reflexologist gathers information on the imbalances found in the feet and transfers this information, via knowledge of the of the location of the reflexes (Anatomical Reflection Theory) and the part of the body involved, to the relevant region of the body, and vice versa. Again this is diagnosis.

c) **Touch and feel**: Thirdly, while working the Reflexologist often picks up imbalances in the reflexes of the feet and via knowledge of the location of the reflexes and the part of the body involved, transfers the felt imbalances to the region of the body, and vice versa. Once more this is diagnosis.

The simple inescapable conclusion is that Reflexologists do in fact diagnose. Honesty is the best policy. It is not diagnosing dis-ease but rather finding the imbalances in the feet (or hands) to the body and the imbalances of the body to the feet (or hands). This is absolutely fine as long as one realises that it does not mean dis-ease but is rather simply a message about the receiver's body. The message of the body is one of an imbalance in an area of the body/feet/hands and vice versa. So what Reflexologists are diagnosing is in fact imbalances that may be physical (and ultimately lead to dis-ease), but are just as possibly emotional, mental and/or spiritual imbalances, and maybe even an energy (chi) imbalance. Therefore, their benefits are for the receiver via the therapist.

Experience indicates that this is extremely useful for the Reflexologist and aids in the treatment given. For this reason alone Reflexology needs to be clear with its students so that they can be made aware of the benefits of such diagnosis while at the same time understanding the dangers in diagnosing only physical imbalances and dis-ease and informing the receivers of this misinformation.

These forms of diagnosis are the standard tools of Reflexologists and should be covered clearly in any training. They are for the Reflexologist, not the receiver. The whole purpose of this form of diagnosis is to make the treatment as specific and accurate for the receiver as possible. So the diagnosis is for the therapist, not the receiver. This is a mistake that some Reflexologists make and it is an important error in judgment for many reasons.

As well, the Reflexologist is assuming that an imbalance noted is a physical one, is relying on the foot map's interpretation of the imbalance, which is not necessarily the case (and in fact often isn't). An imbalance can manifest on a physical level, but it is also just as likely to manifest on an emotional, mental, spiritual or energy level, and so the Reflexologist is on very shaky ground here.

A significant and important point to remember is when a Reflexologist sees or feels an imbalance in the feet, there is no way of knowing for sure what it actually is.

This is one of the major problems with most foot maps and Reflexology training. Reflexology students are taught a map which shows what is where. They are not taught to understand the four-dimensional nature of the human being. When you realise that a human being is four-dimensional and there is depth, it becomes extremely important not to diagnose anything specifically, as it could be anything.

Take for example, a Reflexologist, while working on a receiver, picks up an imbalance in the toes, which is the head and neck reflexes. The Reflexologist looks at their foot map which shows that it is, the brain or the sinuses, or the eye, or … whatever. They then believe that that is what it must be. But there are always options and are a whole range of reflexes in the toes. This is not necessarily correct and is dangerous, and potentially may harm the receiver, the Reflexologist and the profession of Reflexology.

The reality is, on a purely physical level an imbalance in the toes could be anything in the head and neck including the skull (bones), the brain, the mind, the brain stem, the muscles of the head, neck and face, the eyes and seeing, the ears and hearing, nerve impulses from any part of the body, the blood vessels (arteries and veins), the eating and breathing tubes running from the head, certain glands, the neck bones (cervicals), etc. It could be anything from the front of the face and neck to the back of the head and neck and anything in-between. The list is endless. So it is extremely difficult to pinpoint what the imbalance actually is, and this is looking just on a physical level. When one considers the other levels of existence: the emotional, mental, spiritual, and energy (chi), one begins to realise that the options are just about limitless.

Reflexologists should not diagnose an organ or name a disease by giving an imbalance a name, and it is a mistake that many Reflexologists fall into. They pick up imbalances in the feet and diagnose. Giving a label to something is a grave mistake. Reflexologists (and for that matter any natural therapist or health care professional) should never name a dis-ease, or even a particular organ. Why?

Firstly, because some argue that only a medically qualified health care provider has the legal and moral right to diagnose. This may in fact be correct, but there is a more important reason for not diagnosing dis-ease and that is that the Reflexologist then treats a dis-ease and treats a label rather than helping a human being.

The other question here that needs mentioning is that Reflexologists have been known to tell receivers what they have found and plant the seed of disharmony, which may or may not be correct. Furthermore, the Reflexologist risks their professional credibility. If incorrect, they have done harm to the receiver, to themselves and to the profession of Reflexology.

REFLEXOLOGISTS ARE OFTEN ASKED WHEN SOMETHING IS TENDER: WHAT'S THAT?

Initially while learning, and in the early stages of becoming a professional Reflexologist, the tendency is to tell the receiver. This is partly for the giver's learning, so as to gain a better understanding of the feet and the Anatomical Reflection Theory, as well as to convince the giver that Reflexology actually works. This is understandable but it is not a valid reason. What would be better is to simply ask a question. Something like:

"Do you have a problem in this or that area of the body, front and/or back?"

Often this question alone triggers the receiver's memory and they will explain what has been picked up and what they have felt themselves. This is as far as one needs to go, but do take note of this on your consultation sheets (what needs to be done) for present and future reference.

However, the best option here is to downplay the whole process by:

1. Initially, if possible, giving back information the receiver has already given the Reflexologist (from the medical and personal history taken before working). However, the Reflexologist should take note of this as it could be this, but it could also be something else. It is the body's way of giving the Reflexologist a message and that message should be listened to.

2. If this is not possible, the next best option is to state, "It is just an imbalance. Nothing to worry about. It is easily rectified." This statement is neutral and plants no seeds of discontent. It keeps the options open and the chance of healing is increased, or at least it is not decreased.

3. If the receiver does not accept this explanation, the next best option is simply to give a region of the body. For example if it is something in the head/neck region (toes), simply state that it is an imbalance in that area of the body, probably once again something simple, e.g. neck tension.

This is the most that should be conveyed to the receiver, as again it is actually a message to the Reflexologist from the body that it needs help, and should always be followed. Listen to the body, interpret the message if you like and then obey the message. It is as simple as that.

All Reflexologists should do is diagnose an imbalance, which by its very nature is fairly simple to correct, and of no major significance. This phrase is extremely general and neutral and therefore plants no seeds of destructive thought, action or emotion. It is the best option.

One final point on diagnosis is that there are those within the Reflexology professional community, especially Clinical Reflexologists who are from a medical background, who argue that Reflexologists actually do diagnose and that this is wrong. Only those Reflexologists who have specific training in standard western industrial medicine should diagnose and there is nothing wrong with this per se. They reserve the right to themselves. Elitism rings out here, as does a desire to be as good as western industrial medicine. Is this really what Reflexologists and the profession of Reflexology want? Another issue that arises.

But the options that this approach brings are twofold once again, and that is, either:

1. Diagnosing dis-ease by the issuance of a label and therefore treat labels, or
2. Diagnosing imbalances and using these to help the human being.

To conclude then, Reflexology does diagnose in its own unique and useful way and this should be clearly explained, understood and accepted as a natural and necessary part of the practice of Reflexology. The other issues that arise from this, need to be brought out into the open, debated and decisions made about them, for each individual Reflexologist and for the profession of Reflexology. This task lies ahead.

CHAPTER 17
Basic Techniques

The basic techniques of Reflexology are quite simple and there are but a few skills that need to be learned to be able to practice:

1. Thumb walking
2. Finger walking
3. Tip of Thumb
4. Tip of Finger
5. Knuckles
6. Drawing
7. Holding.

The two major techniques are Thumb and Finger walking, with the use of the tip of thumb or finger also extremely useful. There are other techniques which other Reflexology approaches advocate and it is always worth investigating the multitude of techniques once you have learnt the basics for even after completing Reflexology training, your learning should never cease. There is alwayss more to learn. In fact, after becoming qualified is when your major learning occurs; it is then that you begin to develop as a professional, and it is a never-ending process, which in itself brings its own rewards. It is therefore a journey rather than a destination.

In conjunction with these techniques, holding techniques and the Basic Rules of Reflexology are also important to effectively and easily perform Reflexology. (See Chapter 19 and

Chapter 20.)

Let's now look at each of these techniques in detail.

I. Thumb walking

This is the basic technique of Reflexology and you will find it mentioned and described in all Reflexology books. Many of these descriptions contradict one another and so it is sometimes difficult to decide which is the best and what each actually means. It is also a rather difficult technique to explain in words, but is not, with practice, difficult to perform.

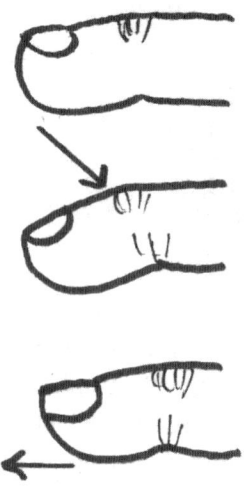

ILLUSTRATION 36: Thumb Walking

Thumb walking, which is sometimes called caterpillar walking, is the major technique designed to make sure you cover all the reflexes of the feet. It is performed by using the first bone of the thumb, and rather than using the tip, it uses the flat of the thumb. This is important, for if you go to the tip of the thumb you will jump and not cover the whole area and more than likely miss small but vital parts of the feet and the reflexes. The reason this technique was developed was to make sure every little bit of the reflex in the feet is covered. You need to realise that the reflexes in the feet are proportional to the body and many are quite small. Therefore, if you go to the tip of the thumb you will miss areas in the feet and perhaps a complete reflex. When you consider that to miss say a millimetre in the feet, you are missing something like a few centimetres in the body, you could completely miss an imbalance, and so it is extremely important to develop thumb walking.

It is designed to take extremely little steps rather than big steps. The best way to do this is to attempt NOT to move the first joint or first knuckle of the thumb. This is actually impossible to do, but the more you try to do it, the better your thumb walking will be.

Thumb walking involves using pressure, as you need to be under the skin to be able to perform it. You start with the thumb flat and then move the first joint up to about an angle of 10% or less and as returning to the flat position, move slightly forward and repeating. This way you are taking very little steps forward each time. NOTE: You do not slide.

Practice is the key to thumb walking as it is for all the techniques. In fact I tell my students to:

"P. P. P. P."

"PRACTICE. PRACTICE. PRACTICE, PRACTICE"

An exercise I would recommend you do as often as you can is to practice your thumb walking on your own forearm. This way you will be able to feel yourself initially taking big steps, but with practice over time, your steps will get smaller and smaller until you can feel a constant steady pressure, much like sliding over the skin, but you are not. You are actually taking extremely small steps.

Also remember that in Reflexology you use both thumbs: right and left. This is something many forget. So you need to develop thumb walking with both thumbs. A relevant aside:

When I first learnt Reflexology, I thought, as I was right-handed, that my right thumb was fine, but that my left was not as good. But I discovered very early that in fact I was fine with my right thumb on the left foot and fine with my left thumb on the right foot, but I felt awkward with my left thumb on the left foot and the right thumb of the right foot. This amazed me and taught me two valuable lessons about Reflexology:

1. It makes one ambidextrous, that is, using left and right hands equally;
2. It integrates the two hemispheres of the brain.

These two advantages of Reflexology are significant, but the disadvantage is that I have become dyslexic. I have great difficulty with right and left. This is due to the fact that as a Reflexologist I face the sole of the feet and therefore right and left is reversed, that is my left hand side is the receiver's right and my right hand side is the receiver's left. Teaching Reflexology has only increased this.

So you need to practice with both thumbs. It will take time and effort but it is worth the effort. The biggest problem when initially learning Reflexology is that you rush. It takes time and effort to master this technique. Slow yourself down and concentrate. Practice as often as you can.

2. Finger walking

Finger walking is basically the same as thumb walking, but of course with a finger instead. You need to choose at least one finger as your main working finger, but also develop at least one other finger as well. I recommend the middle finger, simply because it is the longest and strongest, and then one other, perhaps the index finger.

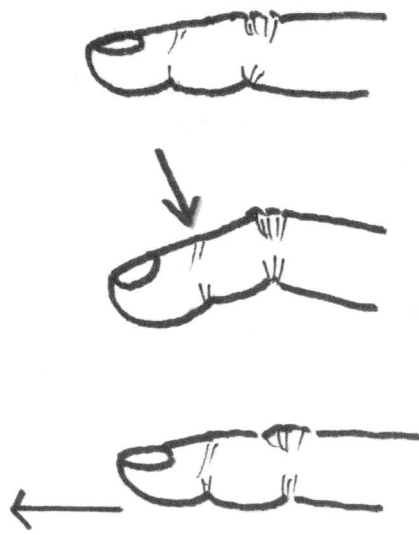

ILLUSTRATION 37: Finger Walking

So, like thumb walking, finger walking is designed to take extremely little steps rather than big steps. The best way to do this is to attempt not to move the first joint or first knuckle of the middle finger. This is actually impossible to do, but the more you try to do it, the better your finger walking will be.

A variation of finger walking occasionally used is walking with your fingers using two or three fingers walking together over an area. There are a few times that this is used, so it is also a variation requiring practice.

Once again, practice is the key to finger walking as it is for all the techniques and so:

"P. P. P. P."

"PRACTICE. PRACTICE. PRACTICE, PRACTICE"

As with Thumb walking, you need to practice as often as you can on your own forearm. Also remember that in Reflexology you use both your right and left middle finger or another finger, so you need to practice with both.

3. Tip of Thumb

The tip of the thumb (or both tips of the thumbs) is also used in Reflexology. This technique is used for accurately working a specific point or, in the case of the Diaphragm Relaxer, a specific line. It is accuracy that is important here. This technique is quite simple, but the difficulty is a tendency to use a dead straight thumb, which leads to the use of the flat of the thumb rather than the tip. You need to hook your thumb so that the tip can be used.

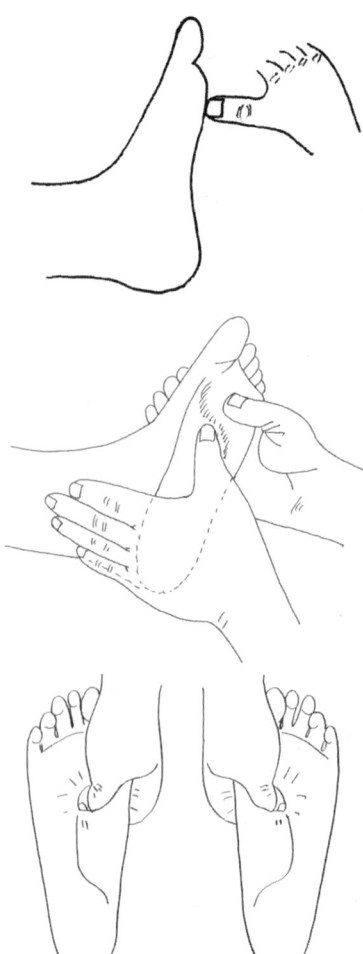

Tip of the Thumb is actually used by bending the first joint of the thumb so that the tip of the thumb is on the spot or line being worked. So, unlike thumb or finger walking where you do not to bend the first joint, in Tip of Thumb technique you do so to an angle of about 45%. Again, either or both thumbs may be used, so both need to be practiced.

ILLUSTRATION 38:
Three Variations of Tip of Thumb

4. Tip of Finger

Sometimes there is a need to use the tip of a finger as well, and usually the index or middle finger. The choice is yours, but the index finger seems easier to use, probably because we are used to pointing this finger at things. Anyway, this technique of using the tip of a finger is rather different from tip of thumb as you can use the tip of your finger dead straight, and come into the reflex or point, directly, at a 90% angle.

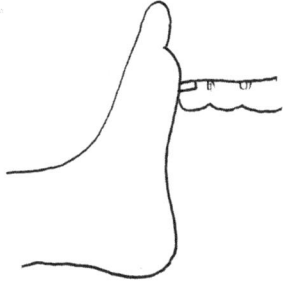

ILLUSTRATION 39: Tip of Finger

5. Knuckles

This is a technique that is not used often, although there are other branches, notably Chinese Reflexology, which uses the knuckles extensively. This is using the inner side of the second knuckle or joint of index finger, in a raking type action over or around a reflex, for example, the inner and outer hip reflexes. It is quite easy to perform and can be done quite quickly.

6. Drawing

This is a technique of using your index finger (or another if you prefer) like a pencil and drawing along a line. Again it is quite simple, but the key is to use the tip of the index finger rather than the flat. Have your finger at 90% to the line you want to draw, and keep it at 90%. That will keep the tip of your index finger doing the drawing. Imagine your finger as a pencil and you want to draw a clear straight line upon the foot or feet. It is as simple as that.

7. Holding

This is a very simple technique of using the tip of your index finger (or another finger) and simply under the skin (but with no pressure) gently holding the point or points. It can be done either on one foot or both at the same time, and is usually done for either four or twelve out-breaths for balancing, or for six out-breaths for treatment.

These then are the techniques that are used in Reflexology. There are others described and used by others and once you have mastered these, you can assess the use of these additional techniques and make your own decision about their effectiveness.

The main techniques used in Reflexology are thumb and finger walking, which need a considerable amount of practice to master. The rest of the techniques are quite easy to learn and perform.

So *"Practice, Practice, Practice, Practice"* thumb and finger walking.

CHAPTER 18
Preparing to work the Feet: What to use and why

One of the advantages of Reflexology is that all you need are your two hands, a pair of feet and the knowledge, especially concerning the practical techniques, to actually perform Reflexology.

One can work anywhere. Short, specific treatments can be applied when out and about, but this is not a complete Reflexology treatment and although it may be effective, should be used only in these sorts of situations. This is one of the advantages of Reflexology: a Reflexologist, once trained and with common sense, can actually work anywhere and at any time.

I have worked in just about every situation you can think of. For me, if someone asks for my help I will give it, and therefore, I have worked in the strangest of places. All you need in these situations is a chair for the receiver, your hands, and a floor to sit on. I have done this more times than I care to remember. What I do in these situations is:

1. Target what they have asked for, and then
2. Balance the whole system.

These two together takes no more than a few minutes. Reflexology states that you must always work all reflexes and both feet. In these situations it is just not possible, and even sometimes in the clinical setting it is not. Experience has taught me that if you tailor what you do to each individual, you cannot always cover everything. This is why I invented the Chi-Reflexology Balancing Sequence, so as to have time to do what is needed, and then in a few minutes balance all the energies of the body at the end.

However, most Reflexologists work in a clinical and therapeutic setting and there are two options here: working in someone's clinic or medical setting, in which case you do not have a great deal of control over the decision-making; or working in your own clinic. I work in my own clinic and therefore have equipment, including a space to work and a warm and inviting environment. It is also preferable to have a reception area and at least one clinic room. The preference for the setting of a clinic varies from clinical and medical to the most common clean and friendly. The choice is largely up to the giver and the type of clinic he/she wants to work in. There are a range of considerations here, including a desk to work at and at least two chairs (one for the Reflexologist and one for the giver); music and candles; posters and artwork; and heating, cooling and lighting, etc.

Remember, your clinic set-up will reflect you and your attitudes and beliefs. As well remember that you also work in your clinic and therefore you must be comfortable in the space, for up to eight to twelve hours per day. So think about what you would like in the space.

A stool is also needed. I would recommend for the Reflexologist to have a swivel and adjustable stool, with a good support for the giver's back, but there are a variety of options such as saddle stool, large inflated ball, etc.

I use a massage table, but the options are either a massage table or recliner chair to work on. The two most common ways of working on a receiver are:

1. With the receiver lying face up on a massage table, with a pillow under the head, a pillow under their knee and a roll to lift the feet up to approximately eye level of the giver; OR

2. With the receiver sitting in a recliner chair, which is raised

when working into a reclined position.

There are advantages and disadvantages in both these options. The choice is ultimately up to you. The Table below summarises the comparison of a massage table vs. a reclining chair.

ILLUSTRATION 40: Table:
Massage Table or Reclining Chair

MASSAGE TABLE	RECLINER CHAIR
1. The receiver is lying down (generally) and therefore more likely to relax and less inclined to talk. Lack of eye contact.	1. With the receiver facing you and able to look at you, the tendency is to talk more.
2. Less portable and mobile. More difficult to do home and out of clinic visits.	2. More portable and mobile. Easier to do home and out of clinic visits: easier to transport and to set up and pack up.
3. The feet are up close to eye level, which makes it easier to work, especially with an adjustable stool.	3. The feet are lower, and it is more difficult to get around the feet.
4. A flat, basically level receiver gains greater benefit from certain techniques such as stretching and vibrating.	4. Certain openings, especially stretching and vibrating, as well as Rocking, are less effective.
5. More permanent fixture.	5. Less permanent fixture and easier to store and transport.
6. The receiver has to get up on the table, which may be more difficult for mature, pregnant, the young and injured receivers.	6. The recliner is a seat in the down position, which is easier for everyone to get into and out of.
7. Normally lay down flat, but with an adjustable end, can sit up if necessary.	7. Are basically always sitting up.

The next significant question is what to use on the feet? Many Reflexologists, especially those also trained in massage, tend to use some form of oil, cream or lotion. Some Reflexologists also clean the feet before working; others give the receiver a footbath.

Looking first at cleaning the feet, I do not clean the feet before a treatment for the follow reasons:

1. It is disrespectful to the receiver. You are indicating, whether verbally or non-verbally (the more powerful) that you consider them dirty. A body therapist would never ask a receiver to have a shower before they would work on them.

2. Hygiene is an excuse that many Reflexologists use to justify their actions. I am not worried about hygiene for myself, but am concerned for the receiver. Cleaning their feet protects me, not them.

3. I want to know the human being as they are. If I clean, or for that matter use any lotion, oil or cream or even give a footbath before treatment, I change the landscape and am unable to know the receiver as they truly are.

These considerations are important to me, and so I have made a conscious decision about how I will work. There is no right and wrong here, it is just a matter of making a conscious decision.

As to lotions, oils and creams, I use nothing on the feet. The main reason for this is, as mentioned above, it comes between me and the receiver, and experience has demonstrated that I do not pick up as much from the feet when there is something used. So it becomes a barrier between me and the feet and therefore the person. Another consideration is, as I diagnose I want to know the person as they are. Lastly such is a moral, ethical and philosophical choice: I accept the human being as they are. And I do not in any way want to introduce a negative into the therapeutic situation. It is my choice.

Lastly, there are footbaths: once again I do not use footbaths at all, and would never use a footbath before a treatment for the reasons mentioned above. It not only relaxes the receiver, but it relaxes and changes the reflexes. However, if your emphasis is on beauty, feel-good and relaxation, then using a footbath could be beneficial for this approach. However, what I do is a treatment and consultation. Part of the problem with the footbaths, is that many Reflexologists have not actually looked at what they do and why. Relaxation is the issue that arises here, and as I do not aim to relax the receiver, it is a consequence of my treatment this is not a consideration for me. (See Chapters 4 and 8 for a more detailed analysis of Relaxation)

Finally I do not work the feet, but the human being through the feet. The feet are my medium into the human being. So I think and work the body, not the feet. Head to buttock, inside and out: a sequence as simple as that and when teaching and presenting I do not even talk about the feet but the body.

There are many issues that one must consider as preparation for performing a Reflexology session, including setting up and running a clinic. And decisions are best made before one begins working so that you can be as professional as possible at the start. It is up to you to think about these issues and make your own decision, consciously, morally and ethically.

"Unto thyself be true."

CHAPTER 19
Holding the Person, Holding the Feet

We all know the importance of touch: it is the basis of all body therapy approaches, including Reflexology. It is well documented that touch is very important, yet we seem to have neglected the consequences of this fact: the importance of not only touching, but how we touch, and the messages conveyed to the receiver by our touch.

We communicate our intentions, attitudes and opinions in many ways. Research has demonstrated that the most powerful form of communication is non-verbal. With this in mind it is important to consider how you hold and support the feet, and therefore how you hold and support the person. Consider for a moment saying something pleasant such as, "You look great today" to someone, while at the same time screwing up your face. Note the perceptions of the receiver. Which sends the more powerful message: the pleasant words, or the non-verbal communication?

With this in mind, would you pick a person up by their head? Would you grab a person around the neck? Would you hold a person's genitalia? Many Reflexologists do, and Reflexology texts describe just these types of actions. What is communicated to the receiver? What does it say about the Reflexologist and their attitudes to Reflexology and to their receivers? As non-verbal communication is the more powerful, these are questions that all Reflexologists need to ask.

Does it really matter how the person is held via the feet? Yes. Why? Because Reflexology is based on the premise that the two feet reflect the human being. If this is so, surely it is important how it is put into practice? If a Reflexologist truly believes he/she is holding the whole person on all levels in their two hands, then how the feet are held and supported should be of paramount importance. How the feet are held also communicates information on a subtle and subconscious level to the receiver: another reason it needs to be an important consideration for all Reflexologists.

> "I do not work the feet, but the human being through the feet. The feet are my medium in to the human being. I work the head and neck (not the toes); the chest (not the metatarsal pad or ball of the feet); the abdomen (not the arch of the feet); the pelvis (not the heel); inside the human being (not the inner aspect of the feet); and the outside and limbs of the body (not the outside aspect of the feet)."

There is another more simple and obvious reason for the importance of how you hold the feet and therefore the person. If you grab the feet (body) you are sending a mixed message. The Refleoxlogist is working two places at the same time. For example, if you grab the head and neck (toes) while working the pelvic region (heel), you are actually sending two messages to the body (head/neck and pelvis) at the same time. This is confusing, disruptive and unclear communications. It is also perhaps one reason why it takes so many treatments to get results: the body has to work out what you are asking it to do. Is it not better to work one thing at a time and therefore send one clear message to the body?

There are many ways of holding the feet that I would not recommend, such as grabbing anywhere, and so if the tips of your support fingers are touching the feet (body) then you are grabbing. Make sure your finger tips of both the working and support hands never touch the feet. This way you will not grab. For me this is a vital aspect of working with another human being. It is of utmost importance that a positive message is conveyed rather than a negative one. So, whenever I talk to receivers and students about the ball of the foot, I call it the chest; when I talk about the heel I call it the pelvic region; I talk about the head and neck rather than the toes, etc. Each reflexologist needs to assess this often-neglected aspect of the science and art of Reflexology. With this in mind I have developed holding techniques based on the above approach.

ILLUSTRATION 41:
Supportive and Nurturing Holding Techniques

1. THUMB ON CHEST/BALL OF THE FOOT: **STANDARD HOLD**

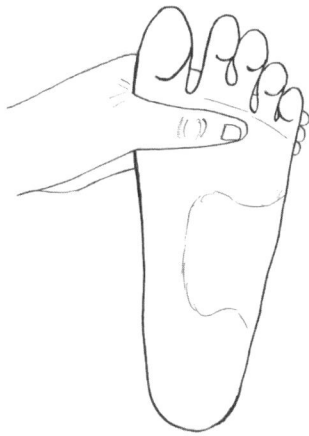

Comments:

This Standard Holding technique is safe and unobtrusive, as very few people are not comfortable being held by the upper chest. Also the chest is a fairly solid structure (ribs) for holding purposes. It is above the breast. The fingers of the support hand are held STRAIGHT across the upper back, and so there is no chance of grabbing and thus working other reflexes.

NOTE: This is the first and number one Holding technique. It is the first you should think of. Go to this, and then, if this will not do, then change to one of the following, or vary this Standard Holding technique.

2. OPEN FIST ON CHEST/BALL OF THE FOOT

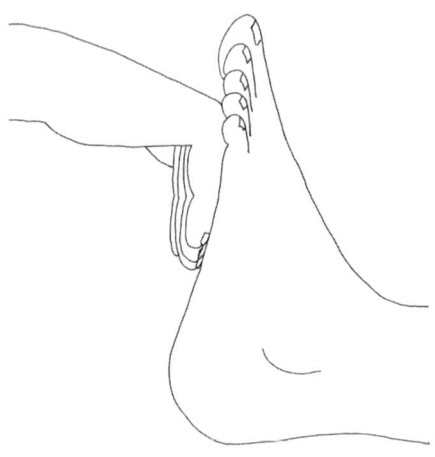

Comments:

This is actually a variation of the Standard Hold, as illustrated above. The knuckles are in line with the top of the shoulders (Shoulder Line) and the fingers are kept straight resting on the abdomen. Again, this is not working or grabbing any other reflexes.

NOTE: The Open fist allows energy to flow, and helps to keep the giver more relaxed (less muscle use and tension).

3. THUMB ON KIDNEY I/TRIPLE BURNER CHI POINT

Comments:

This is a hold that I increasingly use especially when working aspects/reflexes related to Kidney and/or Triple Burner energy. For example, it is an excellent holding technique for working the pelvic region. The fingers are kept straight on the medial/inside so that again one does not grab or work other reflexes/areas of the inner pelvis.

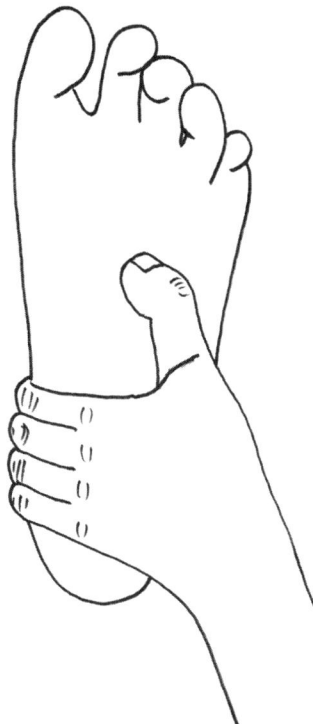

NOTE: This Holding Technique can be reversed, that is the thumb on K 1/Triple Burner point, and the supporting fingers straight on the outside of the foot, when working inside.

I recommend that these three basic holding techniques be used as much as possible while working another area of the person. The first technique involves holding the chest with the thumb, with the fingers of the supporting hand resting straight across the upper back (Do not grab). This technique is what I call the 'Standard Hold' as it is the major method of holding the person and it is the one you should go to first and foremost. The second technique involves using an open fist with the knuckles along the Shoulder Line or top of the chest and the fingers gently down the body/foot. Make sure you do not press the abdomen with the fingers, and especially not the knuckles, as you will be pushing into their major organs. Why an open fist? This is again simple. An open fist allows the chi or energy to flow while a closed fist blocks it. Also, on a physical level, a closed fist increases the muscle tension of the Reflexologist, while an open fist is more relaxed.

ILLUSTRATION 42:
Counter-Productive, Disharmonious Holding Techniques

1. FINGERS OVER THE FACE/TOES

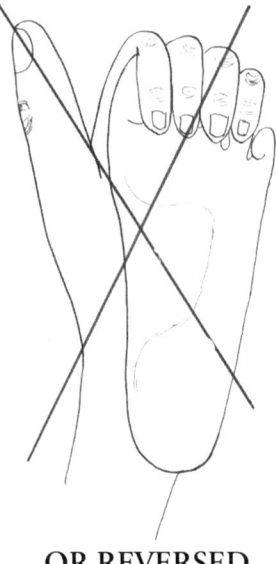

OR REVERSED

Comments:

This is not recommended as a Holding Technique as the giver is firstly covering the face and smothering the person. Also holding the head/neck region puts stress on the neck, a common problem for many receivers, which of course is not wise. The worst variation of this is the holding technique that actually grabs around the neck (base of the toes) as this is strangling the person. Not very relaxing.

This technique is not only working the reflexes of other parts of the body (feet), but also the head/neck, causing both confusion and uncertainty as to what you are doing. Which is it or is it both? It would be better to send a clearer message to the body: one thing at a time.

2. CLOSED FIST ON CHEST/BALL OF THE FOOT

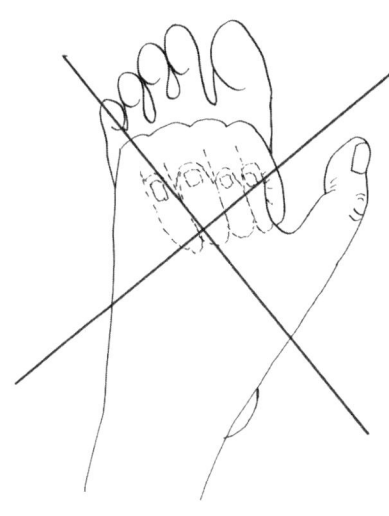

Comments:

This is the variation of the Open Fist Holding Technique and it is not recommended as it prevents the flow of energy and increases muscle tension. So any time you work with a fist, simply open it. It is as simple as that.

3. THUMB ON ABDOMEN/ARCH OF THE FOOT

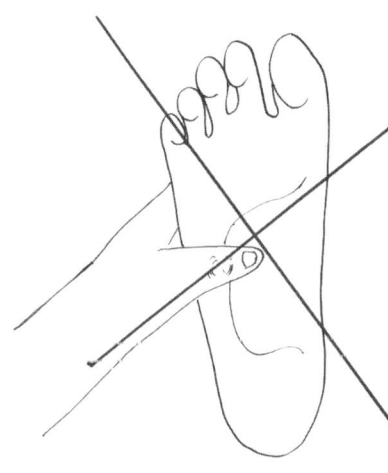

Comments:

This Holding Technique is not recommended as the thumb is pressing into inner organs (abdomen) and at the same time is grabbing the back with the supporting fingers. When using such a hold, the giver is working particular reflexes as well as the abdomen and back reflexes: a minimum of three reflexes at the same time. Extremely confusing and invasive for the body.

4. FINGERS GRABBING ABDOMEN/ARCH OF THE FOOT

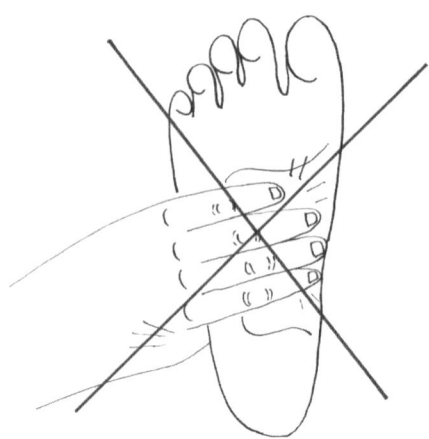

Comments:

This is the reverse of No. 3 above, with the fingers grabbing the abdomen and the thumb grabbing the back.

Not wise.

5. THUMB ON PELVIC REGION/HEEL

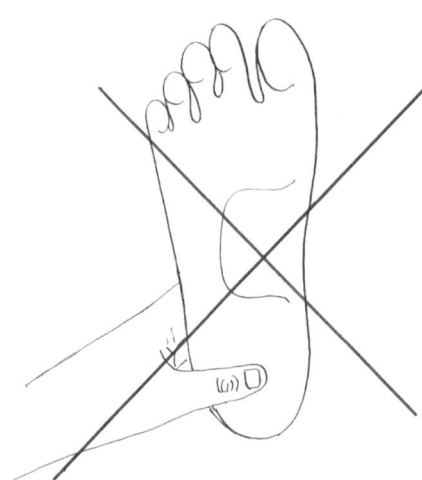

Comments:

This is particularly disharmonious hold, as the pelvic region is the most delicate and most protected part of any human being. This is extremely invasive and if other body therapists grabbed the body in this fashion, there would be legal ramifications. Again, the thumb is pressing into the front pelvic region while the fingers are grabbing the lower back.

Mixed messages to say the least.

6. GRABBING PELVIC REGION/HEEL

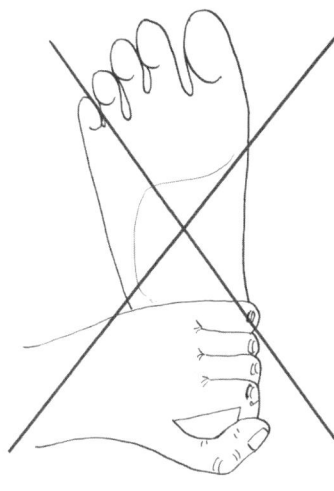

Comments:

Variation of No. 5 above. The difference here is that the whole pelvic region is being grabbed, especially the inside, which is the most delicate and sensitive part of the human body as it is inside the pelvis (for a female inside the uterus and vagina). Not very professional to grab these during a treatment

7. GRABBING THE BUTTOCK/UNDER THE HEEL

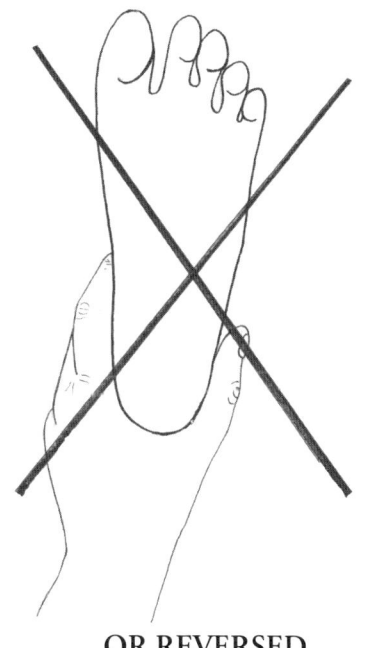

OR REVERSED

Comments:

This holding technique is holding the buttock, while the thumb is pressing into the outer pelvis and the fingers are grabbing the inner pelvis. It is of particular importance as many Reflexologists say that this is such a nice hold and that receivers enjoy it. This may be true. Why? The answer is simple. The giver is holding the receiver by the buttock. It is absolutely fine for a parent holding their child, but it is not an appropriate hold for a Reflexologist. The giver has no right to do this. It may be also a nurturing but de-powering as the receiver is subjected to the authority figure, the giver.

Using these illustrations to guide you, try these holding techniques, both supportive and counter-productive, on the feet first and then on the body. See and feel your response and the receiver's response. It will be quite clear. For example, grab the toes, and then grab the head and face. Press into the abdomen of the feet then press into the receiver's abdomen. Grab the heel, and then grab the pelvic region. Grab around the heel, and then grab the buttocks. How does the giver feel? How does the receiver feel? It becomes quite clear to both that certain holding techniques are comforting, while others are not and in fact are undesirable to the point of being invasive.

As I recommend holding the chest area as much as possible, one question students often ask is, "How do you work the chest area?" I recommend holding the chin or jaw rather than the face, head or neck. This way you are not covering the face (smothering) and you are not grabbing the neck (choking). While not a perfect solution, it is the best alternative I have found and surely this is better than grabbing the face or choking the person. Intent is important here and on a sub-conscious level you are communicating your concern for the comfort of the receiver, which is a positive rather than a negative non-verbal message. Remember, the human being knows on a deep, inner level.

Since non-verbal communication is so significant, ensure you do everything consciously and deliberately. It is not only important how you hold the feet, but also that you work only the area of your intention. To avoid working other reflexes I recommend, as much as possible, placing the fingers of your working hand on the fingers of your supporting hand. By doing this you can gain as much leverage and pressure as you want or need without affecting another area of the person. When this is not practical keep the fingers of your working hand relaxed, but straight, and the tip of your fingers off the body/feet and resting gently on the foot/feet to avoid working anywhere else. With practice, you will find that you do not need to grab the feet to work a reflex. The reason that we grab is that we have been trained from early childhood to grab things, with the fingers and thumb basically parallel. Thus, it is difficult initially not to grab, but with time and effort, you will re-programme your computer (the mind) and you will realise that it is actually not hard at all, and that you do not need to grab for strength. It is a fallacy.

As I emphasise balance as an important part of my work, I believe that the Reflexologist's actions should also be balanced. (See Illustrations below) By this I mean that when I work an area of the foot/feet I balance my own action, as much as possible, with an equal and opposite action, so that the foot/feet do not move unless that is my intention. So if the feet (body) are moving while you are working, then you are not balancing your own actions and the receiver has to balance out your actions by using their muscles, which must create tension and be counter-productive. The foot/feet are stabilised by this approach and do not move at all.

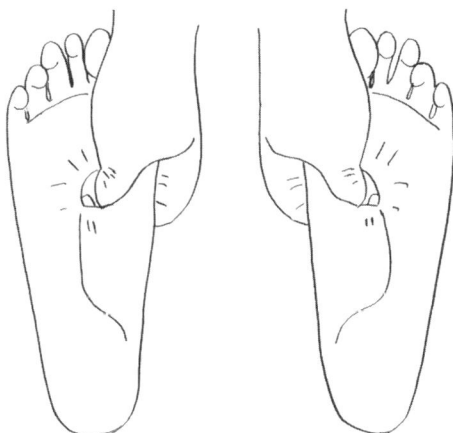

ILLUSTRATION 43: Balancing your own Actions during Reflexology — a) Both Feet Together

For example, as illustrated above, when pressing both the K 1/Triple Burner points, I place my thumb tips on the reflexes and my straight fingers (Do not grab) on the upper back (top of both feet). As I press these two points I balance my own actions by supporting the top of the feet so that the feet do not move. The result is a balanced action. (See illustration b) below.)

Another example, illustrated below, is working the abdomen with the thumb while supporting the body/foot with your other hand on top of the foot and fingers on fingers (i.e. working fingers on support fingers). Again, with a balanced action, the foot does not move.

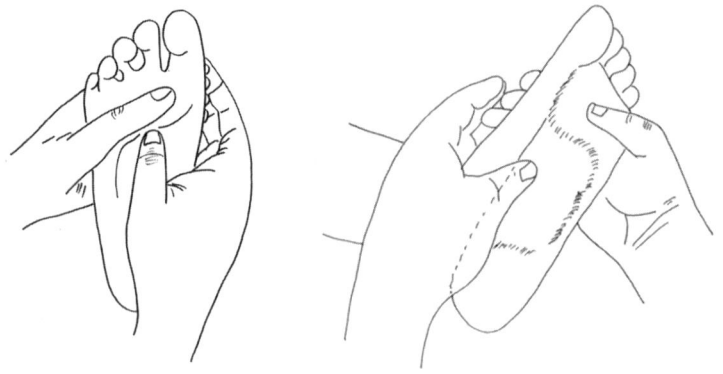

ILLUSTRATION 44: Balance your Own Actions (Fingers on fingers) — b) One Foot

NOTE: The fingers of the working hand are holding the fingers of the supporting hand so that nothing else is worked.

I am increasingly accepting that everything and anything a Reflexologist does during a session has meaning and import. I am consciously, rather than unconsciously, doing things. Everything that is done communicates to the receiver, in some way or another, positive or negative messages. As I want to increase the likelihood of the outcomes that the receiver desires, on whatever level, I am consciously working with the receiver for their benefit. To this end, as a Reflexologist becomes more attuned to the receiver during a session via the above approaches, the Reflexologist knows when they are working with the receiver, or against them.

IN SUMMARY

- Remember the importance of touch, and how we touch
- Give out positive rather than negative messages
- Never grab the feet (body). Place fingers on fingers when working. If not, then straight fingers resting on the side of the foot/feet. That way you will not grab the feet (body)
- Consider how the feet are held and why
- Remember what you are communicating to the receiver
- Use supportive holding techniques for optimum outcomes
- **Standard Hold**: Hold and support via the upper chest area as much as possible
- Balance your own actions/movements
- Work consciously, rather than unconsciously
- Work with the receiver rather than against them

These are the important aspects of touch, how you touch and working the human being through the feet, which are an integral component of the way I perform Reflexology. Each Reflexologist needs to address these questions for themselves. How do you as a Reflexologist hold the person via their feet? What are you doing and why? I believe in Reflexology. I believe I am working the human being via the feet. I respect the person and the process too much to degrade either. Now over to you: the decision is yours.

CHAPTER 20
Basic Reflexology Rules and Treatment Options

The Basic Reflexology Rules that follow comes from a philosophical perspective which has been expounded throughout this work. They are based on the fact that, as Reflexology is a therapy, the Reflexologist always has choices, and the best option is to make these choices consciously and deliberately, firstly for yourself and secondly for the benefit of the receiver.

These rules will be listed in the table below, followed by a brief explanation of those rules that have not already been explained, with the last two sections of this chapter dedicated to the Treatment Options available to the Reflexologist and the methods used: Sedation, Stimulation and Balancing.

Basic Reflexology Rules
ILLUSTRATION 45: List

1 Always work within your own belief system. To do this you must firstly understand and then own your own beliefs.
2 Remember the Hippocratic Oath, respect, desire to help, objectivity and detachment. Promise never to do harm.
3 Work with the body, not against it.
4 **Always** support the foot/feet with supportive holding techniques. **Never grab** the person (feet).
5 Go to **Standard Hold** first and then if necessary adjust or change.

6   Always offer positive messages instead of negative ones. If message cannot be positive, at least eliminate the negative as much as possible.

7   **Balance your own actions**. The feet should not move unless you want them to.

8   Always start with Feet Brushing every time you initially touch the feet, or after you have disconnected for any reason during a treatment.

9   Link your breathing to that of the receiver, and use the receiver's breathing (their natural rhythm of life) throughout treatment.

10 Work across a reflex area and then back as separate action. This is a balancing as well as a working technique.

11 Always work with **fingers on fingers**. If not, then use **straight fingers** of working hand, that way you only work the area/reflex/point you aim to and nothing else.

12 Start with the Left foot, then the Right.

13 AFTER working both feet together, return to the Left foot.

14 **WORK areas of the body together**. Work both halves of the person (feet) together; i.e. work across the feet, left to right and right to left, covering the regions of the body (feet) together.

15 If in doubt, Don't!   Or   If in Doubt, Balance.

16 Once you have connected **do not disconnect**, unless you have to/want to for specific purposes.

17 Move/walk around the person (feet) by moving one hand first to the next place before letting go of the previous place. This keeps the connection.

18 BASIC SEQUENCE of events –   a) **Move**,   b) **Support**,   c) **Work.**

EXPLANATION OF THE RULES

Most of the above rules are either explained elsewhere, or need no explanation, so only the rules that need commenting on here will be listed.

RULE 1: Always work within your own belief system. To do this you must firstly understand and then own your own beliefs.

It is a simple thing to state, but a difficult one is explain and do, but it is extremely important A rule to strive for, knowing full well that you will never fully achieve your aim.

RULE 3: Work with the body, not against it.

I talk about working with the body rather than working with the person, as the aim is to work with the body as against the mind, brain or computer, which is not the body.

RULE 8: Always start with Feet Brushing every time you initially touch the feet, or after you have disconnected for any reason.

SEE Chapter 21 Practical: Openings.

The first thing that should be done to the feet is Feet Brushing, which is introducing your touch to the body. If for any reason, a treatment is interrupted, before continuing perform Feet Brushing, even when demonstrating, doing specific work, or performing a mini-treatment, always Feet Brush first.

RULE 13: After working both feet together, return to the Left foot.

Again this is a necessary rule for all the same reasons as Rule 12 above. It could be reversed if you prefer, as long as you are consistent. The reason is that for learning purposes and once in practice, it is easier to follow the rule, otherwise you might get lost.

RULE 14: Work areas of the body together. Work both halves of the person (feet) together; i.e. work across the feet, left to right and right to left, covering the regions of the body (feet) together.

This is simply working the same reflexes at the same time.

As outlined in the sequence below, working both halves of a reflex at the same time is more therapeutic than working half now and half later. It is also important in that the body knows what you are doing and can follow your movements

The original Reflexology worked all the reflexes on one foot completely and then worked all the reflexes on the other foot. This is how I was taught and I changed it the moment I started working and have been working across the feet for many years. This is also a method that has increasingly been advocated in the Reflexology community.

RULE 15: If in doubt, Don't! Or If in Doubt, Balance.

The first part of the rule: "If in doubt, Don't" is the safety valve if you like. If you are not sure, uncomfortable or hesitant, then I recommend Don't. In other words, err on the side of caution. Later on, as you expand your skills and learn how to balance, when you are not sure, then rather than not doing, you can simply and easily balance the reflex, area or whole body and allow the body to do whatever it needs to do.

RULE 18: BASIC SEQUENCE of events – a) Move b) Support c) Work.

This Rule is extremely important for two reasons.

Firstly, as a learning tool it helps the giver to break the actions up into deliberate segments, that is, always:

- Walk first to where you are going (as outlined in Rule 17 above)
- Work out how to support
- Work out how to work.

As a learning tool this is very useful and allows the giver to break the sequence up into segments for learning purposes. Experience has taught me that most students get lost when they try to put it all together. This Rule will allow you to learn each part of the sequence methodically, which is much easier.

Secondly, this is something I still do to this very day: walk, support and work. It again helps to bring a natural rhythm to what you are doing and is part of the reason that I do not have to try to relax the receiver. It is in itself relaxing, and it is part of the working with the body mentioned above and elsewhere.

Note so many of these rules and other aspects mentioned elsewhere go together: they are all parts of the whole. Together they allow the giver to work with the receiver in a deeper and more trusting way. Nothing is done by accident or without a reason for doing it. These rules are all important aspects of the whole.

BASIC REFLEXOLOGY SEQUENCE

The basic Sequence is a simple one:
1. **OPENINGS** (LEFT foot, then RIGHT, and/or both feet together.)
2. **WORK HEAD TO BUTTOCK**, i.e.
   • **Head and Neck** (Toes: both feet)
   • **Chest and Upper Back** (Ball of the Feet)
   • **Abdomen**, upper and middle (Arch of the feet: both feet)
   • **Pelvis** (Heel: both feet)
3. **REPRODUCVTIVE REFLEXES** (pelvis/heel: Both feet, sole, inside & out)
4. **SPINE/CENTRAL NERVOUS SYSTEM** (Four Lines: Muscles & bones, inner organs, Spine, & muscles of the back), inside the body (Inside of Feet)
5. **LIMBS and OUTER HIP**: Outside of the body (Outside of Feet)
6. **ADRENALS, KIDNEY and BLADDER** (sole: both feet together)
7. **FIGURE EIGHT/INFINITY** to Finish (both feet together)

This then is the basic sequence of events: head to tail, reproductive and inside and out (working both feet together).

This is also covering all the reflexes of the feet and areas of the human being, and is the order you will find the Practical Treatment Techniques, which will be outlined in Chapter 23. It is also the suggested order and sequence which is especially important for learning purposes and perhaps initially when working with receivers.

Alternatively, once you have learnt all the techniques and are comfortable with them and move into practice, the suggested order or sequence would become:

1. Openings (as appropriate to the situation at hand)
2. Working on what the receiver is paying you to do, and related reflexes/areas
3. Working on related reflexes, energies, helper areas, etc.
4. Balancing the whole system, including Figure Eight/Infinite to finish.

This sequence is designed to be therapeutic and specific to the situation at hand rather than simply working all the reflexes all the time.

BASIC TECHNIQUES: Options Available

In the therapeutic setting (as in every aspect of life) the Reflexologist always has a choice. In fact the Reflexologist has many choices, many of which have been discussed earlier in the rules as well as throughout this work.

We always have choices: it is when we think we do not have a choice that problems will soon arise, and harm is very close behind. It is through conscious making of choices that we can decrease the negative in a given situation. This is the only way: ownership and conscious decision-making.

In the therapeutic situation, the Reflexologist (and all body therapists) has a choice of how to work what they find. There are three choices: active (yang), passive (yin) or balance. But the first two choices can be further broken down into two different situations. Therefore there are in fact five choices in any given situation:

1. To stimulate an excess
2. To stimulate a deficiency
3. To sedate a deficiency
4. To sedate an excess
5. To balance, which is where Rule 15 above "If in doubt – Balance" comes from.

So these are the five options that all Reflexologists (and all Body Therapists) have whether they realise it or not. Each of these options will be looked at individually.

1. STIMULATE AN EXCESS

Which increases the imbalance, resulting in the body having to compensate for the increased imbalance: the healing crisis. Often used in standard Reflexology and most body therapies, it is not used in Reflexology as outlined in this work as it creates imbalance in the body and therefore is not working with the body but against it. It makes the body's job harder rather than easier, which does not make sense.

2. STIMULATE A DEFICIENCY

Which obeys the body's message, resulting in gently working with the body and its needs. This makes it easier for the body to strengthen the weakness and move back towards a more balanced state.

3. SEDATE A DEFICIENCY

Which increases the imbalance just like stimulating an excess does. This results in the body having to compensate for the increased imbalance, and possibly a healing crisis. Not recommended, and never used.

4. SEDATE AN EXCESS

Which again obeys the body's message, resulting in gently

working with the body and its needs. This makes it easier for the body to achieve its desired purpose and makes it easier to move back towards a more balanced state. This is the method most commonly used. It is a choice consciously made.

5. BALANCE

The safest method of working is simply to balance, by:
- Pressing gently four times with the receiver's out-breath or
- Holding gently under the skin for four or twelve out-breaths.

These are the two major methods of balancing, but there are others, such as working back and forth as separate actions an equal number of times. Therefore if in doubt, balance.

Now that you know you always have choices, and as a Reflexologist and therapist you have five choices, how do you apply this knowledge and understanding? Quite simply, by using the techniques outlined below as required and requested by the body.

TECHNIQUES: Sedation, Stimulation and/or Balance

There are three techniques mentioned above: sedation, stimulation and balance. These are the three tools that all Reflexologists and body therapists, no matter what techniques they may use, have at their disposal. It is a pity that they do not generally realise this, and that they have these choices and thus options at their fingertips.

NOTE: Thumb and finger walking is a stimulatory technique.

Outlined below is how the Reflexologist can sedate, stimulate or balance any given imbalance found in the feet or for that matter in the body as well.

SEDATION:

1. Locate the exact point of the imbalance then place the tip of your thumb or finger on the exact point. There is **always** an exact point. It is never a region, muscle group or whole reflex area.

2. Define the imbalance, for example: sharp pain.

3. Using the tip of thumb/finger, with gentle pressure under the skin (BUT no pain) gently and slowly circle anticlockwise for six of the receiver's out-breaths.

4. Re-check the point and if it is no longer sharp you have obeyed the body's instructions and nothing more is needed. However, if not, then you may need to repeat the Sedation technique.

NOTE: Once done, leave it. Do not go back or you will change the landscape again.

STIMULATION:

NOTE: Thumb and Finger walking, as well as most other Reflexology techniques are stimulatory techniques.

1. Locate, with the tip of thumb or finger, the exact point. There is always an exact point.

2. Define the imbalance, for example: dull pain.

3. **OPTIONS**:

   a) Using the tip of the thumb/finger, with **strong pressure** under the skin, as deep as you can go, quickly circle clockwise for six out-breaths, if you can. Most likely the pain will become excruciating within seconds. This method is **not** recommended to be used for two reasons:

   i) It causes SHARP pain very quickly and increases the discomfort of the receiver;

   ii) There is ALWAYS an alternative and it is b), below.

   b) Using the tip of the thumb/finger, with strong pressure under the skin, press until you feel the body pushing back and hold for six out-breaths. With experience, you will feel the body pushing back, and as you do slowly release the pressure until the point is filled. An easy and gently way to stimulate.

4. Re-check the point and if it is now sharp or stronger, you have obeyed the body's instructions and nothing more is needed. However, if not, then you may need to repeat the stimulating technique.

NOTE: Once done, leave it. Do not go back or you will change the landscape again.

BALANCE: (NOTE: If in doubt, balance.)

Number of Methods:

1. Press **four** times (for physical and wholistic balance) on a point with your out-breath (linked to the breath of the receiver), that is as you breath out, slowly press and as you breath in release pressure, but do not let go of the point (stay under the skin). Take their full out-breath to press. Do not rush. Slow and steady. Now there is no need to press strongly, as long as you have a rhythm of pressing under the skin a little stronger on your out-breath. This is the major method of balancing.

2. Press THREE times with your out-breath as above (for mental balance). This was once the preferred method but now four times is the better option. It still can be used for mental imbalances or if you (the Reflexologist) want to mentally balance the person, which previously was the reason for its use.

3. Gently under the skin HOLD for four or twelve out-breaths.

4. Doing anything an equal number of times each way/back and forth (as separate actions) will balance e.g. running a spine one way and then the other. However, it is important to disconnect between each movement, otherwise you will scramble the person's energy; that is, go one way, release, then repeat as many times as you would like, then release and repeat in the opposite direction.

Finally, you will notice that there are a number of numbers used in the techniques above and this will be explained in more detail in *Appendix C: Numbers and Reflexology*. However, the Table below summarises this information and explains why certain numbers are used extensively throughout this work.

ILLUSTRATION 46: TABLE: Numbers in Reflexology

NUMBER	EFFECT
2	Emotional Balance
3	Mental Balance
4	Physical and wholistic balance (Due to the four levels of existence: Physical, Emotional, Mental and Spiritual)
12	Spiritual and WHOLISTIC balance (4 X 3)
NOTE – 6	Number of Treatment!

CHAPTER 21
Practical: Openings

Although most Reflexologists call these relaxers and do them at the beginning of a treatment, I see them as Openings. They may be relaxing, but they are also openings: the opening up of the receiver to get things flowing. To this end, for teaching and learning purposes they have been kept at the beginning of the treatment, as most Reflexologists do this. However I would recommend, once you have learnt and are comfortable with these techniques, placing them at the beginning of the appropriate treatment techniques of the same part of the body. To this end then, these would open up that part of the body when the Reflexologist wants to work a particular part which is much more sensible and therapeutic. If necessary or desirable, the openings can also be repeated again after working said area, especially if it is an area or reflex/es that have needed special attention for any particular reason.

Once comfortable with the techniques, I would recommend, as a basic sequence, using a few of these general openings at the beginning of a treatment and then using those appropriate to the situation as needed; that is, you would not do all of these at the beginning of a session, but only if and when they were required. Again, this is about making decisions and working more consciously rather than mechanically. This will help the Reflexologist to tailor a treatment to each individual receiver as well as for each individual treatment on the same receiver.

For the Openings, there are two options available and the choice is yours. These options are:

- Do each Opening on one foot and then repeat it on the other, and so go back and forth from one half (foot) to the other half (foot);   OR
- Grouping of Openings together that relate to the same part of the body and then repeat on the other side of the body (foot). For speed of action this is the better option, but perhaps for learning the first option is the better. To this end I will put in a suggested time to change, but the choice is yours.

One question I am constantly asked is how many times do you do these techniques. The answer is again simple and consistent:

- Four times for balance, (2nd Option: can be 12 times for balance as well) or
- Six times for treatment

1. Feet Brushing

CONNECTING YOUR CHI TO THE RECEIVER'S CHI
Recommended as the first contact to the person/feet. (See RULE 8.)

Draw up, with a definite, medium-type pressure (not too gentle that it tickles, but neither too strong), with your palms and/or back of palms. Avoid using your fingers. (Keep your fingers off the foot/feet as much as possible.) Do both feet together, and stroke up the inside of the feet, disconnect, and then stroke down the inside and disconnect. Follow this up with stroking up the soles, and disconnecting, and then down the sole; stroking down the back, and disconnecting, then finally up the back, and disconnecting. Each movement is a distinct and separate one, yet at the same time it is flowing. The purpose here is to get the receiver used to your touch, which is why it needs to be deliberate rather than gentle, and to balance each surface of the body (feet).

NOTE: To balance each surface, you must disconnect briefly between each direction on the same surface, that is back and forth as two separate actions is a balancing technique. It feels like effleurage (flowing back and forth) but it is not.

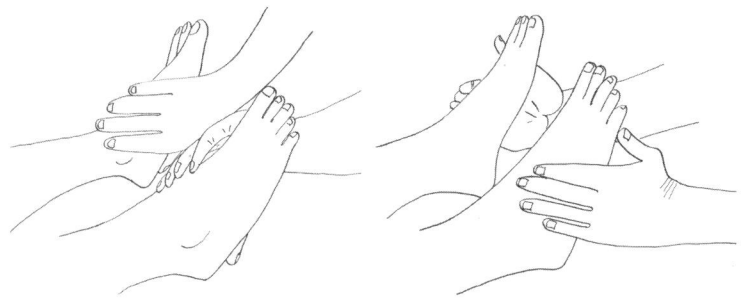

ILLUSTRATION 47: Feet Brushing

After connecting, move to left foot (See RULE 13) and continue Feet Brushing on left foot ONLY, with palms and/or back of palms working front and back together at the same time, and then the inside and outside together, going up and down, disconnecting between directions. This takes you to the left foot to begin the next opening.

2. Pelvic, Sacrum, Hip and Lower Back Relaxer

Put the base of the both palms (natural V shaped hollow of the lower palms) around the ankle bones and cup the ankle-bones, with fingers pointing up the leg.

With medium pressure (stronger if the ankle is tight) do an up and down the leg action (Not a circular action.), quite quickly if you like, so that the toes and top of the foot are waving hello. There should be no rubbing or friction. As long as the foot is waving hello you are getting it right, but if the foot is circling, you are not.

SUGGESTION: Either do left foot then right for each

Opening technique, OR do groupings of same area together on one foot and then the other. For example, do Pelvic, Sacrum, Hip and Lower Back Openings, and Chest Relaxer and Chest Kneading on left foot, then move to the right, and then continue on working back and forth across the feet.

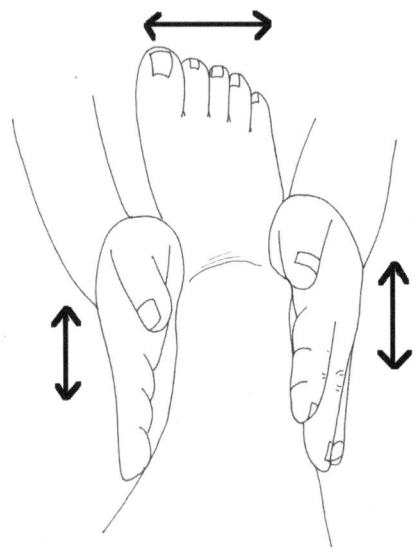

ILLUSTRATION 48:
Pelvic, Sacrum, Hip and Lower Back Relaxer

3. Chest Relaxer

Cup the inside and outside of the chest and upper back area with the middle of both palms, and wobble the hands back and forth, gently and quite quickly if you like. Make sure your outside hand is not on the little toe. You do not want to squash the receiver's head.

This is like putting your hands around the chest and moving back and forth: quite relaxing and opening of the chest area. This is excellent for any chest (especially lung) problems as it loosens up any congestion in this area.

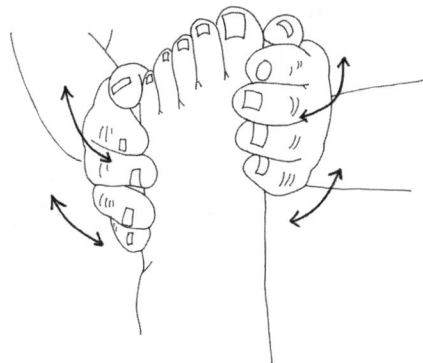

ILLUSTRATION 49: Chest Relaxer

NOTE: Do Left half of person (foot) then Right half (foot) OR No. 2, 3 and 4 (below) and then change feet.

4. Chest Kneading

There are several skills needed for this opening. Firstly, make sure you use an open fist on the chest and that you use your left open fist on the right foot and the right open fist of the left foot. This is important so that you can stretch upwards without twisting the body (foot) that is you are trying to stretch straight up, not sideways. If you use the same open fist on the same foot, the tendency is to push outwards rather than straight up.

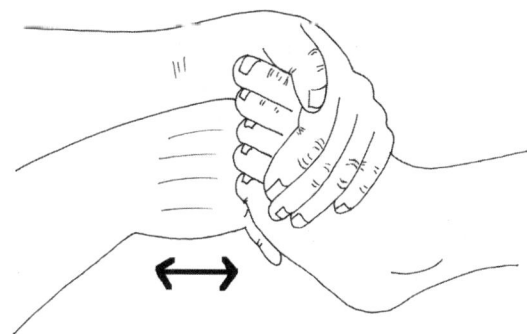

ILLUSTRATION 50: Chest Kneading

Now stretch upwards using the out-breath four times, with each stretch stronger than the last. So stretch one, gentle, stretch two a little more, stretch three medium and stretch four the strongest. Take your full out-breath to stretch (i.e. slowly.). This is important because if you push using your muscles and strong pressure straight away, the body will lock and you will not get the desired result. With practice, you will feel when the body locks and this is as strong as you go. Never force the body to go further than it wants. If the receiver's knee begins to lift up, then you have gone too far.

The second half of this opening is that you cup your other hand over the back (top of the foot). To cup the foot, use the first knuckle (bone) of your fingers and the base of your palm, and you should have a space between your palm and the back of the foot. Between each stretch come back to the resting position (but do not remove your open fist) and give the inside and outside of the chest a little cuddle. It is gentle and supportive. Do not squeeze.

NOTE: Do Left half of person (foot) then Right half (foot), OR No. 2, 3 and 4 (above) and then change feet.

NOTE: This is the opening used to test for the possibility of thrombosis (blood clotting) or Economy class syndrome, which will be discussed in more detail in Chapter 22. *If there is any PAIN, especially in the leg and calf, it is recommended not to continue with the treatment.*

5. Spinal Twist

Place your bottom hand as low as you can go, with thumb on pelvis (sole of heel) region and fingers on the back of foot and a little up the leg, and your other hand immediately above (as close together as possible) in exactly the same position. Lock your bottom hand (strong pressure) so that you can hold the spine (vertebra) still, and twist each vertebra individually. Twist up and down (in a clunking action four times: up/down, up/down), and then move your bottom hand (*NOT your top hand*) up a little. You will bump into the upper hand and by doing this you will take little steps upwards rather than big steps. Remember you are trying to twist each vertebra of the spine, and your bottom hand is holding the vertebra below still, while your top hand is twisting the vertebra immediately above. Do not twist both hands.

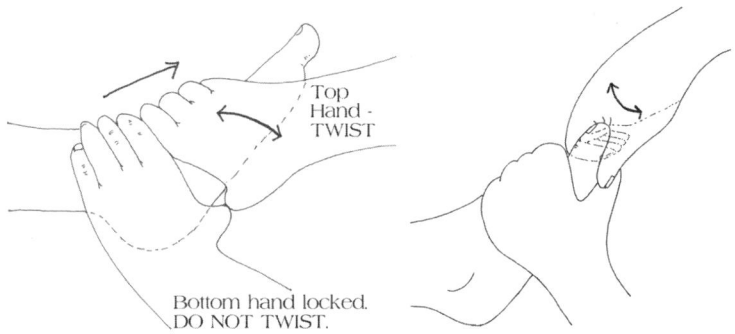

ILLUSTRATION 51: Spinal Twist

Twist strongly in the lumbar region as most receiver's lumbar region is quite stiff (heel and lower arch area), especially men (you can go even stronger), and as you move up your twisting action becomes less strong: medium in mid-back to relatively gentle in the neck as the neck is quite mobile and you do not want to cause any neck problems.

As there are 26 bones in the spine, in theory you should do 26 twists. If you do 20 plus twists you are doing it correctly, as it is impossible to do each vertebra (cervicals) of the neck individually, that is seven twists in second Big toe bone.

Continue twisting upwards until you find that the fingers of your upper (twisting) hand start to hit or push into the back of the head and neck (toes), which is stressing the head and neck. This is approximately around the 1st MPJ joint (i.e. metatarsal phalangeal joint), commonly known as the bunion joint.

Now change your working hand by putting your index

and middle fingers between the Big and second toes, and your thumb under the Big toe. Make sure your thumb is under the Big toe and not on the spine (inner aspect). This will stop you from gently twisting the neck bones (cervicals). See second Illustration above. Continue gently twisting the neck bones (cervicals), moving your support (lower) hand upwards after each twist, until you reach the first joint of the Big toe, which is the top of the spine (C.1) and beginning of the skull. There are seven neck bones, so theoretically seven twists. About four or five is good. Repeat at least four times, working upwards only, i.e. from lumbar to cervicals. For spinal problems repeat six times.

NOTE: Do Left half of person (foot) then Right half (foot).

6. Ankle Gate Opening

This technique actually opens the energies of the ankle and foot and is an opening that I do on every receiver as it opens the energies of the feet and therefore the person. I also do it fairly early in the sequence as the points (Gates) can be quite tender and not all that relaxing.

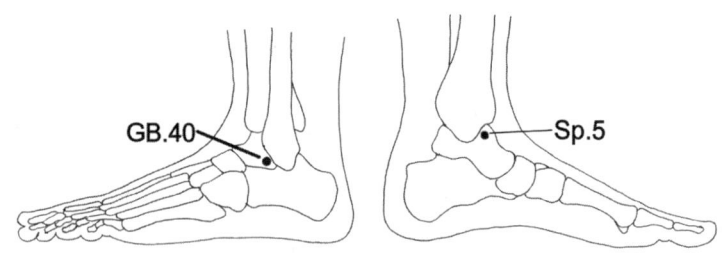

ILLUSTRATION 52: Location of GB.40 and Sp. 5
LATERAL FOOT – GB.40   MEDIAL FOOT – Sp.5

TO LOCATE: Standard hold and wobble the foot back and forth and feel the hollow created. These are the two points, **GB.40** which is located in the depression on the outer ankle in front of the outer ankle; and **Sp.5** which is located in the depression (visible dimple on most people) under the inner ankle crease.

Locate acu-points GB. 40 (outer ankle crease) and Sp. 5 (inner ankle crease). Note that these two points are not directly opposite each other. GB. 40 is lower and Sp. 5 is higher. Locate the two points, and then with the tip of your left thumb and tip of your middle finger clamp the two points fairly strongly. With your right hand hold the Chest area of the foot (Standard Hold) and slowly lift it up and sit it down four times, while holding the two acu-points clamped. When sitting up and stretching down, go as far as the foot will allow

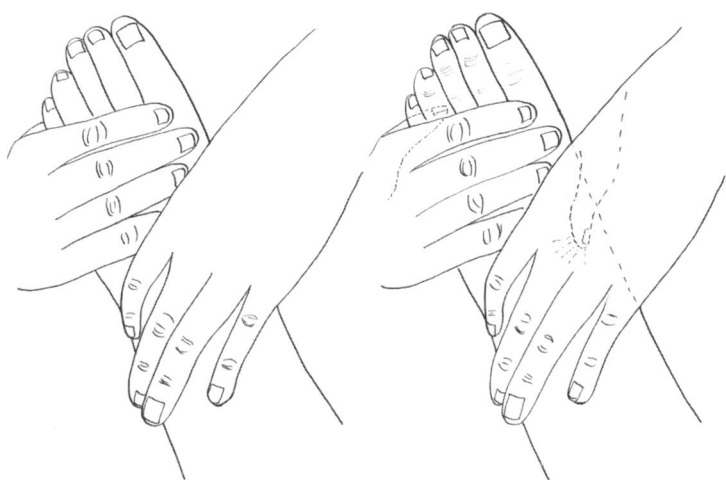

ILLUSTRATION 53: Ankle Gate Opening

Keep hold of the points and with your pressure rotating as the foot rotates, that is as the foot moves outward, press on outside acu-point (GB.40). When the foot is inward, press on Sp. 5. Thus, your pressure rotates with the foot. With your right hand on chest area (Standard Hold) rotate the foot four times in each direction slowly and deliberately.

It does not matter which direction you do first as long as you rotate the foot (and your pressure) an equal number of times each way. This is the actually opening of the Gates of the Ankle, and is a balancing technique.

NOTE: Realise that all Gates have a tendency to be more sensitive than other acu-points, and that if there is an imbalance, it could be a number of things. Do not assume that if a point is sharp that the organ's chi will be as well. Remember there are a number of possibilities, especially with Gates. More commonly, GB. 40 is painful. If this is the case, lessen your pressure on the points while you lift the foot and rotate. Do both sides of the body (feet) before treating.

To treat, first define the pain (sharp: excess or dull: deficient), which is most likely to be sharp. Secondly, check imbalance between the sides of the body (feet), that is, which is the stronger, sharper or more ouch. In theory, no matter what the pain is like, it should be the same both sides of the body, but this is rarely the case.

Gently hold the duller (or less sharp) point with the tip of your index finger and with the other tip of the index finger, gently sedate. (**NOTE**: never rotate both sides of the body together.) Check the side you are rotating for improvement. (It may need to be repeated for another six out-breaths). If it is no longer sharp, check the other side. Quite often, by connecting both points together and working one side while holding the other, it affects both. If this is the case it is an indication that this imbalance is short-term.

However, if it does not balance, it is an indication that the imbalance is rather more long term and you will need to gently rotate anti-clockwise on the other point on the other side of the body.

NOTE: Do Left half of person (foot) then Right half (foot).

7. Diaphragm Relaxer

With Standard Hold and sitting the foot up, use the hooked tip of the thumb of your working hand, and work inside to outside, and then work back. Make sure you use the tip of your working thumb and not the flat. Also, keep your working thumb parallel to the toes, and fingers straight at the side, wherever they are comfortable. Do not grab the foot. You take small steps (a little less than the width of your thumb as you want to make sure you cover it all) across the foot from longitudinal zone 1 to zone 5 and with each step: as you push diagonally upwards at about 45% with the tip of your working thumb in the heads of the metatarsal bones, you pull the chest over, which opens up the diaphragm, as it is up under the ribs.

NOTE: Make sure your supporting hand does not drift up onto the back of the head and neck (toes), as you do not want to stress the neck.

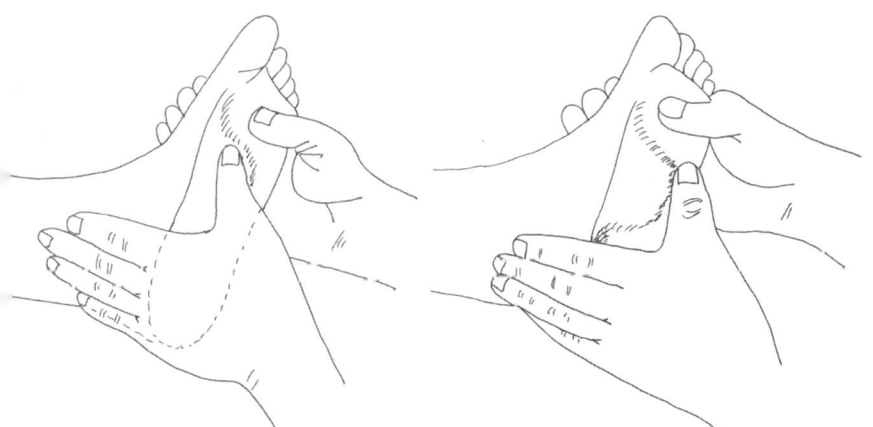

ILLUSTRATION 54: Diaphragm Relaxer
INSIDE TO OUTSIDE and then OUTSIDE TO INSIDE

To come back, you may reverse hands if you like, but it is not necessary and is quicker if you do not. Just pause and then work your way back repeating as above.

NOTE: Do Left half of person (foot) then Right half (foot).

8. Balance K I/Triple Burner (Both feet together)

After the Diaphragm Relaxer, with the tip of both thumbs, locate K. 1. It is located in the hollow, under the second and third toes (zones 2 and 3) just below the diaphragm. Visually if you squeeze the chest area, you will see one major crease down through the Chest and into the Abdomen. Along this crease and immediately under the diaphragm, you will find the hollow, which is K.1.

Once located, place the upside down tips of both thumbs on both K.1s and bring your support fingers of both hands around the inside of the feet and straight across the upper back. Again do not grab. With the receiver's out-breath slowly press into K.1.

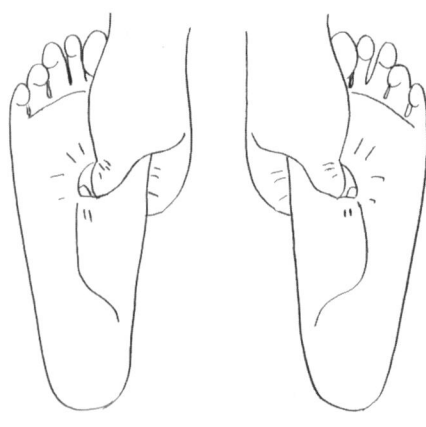

ILLUSTRATION 55: Balance (Both Feet together) K 1

NOTE: Take the full out-breath to press. To balance, press four times with out-breath. Kidney chi is quite often deficient. Do not be fooled by a strong sensation from the receiver. Kidney chi is deep and therefore often intense, but rarely sharp.

To stimulate K.1 rather than strong clockwise rotation, which will cause immediate sharp pain, I recommend holding with strong pressure for six out-breaths each time you press. Strong pressure is a yang technique, and six breaths are for treatment. This is a gentle method of stimulation that causes no pain, and it works. So you can combine the balancing approach (four times) with the treatment technique (hold for six out-breaths). You may find that as you do this each time you do not have to press as deeply, and if so, obey the body's instructions.

9. Head/Neck Opening

Many Reflexology toe techniques actually stress the neck. Look carefully at what is happening to that part of the body.

Perform Standard Hold with thumb on chest and straight fingers on upper back, but a STRAIGHT Index finger (and Middle finger on the Big toe) on the back of the foot/upper back and the straight flat of the thumb underneath actually holding the distal (towards the toes) head of the 1st Metatarsal bone (Big toe long bone).

Start with Big toe, and do each toe (Big to little toe) individually. Once you have the toe end head of the 1st metatarsal held firmly, GENTLY open each toe by **stretching gently upward**, with out-breath, and while holding the stretch, internally rotate the toe bone **four times** in BOTH directions for balance or six times each direction for treatment. The toe should not move, only the bone. The aim is to move **only** the bone of the head/toe you are working. Work inside to out (first to fifth toes).

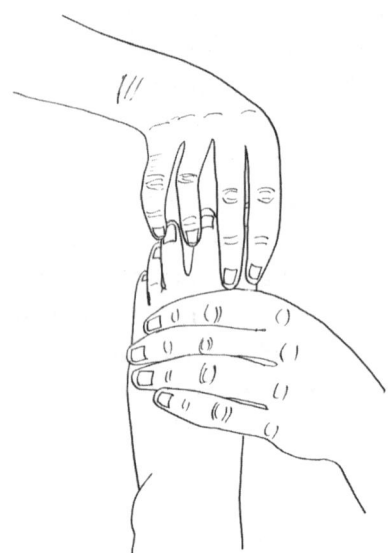

ILLUSTRATION 56: Head/Neck Opening

The key here is to try not to move the toe you are working on. This way it will be an internal rotation and mobilising the bones, and not moving the toe, which is moving the neck around.

NOTE: This is an *Opening*, not working. **Do not** pull or jerk the head/toe. Work with the body, not against it.

Repeat for each toe, moving your Index finger to the next head (towards toe) of the metatarsal bones, from second to fifth. Before stretching (opening the base of the neck) of each toe and rotating, you need to hold the distal heads of the appropriate metatarsal bone still and the third bone of each of the second to fifth toes, otherwise you will not be rotating the bone, but rather the head. This is a mobilisation technique for the foot joints as well as a mobilisation technique for mobilising the base of the neck: C. 7 (last cervical bone) and T. 1 (fist thoracic or upper back bone).

NOTE: Do Left half of person (foot) then Right half (foot).

10. Stretch and Vibrate

A) STRETCH:

Hands under anklebones, and a little up the leg. Make sure you do not slide down into the pelvic region (heel) especially on female receivers.

Breathe in and take the weight of the body/feet and legs, but do not lift them up. **Lock arms**. Breathe out and lean back (use body weight rather than muscle strength). Take your full breath to stretch: slowly. Watch the stretch **open** each joint: Knee, hip, spine, shoulders and neck. The person **should not** slide down the table. Hold stretch until each joint is opened. Can be repeated four or six times.

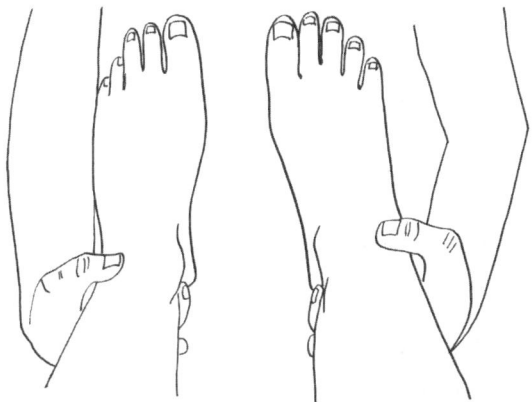

ILLUSTRATION 57: Stretch

B) VIBRATE:

Relax and return feet to resting position. Keep both hands under anklebones, as illustrated above. **The more relaxed you are the better.** Drop your shoulders. **Gently vibrate**; that is, send Chi (energy) up through the legs, torso, neck, head and arms. Do not shake. The **KEY** is the **gentler the vibration the better**: try not to do it. It is so easy. It is an internal vibration rather than an external one. See the vibration pass through everything. Watch what vibrates and what does not. Look for variations in vibration. Do not just stop the vibrating, but rather slowly, gently and naturally allow it to dissipate itself, just as when one throws a pebble into a clear pond, and the ripples created simply spread outward and slowly disappear. This is also important so that you do not shock the receiver on a cellular level.

11. Rocking (Optional) BOTH feet together

This Opening is used for specific purposes, being extremely powerful. It is used in those situations where the person resists relaxing, either due to the person being particularly stressed, or in response to initial consultation.

The aim of this Opening is to achieve the rhythm of life (womb-like fluidity). Like vibrating (above) it can be used for diagnostic purposes. Although you place three straight fingers (index, middle and ring) on the height of both outer ankle-bones, you are actually only using one finger, the middle finger. **Gently** and slowly encourage the person/body to rock rhythmically back and forth (in and out), penetrating the entire person, toes to head. **The more relaxed you are the better.** The more you try not to do it, the better. This may take a few minutes to achieve. The **key** is the gentler and more natural a rhythm, the better. Once the rocking reaches the head, you know you have achieved your aim.

Rocking is extremely difficult to teach and explain, as the rhythm of life that you use is initially your own. So first you must discover your own rhythm. How do you do this? By practice and experience. It is when you lose the rhythm that you realise you had it. So it can only be learnt through experience. Once you have discovered your rhythm, then you can start with that and like fine-tuning a musical instrument you gradually go up and down the scale until you find their rhythm. So you must first discover your own rhythm and then use it to discover their rhythm.

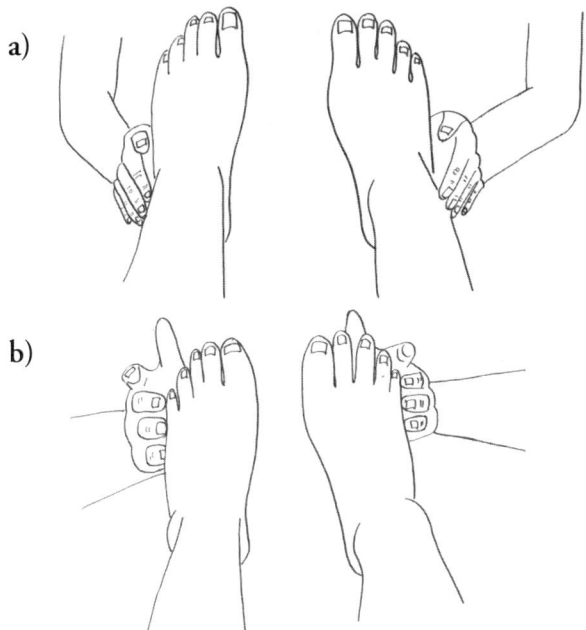

ILLUSTRATION 58: Rocking

Why is this so powerful? You are dealing with cellular memory and the rhythm from the receiver's mother's womb, which is why, if you get it right, they cannot resist it. It is just like taking them back to that time and space when they are most nurtured, protected, warm and safe. This is why it is so powerful. It is, therefore, a technique that I would not recommend for use in public. Both the giver and receiver are vulnerable as their energy has been opened and they are vulnerable to whatever energies are around.

I would also recommend staying at the height of the ankle bones, rather than move up to the little toes, as illustrated in b) above, as this is extremely difficult to maintain the rhythm while moving up the feet. There is in fact no need to do this.

However, if you are drawn to this technique and once you have mastered it, you can attempt to move your three fingers up the outer feet to the tip of the little toes, continuing the rhythmical rock as you go. If you can actually get the receiver rocking from little toe (head) to head (excuse the pun), then it is penetrating all matter.

Once this has been achieved, hold rocking at tip of little toes for four, six or twelve out-breaths, and then rock as you return your three fingers to the anklebones, finishing where you began.

As with Vibrating, but more so: **Do not just stop** the rocking, but rather slowly, gently and naturally allow it to dissipate itself. This is also important so that you do not shock the receiver.

These eleven Openings can be used initially at the beginning of a treatment to relax and for learning purposes. However, other than the Feet Brushing, Ankle Gate Opening, and possibly the Stretching and Vibrating (and if drawn to it – Rocking), I would recommend, once you are comfortable with the techniques, that the other Openings be used at the beginning of working on the related reflexes or area of the body.

So, ultimately you would not have to use all of them, just those that either:

• You are drawn to, and/or
• That are appropriate for a particular receiver and/or situation/imbalance.

Therefore, if you do this, a suggested sequence would be something like this:

1. Always start with Feet Brushing, and Ankle Gate Opening and possibly Stretch and Vibrate (with Rocking optional).
2. Put the rest of the Openings into the treatment sequence before working that part of the body, and possibly again after working said part/reflex/es.
3. Always finish with Figure Eight/Infinity technique (To be outlined in Chapter 23: Practical: The Basic Procedure for a Reflexology Treatment).

CHAPTER 22
Contraindications and Safety Precautions

The list that follows was originally referred to as contraindications, which are any conditions, including dis-ease, that might be harmful to the receiver, the giver or anyone else, especially other receivers; that is to say situations in which you shall not work. However, more recently they have come to be called Safety Precautions: conditions and/or situations, the implications of which the Reflexologist needs to be conscious of in the therapeutic and treatment situations.

The Contraindication/Safety Precaution lists vary between differing schools of Reflexology, which means that all conditions, symptoms and dis-eases with potential risks and/or dangers cannot be listed in depth. No list can cover every possible scenario. Also many lists differ with the degree of danger and range from: Contraindications: you shall not work, through degrees of risk to 'May do harm', 'Keep in mind' and/ or 'Be careful'. Thus it is difficult to generalise about all situations and it is up to the professional Reflexologist to make a decision. However, the list below covers the most common and generally followed basic list of Reflexology Safety Precautions.

Interestingly, in the Reflexology community this issue of Contraindications and Safety Precautions tends to have been largely ignored, with the general process of simply restating, to a great degree, what has come before by either paying brief lip-service to the issue, or simply following the general consensus with little detailed discussion. There are of course exceptions to this with some Reflexologists beginning to question the validity of many of these Contraindications and Safety Precautions.

Something that needs to be kept in mind here is the axiom: Do not diagnose and treat dis-ease. It would also be wise for Reflexology students, early in their professional development to err on the side of caution and to follow these Safety Precautions, although, with common sense, experience and knowledge, the risk decreases significantly. Regardless always keep in mind: *If in doubt, don't.*

Before continuing, it is important to acknowledge here that each individual Reflexologist in any given situation or presenting symptoms must decide for themselves their own personal limitations. The decision is theirs: to work or not. The best advice is simply: unto thyself be true, and honesty is the best policy.

The key to this whole question is quite simple: If in doubt, don't. When you are not comfortable or unsure of the best course of action, err on the side of caution. Again honesty arises here:

- Initially decide yourself whether you will offer your services to the receiver
- Simply state what you understand to be the case and/or your concerns, and give the receiver the option
- Where necessary consult with their health care provider directly yourself or through the receiver.

Remember, there are always options.

Safety Precautions
ILLUSTRATION 59: List

1. Current Foot Injuries, including recent fractures or breaks
2. Diabetes
3. Thrombosis, Economy Class Syndrome or history of blood

clotting (TEST: soreness in calf muscle when foot raised, i.e. Chest Kneading Opening)

4. Inflammation conditions of the Lymphatic and/or Vascular systems

5. Pregnancy: First Trimester (three months) or any history of reproductive problems

6. Unstable Blood Pressure (High or Low Blood Pressure is not a problem)

7. Heart conditions

8. Contagious or infectious diseases

9. Cancer, especially Lymphatic cancer

10. Receivers who have had a donor organ operation within the last six months

11. Dry scaly skin conditions (reflects emotional distress)

12. Psychologically disturbed people and mental illnesses

13. Babies and Infants under the age of two years old

14. Mature people and those in palliative care

15. Heavy and long-term drug use, including prescribed drugs

16. Irresponsible individuals

The first comment worth making here is that the majority of this list actually comes from Massage Therapy and so if you consider Reflexology to be a form of massage then perhaps these may apply. Perhaps the logic is that all body therapies have the same contraindications and safety precautions. But the question is: Is Reflexology a form of massage? If not, as this list comes from massage, then it brings them all into question.

One final point is that many of these situations call for common sense. However, with diagnosed medical conditions there are other ethical, moral, professional and legal considerations which arise. The legalities vary from country to country, and even within countries, so it would be wise to find out your legal position for yourself. The Reflexology training institutions and professional organisations are a good starting point. But always remember: never fail to respect the rights of the individual and your professional concern for them.

Next, let's look briefly at each of these safety precautions and their implications and applications to the practice of Reflexology.

1. CURRENT FOOT INJURIES, INCLUDING RECENT FRACTURES OR BREAKS

Common sense would indicate that it would be wise not to have Reflexology, especially any deep-tissue type Reflexology, if there are recent foot injuries, including broken bones. These may, during the healing process, do more harm than good. However, depending on the damage and location of the injury, it is possible to still work some of the foot reflexes, especially those that may assist in the healing process of the current injury. The Reflexologist needs to carefully assess the situation before proceeding.

2. DIABETES

Diabetes is a serious illness, with various different types that need to be taken into consideration. Diabetics should be under the care of a health professional, and if this is the case, and the individual is being responsible, then there is no major problem. Remember though never treat a dis-ease.

3. THROMBOSIS, ECONOMY CLASS SYNDROME
OR HISTORY OF BLOOD CLOTTING

Again, never treat a dis-ease is the first point to be made. Secondly much of the explanation and justification for this is questionable. The reason this is listed is the theory that Reflexology stimulates the circulatory system (blood) and therefore if there are blood clots, especially in the leg and foot, then Reflexology may move the clots, which in turn may increase the likelihood of the blood clot causing a problem.

The test for the possibility of blood clots is the Chest Kneading Opening. Again theoretically, when stretching the foot upwards towards the torso, if there is any sharp pain in the leg, especially the calf, there is the possibility that the pain is the result of a blood clot or clots. This is not guaranteed and there are other reasons for possible pain in the leg other than blood clots. So, firstly, no Reflexologist should assume that this is definitely the result of blood clotting. However, the standard response is to err on the side of caution and therefore do not work. But Reflexology may actually help.

If the receiver is either on blood thinning medication or has been cleared of the problem, then there is no problem working.

4. INFLAMMATION CONDITIONS OF THE LYMPHATIC AND/OR VASCULAR SYSTEMS

This is rather an interesting assertion when one considers that the first and major defence mechanism of the body is inflammation, so there are many reasons why there may be inflammation. One must ascertain what type of inflammation and why before making a determination and Reflexology may help many instances of inflammation.

Theoretically the reason this is mentioned (and especially Lymphatic and/or Vascular inflammation specifically) is the concern that Reflexology stimulates the circulatory system (blood) as well as the lymphatic (fluid) system and therefore by stimulating the movement of blood and lymph, it may, in theory, make the situation worse.

Depending on the location of the inflammation, either in the body or the feet, then Reflexology can be of assistance. However, if the inflammation were in the feet (and possibly the body as well), then theoretically it would be better to avoid working the inflamed area of the foot/feet.

5. PREGNANCY: FIRST TRIMESTER (3 MONTHS) OR ANY HISTORY OF REPRODUCTIVE PROBLEMS

This is the standard assertion of both massage and Reflexology. The assumption here is that the first trimester is early in the pregnancy and that miscarriages are more likely to occur, and so theoretically Reflexology can bring on a miscarriage. However, this is questionable.

But perhaps initially while learning and early in one's professional development: err on the side of caution. Once you are experienced and have an understanding of the process of pregnancy, then there are no problems working from pre-conception through to post-natal, and in fact medical research is increasingly indicating the benefits of Reflexology in pregnancy, especially when there are no complications. In fact there is a significant specialist area of Reflexology called Maternity Reflexology, an area where Reflexology is making major inroads into the health care system.

Another point worth mentioning here is that Reflexology receivers have been pregnant (1st trimester) without even knowing it, and so it is sometimes very difficult to avoid this situation. So far there is no evidence that Reflexology has caused any problems as a consequence whatsoever, yet very deep Reflexology approaches are more risky and should be avoided.

Once again, with experience, knowledge and common sense, and the fact that this is a natural process rather than a dis-ease, this is not a problem unless there are medical reproductive problems and certain other problems that arise during pregnancy which require specialist intervention. So, unless this is the case, then there should be no problems with Reflexology during pregnancy.

6. UNSTABLE BLOOD PRESSURE
(HIGH OR LOW BLOOD PRESSURE IS NOT A PROBLEM)

This is a serious medical condition and therefore would not arise. An individual with unstable blood pressure would be extremely ill and either in an ambulance or in hospital. However, high (Hypertension) or low (Hypotension) blood pressure, although worth taking into account of course, is not a problem for Reflexology.

7. HEART CONDITIONS

This contraindication comes from Chinese Reflexology, as it is a deep-tissue approach which puts extra strain on the heart of the receiver. Chinese Reflexologists will not work if the Heart reflex or energy (chi) is excessive, or if there is any history of any heart conditions. So, with a deep-tissue approach this needs to be taken into account.

8. CONTAGIOUS OR INFECTIOUS DIS-EASES

Firstly contagious or infectious dis-eases range from the common cold to HIV and Aids, so it is a little difficult to generalise. The first question is a choice of the Reflexologist: Will the Reflexologist work on a receiver with certain contagious or infectious dis-eases? The choice is his/hers. Some Reflexologists may make a moral decision not to work on some of these conditions, and they have this right. Others (myself included) will work on an individual who asks for help and therefore I will take the risk. It is my choice. So there is no right and wrong here, just simply a decision which has to be made consciously by the Reflexologist.

However, if one were to strictly follow this as a contraindication, then there would be very few receivers ever worked on, as most have some form of contagious or infectious dis-ease at one time or another.

The major question here that the Reflexologist needs to answer initially is for him/herself and then for other receivers is the risk assessment of cross-contamination. Legal and Occupational Health and Safety issues arise here. As long as appropriate precautions and sanitation is maintained between Reflexologist and receiver, as well as between treatments, this is not a major problem, but is something that must be borne in mind.

9. Cancer, especially Lymphatic cancer

The question of cancer is an increasingly prevalent issue. This again arises from massage, and perhaps is based to some degree on fear. In the past, especially with Lymphatic cancer, the theory was that Reflexology, as it stimulates the blood and lymph, could make the situation worse. Current thinking on this issue is changing and increasingly those within the health care system are encouraging people to have Reflexology as they have observed the benefits. This is a debatable issue at this stage and in a state of flux. For example, in Australia, cancer support groups are asking for Reflexologists to work on cancer patients.

10. Receivers who have had a donor organ operation within the last six months

The theory behind this safety precaution is that the receiver of a donor organ needs time for their body to recover from the operation and for their anti-rejection medication to be adjusted and to settle down. After any operation, especially major surgery, it would be extremely wise to err on the side of caution and initially work very carefully, especially on the affected reflex/es.

11. Dry scaly skin conditions (reflects emotional distress)

Let's assume this assumption is correct. Why not work? Is this assumption correct? Dry scaly skin conditions reflect emotional distress and Reflexology cannot help those with emotional distress. This is what this is actually saying. Who isn't to some degree or another emotionally distressed? If Reflexologists were to follow this advice then they would have very few receivers.

12. Psychologically disturbed people and mental illnesses

If one followed the principal of not working on psychologically disturbed people, again there would be very few receivers of Reflexology. Who isn't to some degree or another 'psychologically disturbed'? There are issues, such as drugs/medication, that need to be taken into consideration when working on mental imbalances, but with such precautions and common sense, Reflexology can help.

13. BABIES AND INFANTS UNDER THE AGE OF 2 YEARS OLD

There are those who argue that, as the body of a baby is still developing internally (as well as externally) and that all the inner organs are not fully developed, Reflexology should not be performed on infants under two years of age. Perhaps it would be wise not to perform a full Reflexology treatment on infants, but that does not mean that Reflexology is not beneficial.

14. MATURE PEOPLE AND THOSE IN PALLIATIVE CARE

There are certain issues that need to be considered when working on mature receivers, but otherwise Reflexology can be of great benefit to them. In fact, the Palliative Care area of the health care system is one where Reflexology is consistently making inroads.

15. HEAVY AND LONG-TERM DRUG USE, INCLUDING PRESCRIBED DRUGS

Firstly, heavy and long-term drug use; whether as prescribed drugs or illegal drugs, need to be defined. Heavy here refers to a cocktail of drugs. This is most common in mature people where they are taking drugs to counteract the side effects of other drugs. This is an issue where Reflexology does not so much effect the drugs as such, but its effectiveness is decreased to the extent to be purely symptomatic, that is, the receivers gain minimum benefit from their aches and pains but that is all. Rather than counteracting the drugs, the tendency is to decrease the effectiveness of Reflexology.

Strictly speaking, by the Chinese definition of long-term or chronic, in this case it is anything the body cannot throw off within two weeks (14 days). My experience is that short-term is anything from six to eighteen months, and therefore up to this length of time there are no major problems with having Reflexology.

Long-term, on the other hand, would definitely be anything over eighteen months, and could be as soon as six months. Nothing should be taken for the rest of the life. In the long-term anything taken indefinitely will cause imbalance in the body, Again, experience shows that the effectiveness of Reflexology is decreased and it becomes more symptomatic.

One group of drugs worth mentioning is drugs used in mental imbalances which tend to be suppressants, that is, they suppress the natural body responses. If this is also long-term, then there is a pattern that some times develops worth noting. A fluctuation from polar opposites occurs: after one treatment the receiver feels absolutely fantastic and the next down in the dumps or depths of despair. Now this scenario does not always happen but it is worth knowing of and warning receivers about the risks of Reflexology for those who have been on long-term medication. In the short-term, every second treatment the receiver will have an increase of the symptoms that they have been suppressing, which is the body's attempt at homeostasis or balance. It is a short-term reaction to a long-term problem.

16. Irresponsible Individuals

These are the individuals who do not take responsibility for their own health and wellbeing but rather either place the responsibility on their doctors, health care provider or Reflexologist, or they are just generally irresponsible about their health and wellbeing.

As the person concerned is responsible for their own health and wellbeing, this is a major concern and these individuals need to be educated to realise this.

So to reiterate, the options are:

1. Initially, each individual Reflexologist must make their decision about the treatment based on their knowledge, experience and belief system. You have a right to offer your services or not.

2. Secondly, empower the receiver by honestly explaining your concerns and those of the profession, and giving them a choice.

3. Thirdly, consult with the receiver's other health care professionals.

4. Finally, consult with another member of the receiver's family, especially in the case of the young and possibly the mature, if for various reasons they are not capable of making the decision.

For me the decision is simple. I will give my help to anyone who asks. The choice is theirs. It is their health and wellbeing, and as I offer assistance and help if asked, I feel obliged to give assistance. The only receivers that I choose not to work on are those who have had an organ transplant. My choice. I am not so much concerned for my own safety but rather the safety of others. This is what is paramount to me. I choose to take the risk if asked. My choice and the consequences are mine.

To conclude, these then are the contraindications/safety precautions which all Reflexologists need to make decisions about. The list of course is not complete nor does it cover every possible scenario, which is why each Reflexologist must learn to think on their feet by being honest first with themselves and second with the receiver, thus making decisions with wisdom and compassion and always keeping the Hippocratic oath: I shall do no harm, foremost in their minds and, If in doubt, don't.

There are no absolutes here. The truth is there is more we do not know than we do, and so we are all learning as we go along. There are those who would like a nice neat little package that they can present the general public, the Reflexology profession and the health care system, but this is just not possible. Reflexology is expanding and learning all the time and no two Reflexologists are the same. This is both a strength and a weakness, which I for one, do not wish to change. The mechanic vs the artist comes once more to mind.

CHAPTER 23
Practical: The Basic Procedure for a Reflexology Treatment

The basic sequence of working is:

1. **Openings**
2. **Work Head to Buttock**, i.e.
   - Head and Neck (Toes): both feet;
   - Chest (ball of the feet): both feet,
   - Abdomen: upper and middle (arch of the feet): both feet;
   - Pelvis (heel): both feet;
3. **Reproductive Reflexes** (Pelvis/Heel): Sole, Inside and outside: both feet together;
4. **Inside the body** (feet): Inside the body (Spine/Central Nervous System): both feet
5. **Outside of the body (feet)**: Outside of the body (Limbs and outer Hip): both feet;
6. **Kidney, Adrenal and Bladder**: both feet;
7. **Figure Eight/Infinity** to finish: both feet together.

This then is the basic sequence of events: head to tail, reproductive and inside and out (working both feet together). It is a simple and easy sequence to remember and follow. This also covers all the reflexes of the feet and areas of the human being and is the order in which you will find the practical treatment techniques outlined below. It is also the suggested order and sequence especially important for learning purposes and perhaps initially when working with receivers. **NOTE**:

Always work the same reflexes (both feet) at the same time, which is much more therapeutic, e.g. working all head techniques on one foot and then the other before moving on, and so on.

1. OPENINGS: (See Chapter 21)

- Feet Brushing
- Pelvic, Sacrum, Hip and Lower Back Relaxer
- Chest Relaxer
- Chest Kneading
- Spinal Twist
- Ankle Gate Opening
- Diaphragm Relaxer
- Balance Kidney 1/Triple Burner
- Head/Neck Opening
- Stretch & Vibrate
- Rocking (Optional)

2. WORKING THE HEAD:

2.1 HEAD: BOTTOM OF ALL TOES

a) Inside to Outside:
- STANDARD HOLD, but move support fingers up to the back of the head (top/back of toes). Make sure your support fingers are behind the toe you are working on (always support and balance your own actions). Keep support thumb on the upper chest.
- Ensure working fingers are on top of support fingers
- Thumb Walk down ONLY (*SEE Illustration below*)
- Big toe: five to six lines down each big toe.
- Other toes: three to four lines down each toe. Four times for balance or six times for treatment.

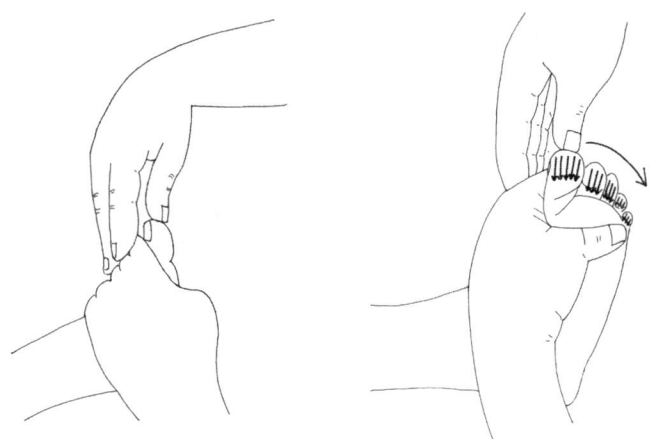

ILLUSTRATION 60: Head/Bottom of Toes

2.2 HEAD: UP OF ALL TOES

b) Outside to Inside: EITHER:

1. REVERSE hands and repeat (as for above) working (Little toe to Big toe)   *OR*

2. Simply drop working hand down, keeping fingers straight at the side and thumb walk up each toe, keeping working thumb parallel to the toe being worked on. Make sure your support fingers are up behind the head (Top/Back of toes)

SUGGESTION: Either:

1. LEFT Foot: Bottom of toes and THEN RIGHT foot: Bottom of toes;   *OR*

2. Do LEFT Foot: Bottom of toes, THEN Up All Toes, and THEN Press/Squeeze Inside & Out; **THEN** LEFT Foot (same techniques), i.e. stay on Left Foot until 2.1, 2.2 & 2.3 is done, then move to RIGHT FOOT & repeat all (2.1, 2.2 & 2.3)

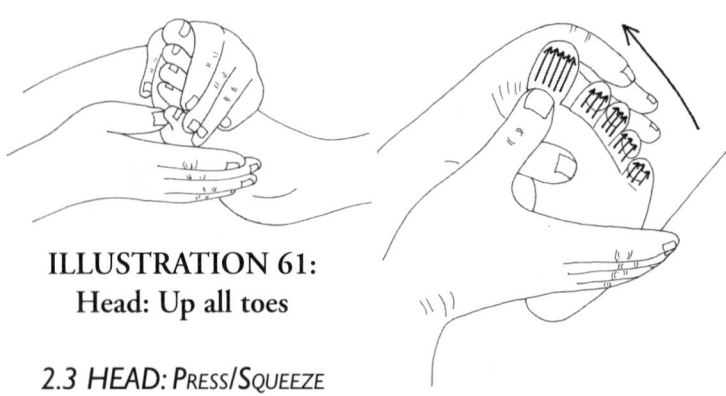

ILLUSTRATION 61:
Head: Up all toes

2.3 HEAD: *PRESS/SQUEEZE*

INSIDE AND OUTSIDE OF EACH TOE

SUPPORT HAND: Thumb on toe pad, sitting toe outwards, and fingers straight at the side. DO NOT GRAB. Use tip of thumb and side of Index finger, inside and outside of Big toe. PRESS (Squeeze) inside and outside of each Toe, working up to either side of the base of the toenail. DO NOT go above the base of the toenail, as damage could be done to the cuticle Big toe to Little toe **ONLY**. Four times for balance or six times for treatment.

SUGGESTION: LEFT Foot & then RIGHT Foot *OR* Stay on LEFT Foot until 2.1, 2.2 & 2.3 is done, then move to RIGHT Foot and repeat all.

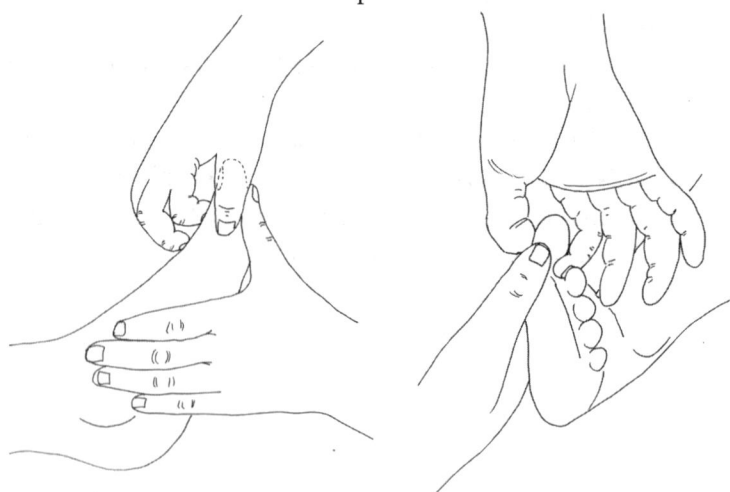

ILLUSTRATION 62: Head Press/
Squeeze Inside and Outside of each toe

2.4 HEAD: Top and bottom: Palm front and back of head

BOTH FEET Together: with **FLAT** (straight) thumb underneath and **FLAT** (straight) index finger (all toes index finger ONLY except Big toe: index & middle fingers: as illustrated) on Top/Back of body (feet). DO NOT PINCH.

PALM front and back of each toe from bottom to top and from Big to Little toes. Stop at top of each toe when you can pull your index finger and thumb together (about on the toenail), and squeeze for four or six out-breaths, then move to next toe.

REMEMBER to keep your fingers and thumb working STRAIGHT, which will stop you from pinching rather than palming. Four times for balance or six times for treatment.

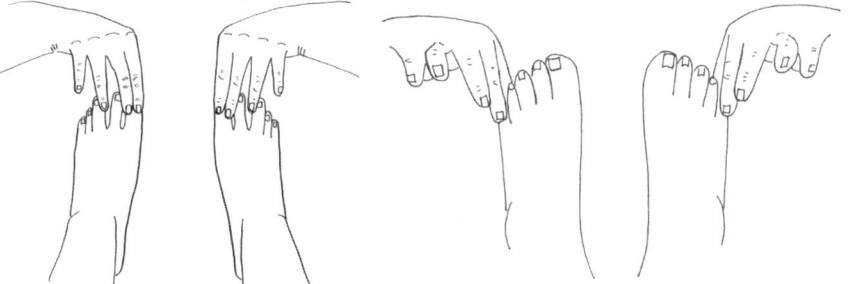

ILLUSTRATION 63: Head: Top & Bottom: Palm Front & Back of Head

2.5 BALANCING THE MAJOR GLANDS: BOTH Feet Together

ILLUSTRATION 64: Balancing the Major Glands

a) Pineal Gland (Crown Chakra): BOTH feet together

Right on the top inner corner of the Big toe beside the top on the toenail, use the side of BOTH your index fingers, and HOLD gently for 12 out-breath breaths.

NOTE: Some argue Pineal gland should be treated for insomnia; BUT recommended that you only balance and you DO NOT TREAT, only balance it.

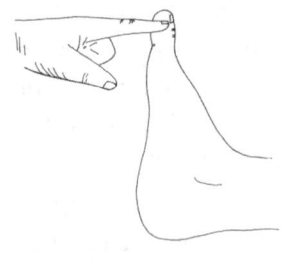

b) Pituitary Gland (Brow Chakra): BOTH feet together

On the medial aspect of the feet, below the base of the Big toenail and above the 1st joint of the Big toe. HOLD the side of both Index fingers, gently for 12 out-breaths.

NOTE: Recommended to balance Pituitary gland on everyone, but you may wish to treat as well or instead: See 2.6.

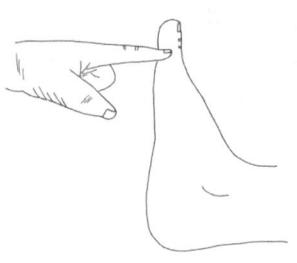

c) Thyroid/Parathyroid Gland (Throat Chakra): BOTH feet together

On the inside of the feet, at the base of the Big toe & above the 2nd joint (MPJ: Metatarsal phalangeal joint) of the Big toe. HOLD the side of both Index fingers, gently for 12 out-breaths to balance. **NOTE**: Recommended to balance Thyroid/Parathyroid gland on everyone, but you may wish to treat as well or instead: See 2.6.

2.6 TREATING THE MAJOR GLANDS: *BOTH FEET TOGETHER*
ILLUSTRATION 65: Treating the Major Glands

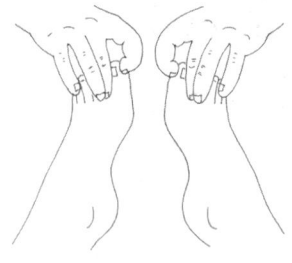

a) Pineal gland, Pituitary Gland & Thalamus/Hypothalamus: BOTH feet together

SUPPORT with thumb and middle fingers together at the base between both Big & 2nd toes. HOOK fingernail (very small) of BOTH index fingers around onto reflex

Straight in (90 degrees) = Thalamus/Hypothalamus
Towards sole (75 degrees) = Pineal gland
Towards back (75 degrees) = Pituitary gland
Stimulate or Sedate as needed for six out-breaths.

b) Thyroid/Parathyroid Gland (Throat Chakra): BOTH feet together

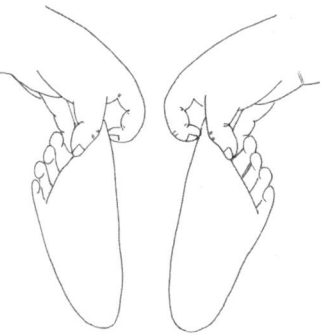

SUPPORT with thumb and middle fingers together at the base between both Big and 2nd toes. HOOK tip of BOTH index fingers around onto Thyroid gland reflex. You can use your fingernails.

Stimulate or Sedate as needed for six out-breaths.

3. NECK & SHOULDERS:

3.1 WORKING THE SHOULDERS (WALKING THE RIDGE)
ILLUSTRATION 66: Working the Shoulders

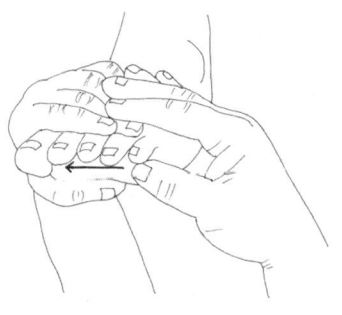

STANDARD SUPPORT: Make sure fingers stay on the Upper Back rather than the back of the neck. The tendency is to drift up. Working fingers on on support fingers, with FLAT thumb on Shoulder Line, thumb walk across from outside to inside of the four toes (NOT the Big toe)

Four times for balance or six times for treatment.

3.2 WORKING THE NECK
ILLUSTRATION 67: Working the Neck

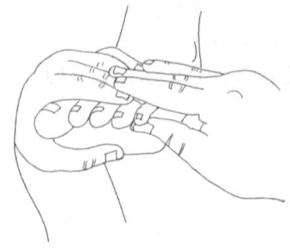

STANDARD SUPPORT but move support fingers up to the back of the Head/Neck (back of toes). Working fingers on support fingers, with FLAT thumb on the Neck (under toe pads), thumb walk across from outside to inside of four toes (NOT the Big toe). Four or six times.

3.3 WORKING BACK ACROSS SHOULDER FIRST
AND THEN NECK
ILLUSTRATION 68: Working back across Shoulder & then Neck

REVERSE HANDS and repeat walking Shoulders and Neck (i.e. 3.1 & 3.2 above). Working fingers on support fingers, and as you thumb walk across Shoulder (and then Neck), allow working hand to pivot over the Big toe. LEFT Foot & then RIGHT Foot, i.e. 3.1, 3.2 & 3.3 on LEFT Foot and then 3.1, 3.2 & 3.3 on RIGHT Foot.

3.4 SHOULDER (BOTH FEET TOGETHER) OPTIONAL/ALTERNATIVE
ILLUSTRATION 69: Shoulder (both feet together)

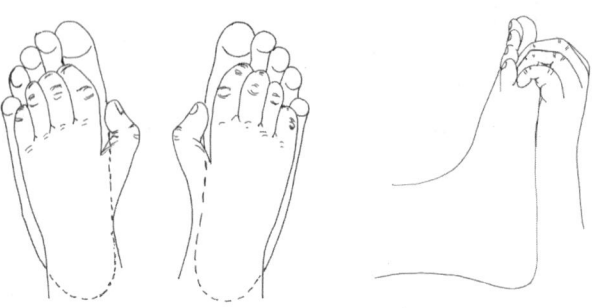

OPTIONAL, ALTERNATIVE, or EXTRA. BOTH Feet Together.

Place hooked finger tips between each toe as much as you can but DO NOT force toes apart and:

1. Play the Piano, i.e. press between each toe both sides at the same time with the same finger (inside to outside)

2. **Sit feet completely up** and HANG and pull downward with all eight fingers at once and HOLD for four or six outbreaths.

Side View, NOTE: Fingers cupped or hooked between the toes. DO NOT force the toes apart.

4. CHEST:

4.1 CHEST

ILLUSTRATION 70: Chest

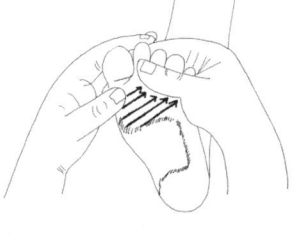

a) Inside to Outside:

STANDARD support, but turn to side of thumb and move upwards along the jaw (base of toe pads). Keep support fingers on Upper Back, **NOT back of head**. Be careful of tendency to drift up with support fingers. SIT foot up. Fingers on fingers and thumb walk diagonally upwards across Chest. Make sure you cover the whole Chest area. Better to overlap than under lap.

b) Outside to Inside:

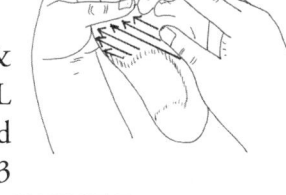

REVERSE HANDS and repeat (as above) but from outside to inside. Four or six times.

SUGGESTION: LEFT Foot & then RIGHT Foot, *OR* ALL Chest treatment LEFT Foot and then RIGHT, i.e. 4.1, 4.2 & 4.3 LEFT Foot then 4.1, 4.2 & 4.3 on RIGHT Foot.

4.2 CHEST:Working the Zones
ILLUSTRATION 71: CHEST: Working the Zones

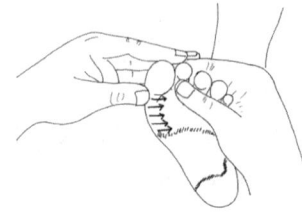

a) Working in under the Big toe:

STANDARD support, but turn to side of thumb and move upwards along the jaw (base of toe pads). Keep support fingers on upper back, **NOT back of head**. Be careful of tendency of support fingers to drift up. SIT foot up. Fingers on Fingers, thumb walk in under Big toe (Zone 1 of chest).

Four times for balance or six times for treatment.

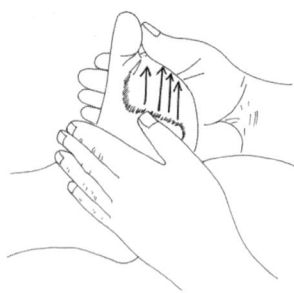

b) Inside to Outside:

STANDARD support, but turn to side of thumb and move upwards along the jaw (base of toe pads). Keep support fingers on upper back, **NOT back of head**. Be careful of tendency for support fingers to drift up. SIT foot up. After a) above, drop working hand down to side of foot (straight fingers) and thumb walk up between each toe of the chest. (Inside to Outside). Four times or six times.

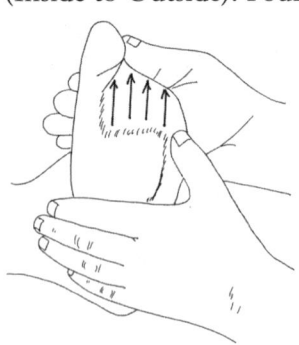

c) Outside to Inside:

STANDARD support, but turn to side of thumb and move upwards along the jaw (base of toe pads). Keep support fingers on Upper Back, **NOT back of head**. Be careful of tendency for support fingers to drift up. SIT foot up. After b) above, simply pause and then thumb walk up between each toe of the chest. (Outside to Inside) Four or six times.

4.3 CHEST: Upper back
ILLUSTRATION 72: CHEST: UPPER BACK

One Foot and then the other:
SUPPORT with Open Fist & working thumb on back of palm. Finger walk down between the bones (metatarsals) of the upper back, inside to outside, THEN **pause**, and work back down between the bones, outside to inside. Four times or six times.

LEFT Foot and then RIGHT Foot.

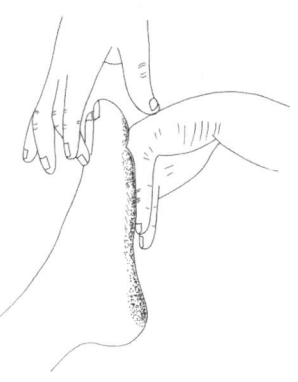

ILLUSTRATION 73: CHEST: Upper Back (Alternative)

ALTERNATIVE: Both Feet Together
SUPPORT with BOTH thumbs on the chest/ball of the feet. Sit feet up and finger walk down between the bones:

i) Inside to outside, and **pause**, THEN

ii) Return: outside to inside.

Four times or six times.

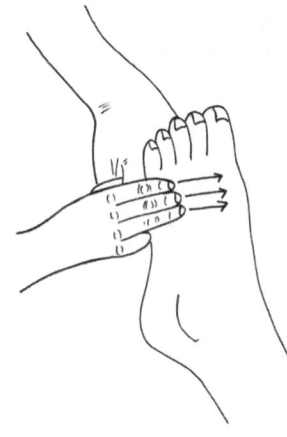

ILLUSTRATION 74: Working the Upper Back

Working the Upper Back
SUPPORT with Open fist. Thumb of working hand on support fingers, finger walk (with two or three fingers) across upper back: inside to outside, and THEN REVERSE HANDS and finger walk outside to inside.
Four times or six times.
LEFT Foot, and then RIGHT Foot.

5. ABDOMEN AND PELVIS:

DIAPHRAGM TO BUTTOCKS

ILLUSTRATION 75: Diaphragm to Buttocks

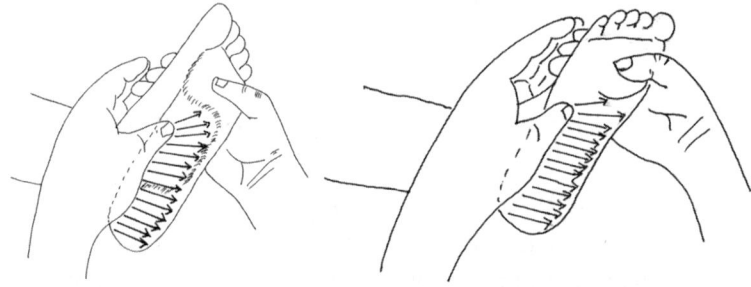

STANDARD SUPPORT, but support fingers move down the back/top of foot, each time you return to inner aspect to begin a new line, so that when you get to the pelvis, you can have fingers on fingers for as long as possible: Thumb walk diagonally upwards and across the abdomen, working down towards the buttocks. Fanning action: start out diagonal and end up (in pelvic region) straight across. Inside to outside. Four times or six times. THEN REVERSE hands and thumb walk back (working diagonally upwards and across) down to the buttocks. Outside to inside. Four or six times. LEFT Foot and Then RIGHT Foot.

    a) **Pelvis, with Fingers on Fingers** (preferred option) but if unable to then

    b) **Pelvis, with Straight Fingers** STANDARD SUPPORT with straight fingers resting on the ankle and up the leg.

ILLUSTRATION 76: Diaphragm to Buttocks: Fingers on fingers or Straight fingers

a)   b)

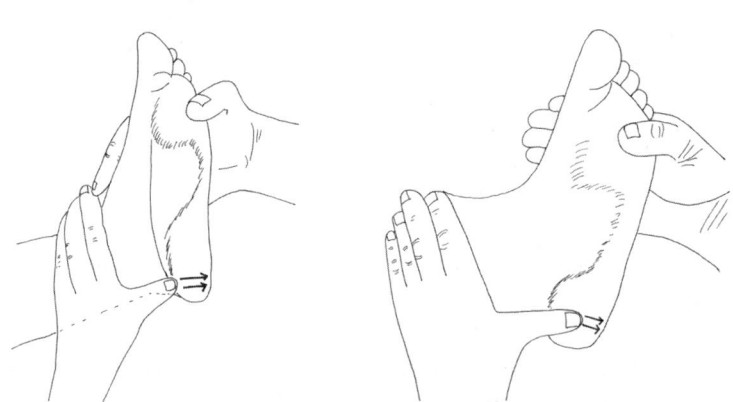

6. LARGE INTESTINES:

ILLUSTRATION 77: Rectum and Anus

A) *Rectum, Anus & Sigmoid Colon: Inside*

TO BALANCE: Drawn down Sigmoid to Anus, four times.

TO TREAT: STANDARD HOLD. Stimulate or sedate in direction of flow six times.

LEFT FOOT then RIGHT.

ILLUSTRATION 78: Large Intestines

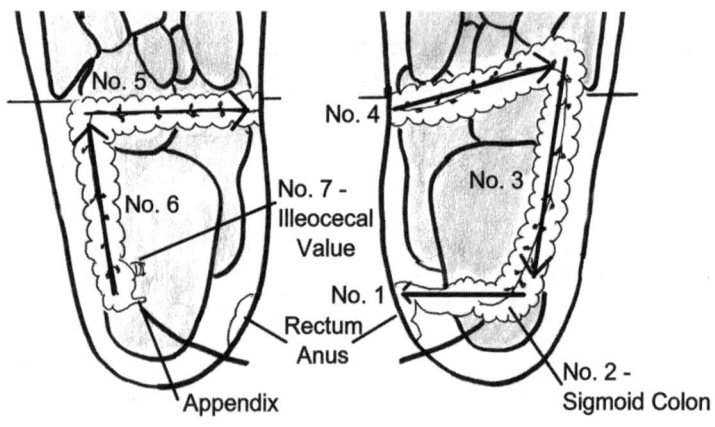

B) *The Whole Bowel:*

Work in direction of flow, i.e. towards the anus, but in sections from anus back, i.e.

No. 1: Straight across below Heel Line

No. 2: Sigmoid Colon (Illustrated below)

No. 3: Descending Colon

No. 4: 1st half of Transverse Colon

No. 5: 2nd half of Transverse Colon

No. 6: Ascending Colon

No. 7: Illeocecal Value (Illustrated below)

TO BALANCE: Draw gently in direction of flow each section in above order four times.

TO TREAT: Stimulate or sedate in direction of flow each section six times, or until clear for six times. REPEAT sections if necessary.

- **Sigmoid Colon (No. 2):** STANDARD SUPPORT Locate Sigmoid Colon (Left foot): + on sole of pelvis/heel and one thumb out and down one thumb. PRESS with tip of thumb, thumbnail parallel to toes: Stimulate or sedate as needed. Six times or for six out-breaths for treatment.

- **Ileocecal Value (No. 7):** Locate Ileocecal Value (Right foot: under 4th toe towards 5th toe, and a little below half way down from heel colour change or Heel Line. PRESS, with tip of thumb, thumbnail parallel to toes (i.e. vertical thumb nail). Stimulate or sedate as required: six times or for six out-breaths for treatment.

**ILLUSTRATION 79: No. 2 Sigmoid Colon
and No. 7 Ileocecal Value**

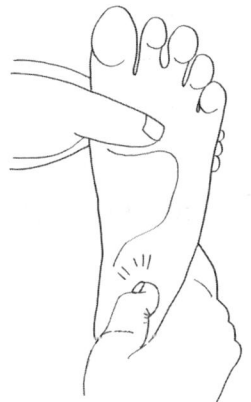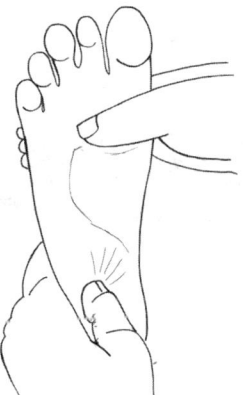

7. REPRODUCTION:

7.1 *LOCATION* OF *INNER* AND *OUTER* *REPRODUCTIVE REFLEXES*

ILLUSTRATION 80: Male and Female Reproductive Systems

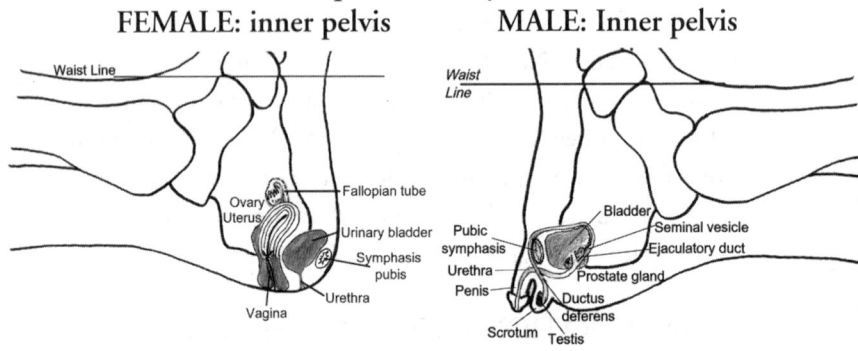

FEMALE: inner pelvis

MALE: Inner pelvis

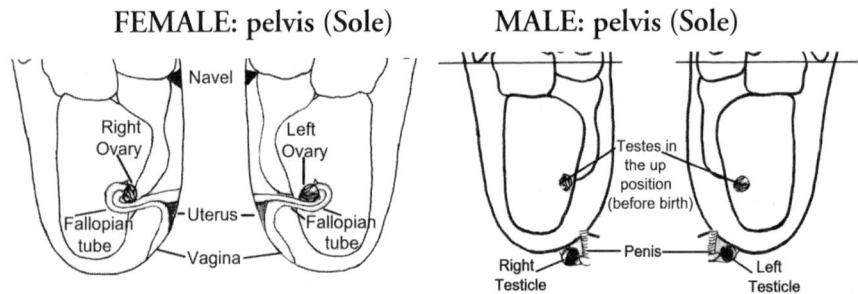

FEMALE: pelvis (Sole)

MALE: pelvis (Sole)

HELPER POINT

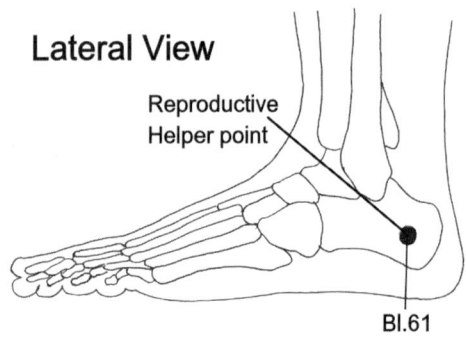

7.2 PELVIC OPENING: REPRODUCTIVE REFLEXES
ILLUSTRATION 81: Pelvic Opening

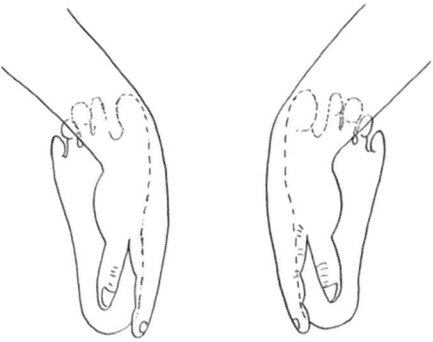

PELVIC OPENING: BOTH feet together

Fingers straight covering the whole inner pelvis (sacrum, rectum/anus, uterus, vagina, bladder) and thumbs resting on Ovaries (sole) in the pelvis/ heel. Using forearms across the chest stretch feet upwards and HOLD for 12 out-breaths for balance. For rest of Reproductive DO NOT LET GO. Take pressure off and walk to next Technique.

7.3 REPRODUCTIVE: LEFT FOOT: INNER FEMALE AND MALE
ILLUSTRAION 82: Inner Reproductive (Left Foot)
FEMALE: Inner left half of uterus and ovary
MALE: Inner left half of prostate and seminar vesicle.

Use tip of index or middle finger, place it on inside left half of reproductive reflexes on LEFT Foot. HOLD for six out-breaths: stimulating or sedating GENTLY as required.

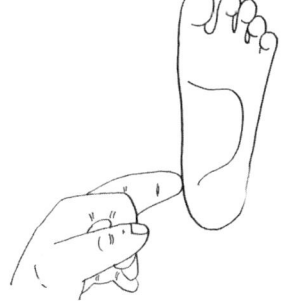

NOTE: As this is gentle, there is no need for support.

7.4 REPRODUCTIVE: INNER FEMALE AND MALE (BOTH FEET)
ILLUSTRATION 83: Inner Reproductive (Both feet)

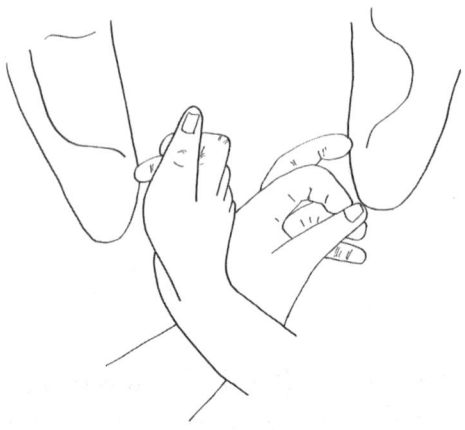

BOTH feet together. Comparing both inner halfs. Use tip of index or middle finger, place it on inner reproductive reflexes on Right foot, and tip of left index or middle finger on inner reproductive reflexes on Left foot. HOLD both points for six out-breaths: stimulating or sedating GENTLY as required.

7.5 REPRODUCTIVE: RIGHT FOOT: INNER FEMALE AND MALE
ILLUSTRATION 84: Inner Reproductive (Right foot)

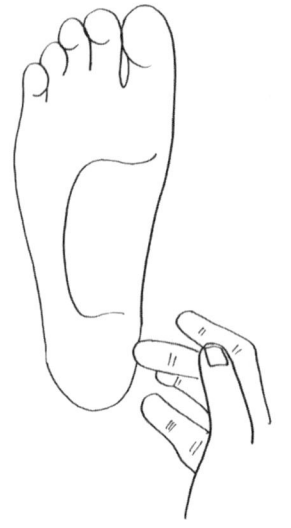

FEMALE: Inner right half of uterus and ovary

MALE: Inner right half of prostate and seminal vesicle.

Use tip of index or middle finger, place it on inside left half of reproductive reflexes on Right Foot. HOLD for six out-breaths: stimulating or sedating GENTLY as required.

7.6 REPRODUCTIVE: SOLE: OVARIAN SACK OR TESTES
IN THE UP POSITION
ILLUSTRATION 85: Sole Female & Male Reproductive Reflexes

BOTH feet together.
FEMALE: Both ovaries
MALE: Both testes in the up position

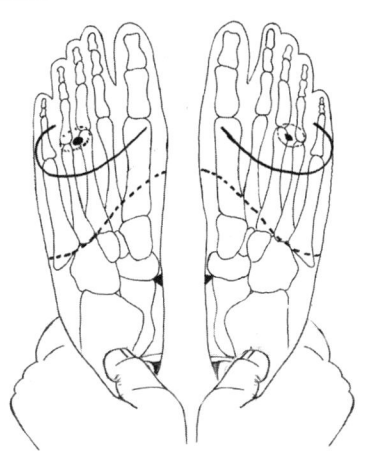

Tip of both thumbs with vertical thumb nail.

HOLD for six out-breaths: stimulating or sedating GENTLY as required.

ALTERNATIVE: Left foot and then Right. (Not illustrated)

7.7 REPRODUCTIVE: SOLE: MALES TESTES AND PENIS
ILLUSTRATION 86: Sole Male Reproductive Reflexes

BOTH feet together.
Use tip of index or middle finger, place it on inner teste and penis on Right foot, and tip of left index or middle finger on inner teste and penis on LEFT foot. HOLD for six out-breaths: stimulating or sedating GENTLY as required.

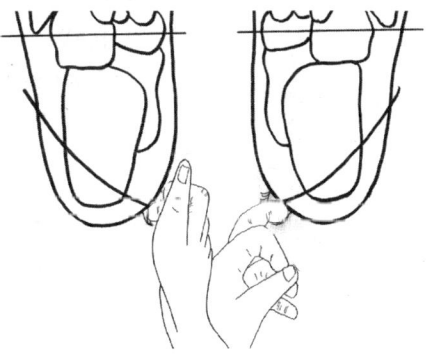

ALTERNATIVE: Left foot and then Right. (Not illustrated.)

7.8 REPRODUCTIVE – HELPER POINTS (BL.61):TWO OUTER POINTS
ILLUSTRATION 87: Outer Helper Points

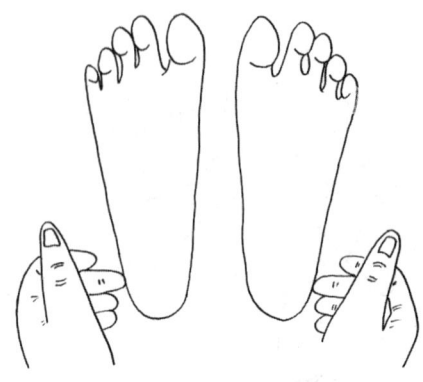

Use tip of index or middle finger, place it on Helper point on Left foot, and tip of index or middle finger on Helper point Right foot.

HOLD both points for six out-breaths: stimulating or sedating GENTLY as required

NOTE: Treatment (six) and Balance (four or twelve)

ALTERNATIVE: LEFT foot, then RIGHT (not illustrated)

7.9 REPRODUCTIVE: DRAW UP BLADDER MERIDIAN
ILLUSTRATION 88: Bladder Meridian

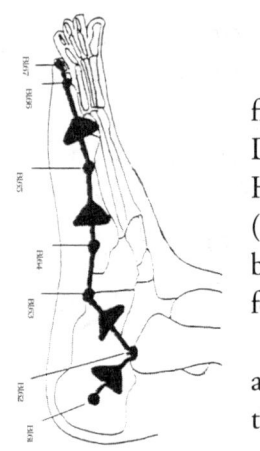

BOTH Feet Together.

With tip of BOTH index or middle fingers, and using them like a pencil, DRAW up from Outer Reproductive Helper point (Bl. 61) to tip of Little toe (Bl. 67: above first joint and below the base of the little toenail) and hold for four out-breaths.

RELEASE and return to beginning and REPEAT three times. A total of four times.

NOTE: Each time you release, move away from the little toe by falling off, i.e. roll out and down. DO NOT FLICK or draw upwards. DO NOT take energy out or deplete the body. Rather fall out and down and away, making a large circle away from the outside of the feet. This way you will not deplete the body, but simply get energy flowing.

8. INNER AND OUTER PELVIS:

START at Ankle Gate points, i.e. GB.40 (outside) and Sp. 5 (inside). With both middle fingers, finger walk up the inner and outer pelvis (ankle cease) until just before pinching the skin, then release one middle finger and slide over with the other to where you started on other side. REPEAT, but this time just before pinching remove other middle finger and slide on the other side to where you began.

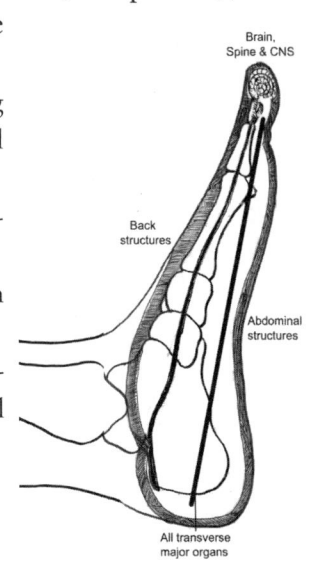

NOTE: This is doing the technique ONCE. Repeat a total of four or six times. LEFT Foot and then RIGHT.

ILLUSTRATION 89: Inner & Outer Pelvis

9. INSIDE THE BODY:

NOTE: There are actually four lines worth working both up and down on the inside of the feet (See Illustration 34: Physical Foot Chart, Inside of the Body View, Chapter 13), and they are, from the front (sole) to the back (back/top of the foot):

1. Front structures of the body, including skin, deep and superficial abdominal muscles and bones
2. All the major inner organs that transverse the body
3. the Spine and Central Nervous system (bones of the feet)
4. The back structures of the body, including skin and both deep and superficial muscles.

ILLUSTRATION 90: Four lines of working on the inside of the feet/body

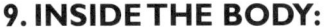

NOTE: The techniques for the other three lines are the same as for the Spine/Central Nervous system, explained below.

9.1 SPINE/CENTRAL NERVOUS SYSTEM: WORKING UP.

ILLUSTRATION 91: Spine/CNS

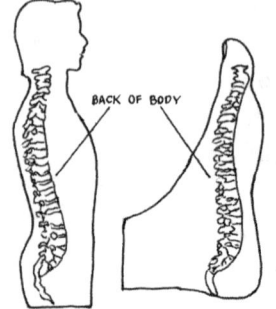

Working up the Spine: Coccyx to Cervicals

Firstly, in order to perform this technique you need to get your own body in the right position. Turn to face the inside of the foot you are working on (Start on the Left foot).

STANDARD SUPPORT. Thumb on coccyx (joint between calcaneus/heel and talus bones), and slightly underneath the heel (coccyx). Point working thumb in the direction of working and work up. Straight fingers on the outside heel. DO NOT GRAB.

ILLUSTRATION 92: Working up the Spine/CNS

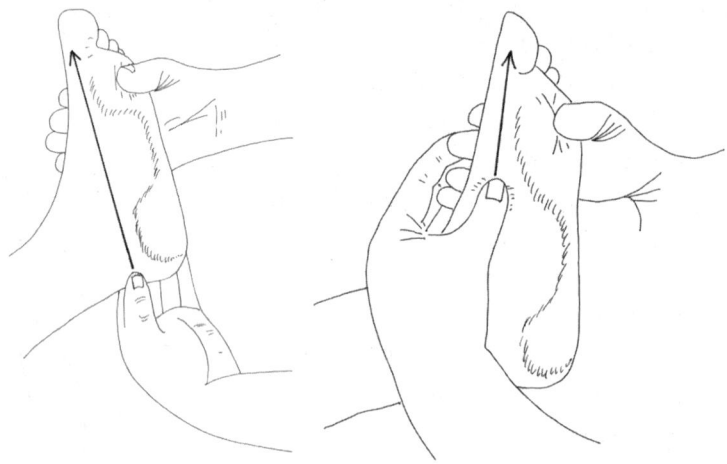

Thumb walk up spine, allowing working fingers to slide out from outside and underneath, until just before you are stretching; THEN **STOP, and leave working thumb where it is** and move working fingers from under the buttock/heel and at the same time bring your support fingers down the back, so that you can put working fingers on support fingers; THEN pointing thumb in direction of working (towards the neck/Big toe), thumb walk up to the top of the neck (cervicals), i.e. 1st joint of the Big toe. Four or six times.

9.2 SPINE/CENTRAL NERVOUS SYSTEM: WORKING DOWN
ILLUSTRATION 93: Working down the Spine/CNS

Working Cervicals (neck) to coccyx
REVERSE hands. SUPPORT HAND: Open and flat hand on sole. Make sure your knuckles are on the upper chest/ball of the foot and NOT on the abdomen/arch of the foot. Keeping working fingers STRAIGHT on the Back/top of foot, and without grabbing, thumb walk down the Spine.

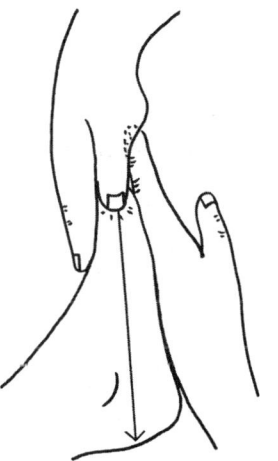

Four or six times.

LEFT Foot and then RIGHT Foot.

OPTIONAL: SPINAL TWIST after (and possibly before) working the Spine/ Central Nervous System.

10. OUTSIDE: SHOULDER AND ARMS:

ILLUSTRATION 94: Shoulder & Arm

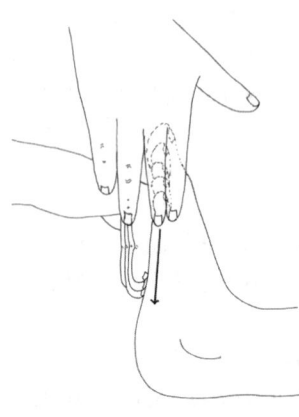

a) Shoulder Tip to Elbow (Humerus/ 5th Metatarsal bone):

SUPPORT with Open Fist on chest. Knuckles in line with Shoulder Line.

With middle finger, finger walk down between the two heads of the 5th Metatarsal bone (humerus bone of arm), from bump to bump, with middle finger half on bone and half under bone (towards sole, but still on the outside). Four or six times.

NOTE: Upper bump (distal head of 5th Metatarsal) is Shoulder joint and the second or lower bump (proximal head of 5th Metatarsal) is the Elbow.

b) Elbow to Shoulder Tip:

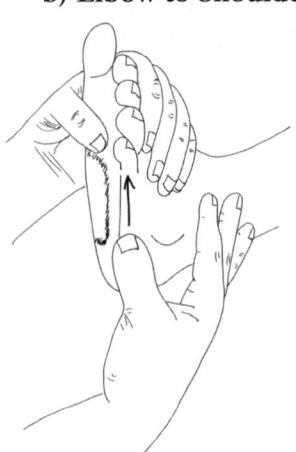

REVERSE HANDS. STANDARD SUPPORT or SUPPORT with Open Fist on Chest (Not illustrated). From lower bump (Elbow), thumb walk (with STRAIGHT fingers resting against foot) up to upper bump, again half on bone and half under bone (5th Metatarsal = humerus bone).

Four or six times.

LEFT Foot and then RIGHT Foot

11. OUTSIDE: Lower Limb

ILLUSTRATION 95: Lower Limb

a) Working Up over Leg:
Triangular area from lower bump (head of 5th Metatarsal) to bottom corner of outer pelvis/heel: hip joint, i.e. femur joining with pelvic bones.

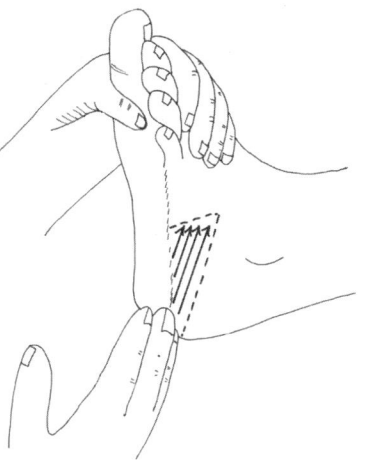

STANDARD SUPPORT. With two or three fingers (index, middle & ring) finger walk upwards in every direction, overlapping Leg Reflex (i.e. change upward direction each time you go over this area).

Four or six times.

b) Working Down over Leg:
REVERSE HANDS SUPPORT with open fist.

With two or three fingers (index, middle & ring) finger walk downwards in every direction, overlapping Leg Reflex. Again change downward direction each time. Four or six times.

LEFT Foot and then RIGHT Foot.

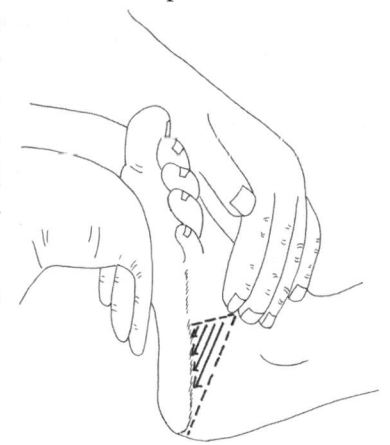

12. OUTSIDE: Outer Hip

OUTER HIP
ILLUSTRATION 96: Outer Hip

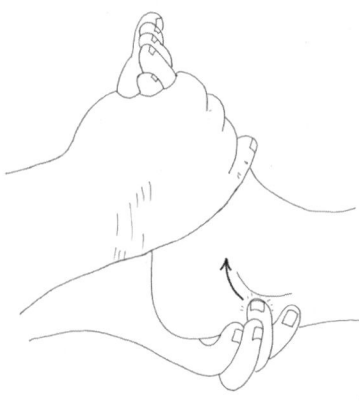

a) Working Up around Outer Hip:

STANDARD SUPPORT. With working hand underneath around the Achilles Tendon (but not grabbing), and working thumb resting gently up the leg, using middle finger, finger walk up and around the outer hip/ankle bone.

Start finger walk from under anklebone and keep side of working middle finger against the anklebone. Once you are stretching you have gone far enough. Four or six times.

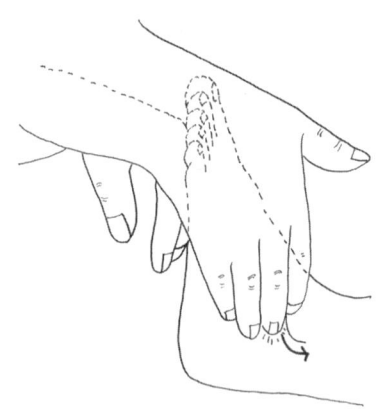

b) Working Down around Outer Hip:

REVERSE HANDS. SUPPORT with Open Fist.

Using middle finger, finger walk down and around the Outer Hip/Ankle bone. Start finger walk from GB.40 point and keep side of working middle finger against the hip/anklebone. Finger walk down and around the corner. Once you have rounded the corner you are finished. DO NOT finger walk up the leg AT ALL. Four or six times.

LEFT foot and then RIGHT foot.

INNER & OUTER HIP *TOGETHER*
ILLUSTRATION 97: Inner & Outer Hip Together

ALTERNATIVE or as an Opening

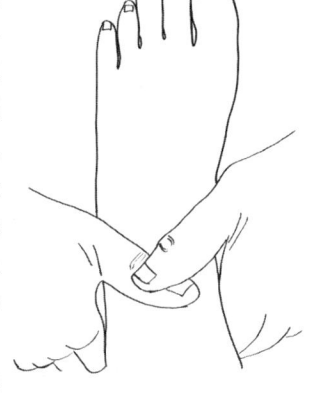

With thumbs crossed over the ankle crease and using inner side of 2nd knuckle of BOTH index fingers, rake quickly around inner and outer hip reflexes, one direction and then back, equal number of times, e.g. 12 one direction and 12 back in the other direction. Can be done as a once over lightly for hips, as an opening, or before/after treatment: No. 12 above.

NOTE: For treatment: Can work inner hip as well as above (same techniques).

13. KIDNEYS AND ADRENALS:

ILLUSTRATION 98: Kidneys

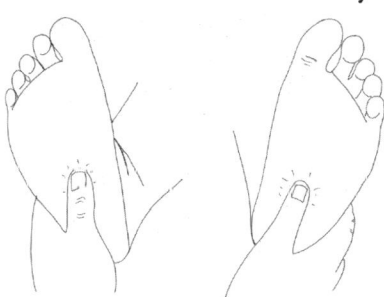

A) KIDNEYS: BOTH FEET TOGETHER

TO LOCATE: There are two options:

1. Under 2nd and 3rd toes, and in line with the lower bump (proximal head of 5th Metatarsal) with the FLAT of thumb pad; *OR*

2. With thumbs relaxed and parallel with index fingers and fin-

gers STRAIGHT, find bump and slide both hands under the bump up feet/leg & FLATTEN thumb.

HOLD with strong pressure (usually needs stimulating) for four or six out-breaths.

ILLUSTRATION 99: Adrenals

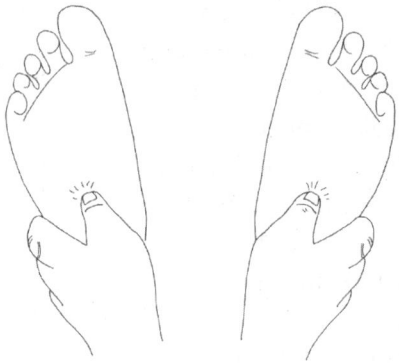

B) *ADRENALS:* **BOTH** *FEET TOGETHER*

From previous positions, raise BOTH thumbs directly above to tips onto Adrenals. Adrenals need both stimulating (need energy: exhausted) but you do not want to stimulate as gland will produce more adrenaline; and so sedating and nurturing, therefore HOLD, gently varying your pressure until BOTH feel closer to the balanced state.

Recommended to do this for 12 out-breaths

ILLUSTRATION 100: Kidneys to Bladder (Ureter Tubes)

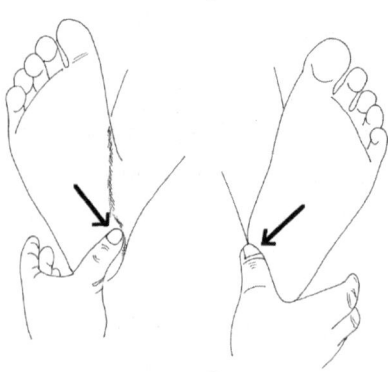

c) Draw Down from Kidney to Bladder (Ureter tubes):
BOTH feet together.

Draw straight down with tip of thumbs (as a pencil) from Kidneys to Bladder. Four or six times.

14. INFINITY/FIGURE EIGHT: Both Feet Together

ILLUSTRATION 101: Infinity/Figure Eight

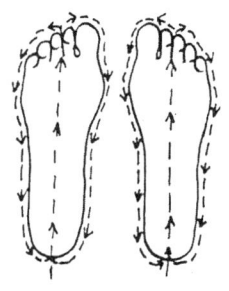

TO FINISH: Figure Eight/Infinity around BOTH feet together. *Tai Chi/ balanced actions.*

NOTE: The middle bone of the middle finger is the one doing the drawing and so it MUST always stay in contact with the feet. Your other fingers simply follow.

START with straight middle fingers and the middle bone of the middle fingers on the centre of BOTH feet underneath on front of the buttock. Draw up the centre of both feet (to 3rd toes: slightly outward), then cup fingers on top of the toes and draw down the outside of both feet in cupped position.

At outside of the outer pelvis/heel straighten fingers and as you do turn underneath back to where you started and then draw up the centre of both feet again.

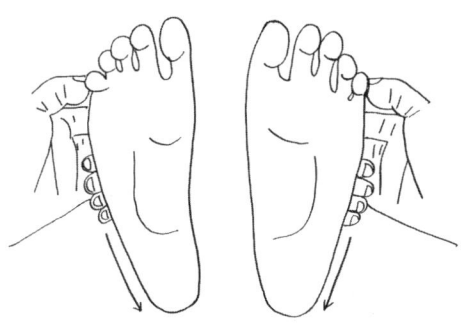

STRAIGHTEN FINGERS and turn fingers away from yourself (palms upward), and draw down inside of both feet, turning the fingers under at the centre of the bottom (palms downward), back to where you started.

THIS IS COMPLETING THE TECHNIQUE ONCE.

Repeat whole sequence **THREE** more times. A total of **FOUR** times.

Finish by drawing up the centre of BOTH feet, and coming off the feet on the chest/ball of the feet rather than the toes to prevent you from flicking.

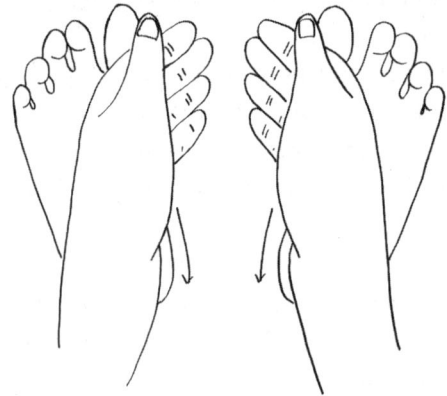

CHAPTER 24
Summaries of the Sequence

There are two different types of summaries of the Basic Procedure for a Reflexology Treatment (Chapter 23) as different people learn in different ways. The first is a written summary, outlining the techniques in words, and the second is a visual summary.

In conjunction with the outline in the previous Chapter, the written summary is designed to work through to learn the actual techniques, and so is more detailed than the second summary. The second summary is designed as a brief overview to be used once you have learnt the actual techniques and you are comfortable with them and to learn and remind you of the techniques as well as the sequence of events: head to tail, reproductive, inside and out.

WRITTEN SUMMARY OF THE BASIC PROCEDURE FOR A REFLEXOLOGY TREATMENT

OPENING TECHNIQUES

1 Feet Brushing

Up and down each surface (front, back, inside and out), using palms. Disconnect between directions on each surface.

2 Pelvic, Sacrum, Hip and Lower Back Relaxer

Palms around ankle bones: up and down leg. Get the foot waving hello. No Chinese burns.

3 Chest Relaxer

Palms on outer and inner chest: Cuddle the chest.

4 Chest Kneading

Open fist and hand on top to cuddle. Stretch and cuddle four times.

5 Spinal Twist

Bottom hand locks (and move bottom hand ONLY), top hand twists: 26 steps. (20+ steps is good)

6 Ankle Gate Opening

GB. 40 (outside) Sp. 5 (inside) Lock points, up and down four times and then four circles each way (rotate pressure with foot).

7 Diaphragm Relaxer

Tip of thumb, pull chest over as push thumb up: inside to out and back. Make sure your support fingers DO NOT slip up on to toes.

8 Balance K.1/Triple Burner

Tip of thumb, press four times with out-breath on both points (feet) together.

9 Head/Neck Opening

Hold metatarsal head still (strong pressure) and rotate the bone, NOT the toe (four or six times each direction) All toes.

10 Stretch and Vibrate

BOTH feet together. Stretch: hand under ankle and on leg, use body weight and lean back slowly. DO NOT PULL.

11 Rocking (Optional)

Both feet together. Middle fingers (three fingers) on outer ankle bones: rocking action. DO NOT just stop the rocking.

HEAD/NECK: ALL TOES: Left Foot then Right.

2.1 Thumb walk down all Toes

Standard Hold, but fingers up behind head/toes. Fingers on fingers. Thumb walk down ONLY and work Big to Little toe: four or six times.

2.2 Thumb walk up all Toes

REVERSE hands and repeat (Little to Big toe): four or six times.

2.3 Press/Squeezing inside and out of all toes

Support Hand: thumb on back of toes, fingers straight at side. Tip of thumb and tip of Index finger press and move up each toe to base of toenail: four or six times Big to Little toe ONLY.

2.4 Front and Back of all Toes

Both feet together, Big toe to Little toe, palm up and pinch at top.

2.5 Balance Glands

Pineal, Pituitary, Thyroid: HOLD for 12 out-breaths.

2.6 Treating Pituitary and Thyroid Glands

BOTH feet together. Support with Thumbs and Middle fingers between Big and 2nd toes. Work with Index fingers: stimulate or sedate as required for six out-breaths.

NECK/SHOULDERS: Left Foot then Right.

3.1 Working the Shoulders

Support fingers on upper back (not Toes). Thumb walk outside to in, four or six times, then

3.2 Working the Neck

Support fingers up behind head/toes. Thumb walk, outside to in, four or six times, then

3.3 Working Back across Shoulder and Neck

Reverse hands and come back other way on Shoulder and then Neck. Remember bring hand over Big toe: four or six times.

3.4 Working the Shoulders (Optional Extra)

BOTH feet together. With claw fingers, play piano and then hang from the shoulders.

CHEST: Left Foot then Right

4.1 Criss-cross Chest

Standard Support, thumb on (Chin/jaw/toe pads), fingers on

upper back. Fingers on fingers and thumb walk across chest. Work diagonally upwards across chest inside to out, then reverse hands and work outside to in.

4.2 Working the Zones

Standard Support, thumb on chin/jaw, fingers on upper back. Fingers on fingers, first work from base of Big toe (Neck) down to diaphragm (Zone 1), then work with thumb walk up between the bones, inside to out, from Zone 1 to Zone 5; THEN Reverse hands and work up between bones, outside to in (Zones 5 to 1)

4.3 Upper Back/Top of Foot

Support with an open fist on chest. Work finger walk with Middle finger down between zones inside to out and then outside to in.

Upper Back: Alternative

BOTH feet together. Support thumbs on Chest.

Working Upper Back

Support Open fist. Working hand thumb on support fingers. Finger walk (two or three fingers) down only, in to out THEN reverse hands and finger walk out to in. Four or six times. Left foot then Right.

5. ABDOMEN/DIAPHRAGM TO BUTTOCKS:
Left Foot Then Right

STANDARD SUPPORT, with straight fingers moving down back (small steps). Thumb walk fanning action: start off diagonal and end up (pelvis) straight across. Overlap, don't under-lap. Work inside to out, then reverse procedure outside to in. Work major organs. Pelvis: either fingers on fingers or straight fingers.

6. LARGE INTESTINES (Both feet together)
Inside Body (Foot)

SIGMOID COLON, RECTUM and ANUS:
Balance: Draw four times from Sigmoid down to Anus.

Treat: as below

The whole Bowel

Work in direction of flow (towards anus) BUT in sections from anus backwards:

No 1: Straight across below heel line,

No 2: Sigmoid Colon,

No 3: Descending Colon,

No 4: 1st half of Transverse Colon: Left foot,

No 5: 1st half Transverse Colon: Right foot,

No 6: Ascending Colon,   and

No 7: Ileocecal Valve.

To Balance

Draw each section gently in direction of flow: four times (Leaving out Sigmoid Colon) but doing Ileocecal Value.

To Treat

STANDARD SUPPORT. Thumb walk each section in direction of flow: six times, plus No. 2 Sigmoid Colon and finish with No. 7 Ileocecal Value.

7. REPRODUCTIVE REFLEXES (INSIDE & OUTSIDE): BOTH FEET

7.1 Location

Inside and outside point/reflexes plus sole ovary reflex.

7.2 Pelvic Opening

BOTH FEET TOGETHER. Place thumbs gently on sole ovaries, and straight fingers covering the inner pelvis/heel. Use arms and body weight to sit the feet upright, and hold for 12 breaths. Opening and nurturing of pelvic region.

7.3 Left Foot

Finger tip LIGHTLY only, hardly any pressure at all. Touch inside reflex of LEFT FOOT for six out-breaths (stimulate or sedate), then

7.4 Inner Female and Male

Finger tips touching both inner reproductive reflexes (six breaths) stimulate or sedate, then

7.5 Right Foot
Touch inside reflex of RIGHT FOOT for six breaths (stimulate or sedate), then

7.6 Sole: Ovaries or Testes
BOTH FEET TOGETHER. Tip of both thumbs on ovary/testes for six out-breaths (stimulate or sedate), then

7.7 Sole: Male Testes
BOTH FEET TOGETHER. Tip of Index or middle fingers on reflex for six out-breaths (stimulate or sedate), then

7.8 Helper Points (Bl.61)
BOTH FEET TOGETHER. Tip of Index or Middle fingers on outside Helper points (Bl.61) for six breaths (stimulate or sedate), then

7.9 Bladder Meridian
BOTH FEET TOGETHER. Finger tip: To finish draw up from both outer points to tip of little toe, four times. Fourth time hold for four out-breaths. DO NOT FLICK OFF end of little toe.

8. INNER AND OUTER PELVIS: *LEFT* THEN *RIGHT* FOOT.
Work up in ankle crease with both middle fingers. Work with BOTH middle fingers towards center until a ridge of skin appears, then slide down ankle crease. Repeat again and slide vertical finger down other side of ankle crease. Total four or six times.

9. MEDIAL: INSIDE THE BODY: LEFT THEN RIGHT FOOT.
NOTE: 4 lines of inner aspect of foot: Back, spine (CNS), inner organs and abdomen.

9.1 Working up Spine: Coccyx to Cervicals
STANDARD SUPPORT. Thumb on coccyx, straight fingers underneath. Thumb walk up spine. Stop and bring fingers up (fingers on fingers), and continue up to base of neck.

9.2 Working Down Spine: Cervicals to Coccyx
REVERSE HANDS. Support: opened back of hand/arm.

Thumb walk down spine. Straight working fingers. DO NOT GRAB.

10. SHOULDER AND UPPER ARM: LEFT THEN RIGHT FOOT:

Support: Open Fist. Middle finger, finger walk down between bumps of Fifth Metatarsal bone, on outside of foot. Work with middle finger half on bone, half under bone. REVERSE HANDS and thumb walk up with thumb half on bone and half under bone.

11. KNEE. LEG, HIP AND LOWER BACK: LEFT THE RIGHT FOOT:

Triangle area on outer heel/foot from base of Fifth Metatarsal bone (lower bump) down to front of hip/buttocks. STANDARD SUPPORT. With two/three fingers, finger walk upwards in every direction. REVERSE HANDS (Support Open Fist) and two/three fingers, walk downwards in every direction.

12. HIP: LEFT THEN RIGHT FOOT.

STANDARD SUPPORT. Middle finger walks up around outer ankle bone. REVERSE HANDS (Support Open Fist) middle finger walks down around ankle bone.

ALTERNATIVE or OPENING: Inner and Outer Hips: Rake inner Index finger knuckles quickly around inner and outer hips (anklebones), equal number of times both ways, e.g. 12.

13. KIDNEYS AND ADRENALS : BOTH FEET TOGETHER.

a) Kidneys

To locate, place four straight fingers of BOTH hands below waistline bump on outside of feet let thumbs fall flat = **Kidneys**. Stimulate for six out-breaths, then

b) Adrenals

Raise to tip of thumbs for **adrenals**. Leave tip of thumbs on Adrenals to balance for 12 breaths.

c) Kidney to Bladder

Both feet together: Draw straight down from Kidneys to Bladder: four or six times.

14. FIGURE EIGHT/INFINITY: Finish with BOTH feet together.

Draw up, center of both feet, cup fingers and draw down outside, straightening fingers underneath (on buttocks), draw up center of both feet, turn fingers toward each other and palms upwards, and draw down inside and underneath (on buttocks). This is completing technique once. REPEAT THREE more times, a total of FOUR times. Then to finish, draw up center of both feet, and disconnect on chest rather than toes (stop from flicking).

This then is the written summary.
Following is the Visual summary

VISUAL SUMMARY OF THE BASIC PROCEDURE FOR A REFLEXOLOGY TREATMENT

I. OPENING TECHNIQUES

1 Feet Brushing

2 Pelvic, Sacrum, Hip and Lower Back Relaxer

3 Chest Relaxer

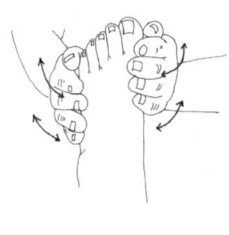

4 Chest Kneading

5 Spinal Twist

Top Hand - TWIST

Bottom hand locked.
DO NOT TWIST.

6 Ankle Gate Opening

7 Diaphragm Relaxer

8 Balance K.1/Triple Burner

9 Head/Neck Opening

261

10 Stretch and Vibrate

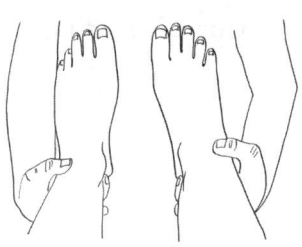

11 Rocking (Optional)

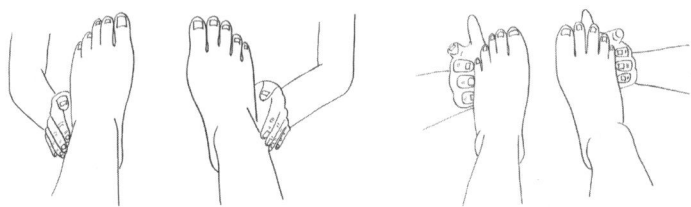

2. HEAD/NECK: ALL TOES: LEFT FOOT THEN RIGHT
2.1 2.2 2.3 2.4 2.5 and 2.6

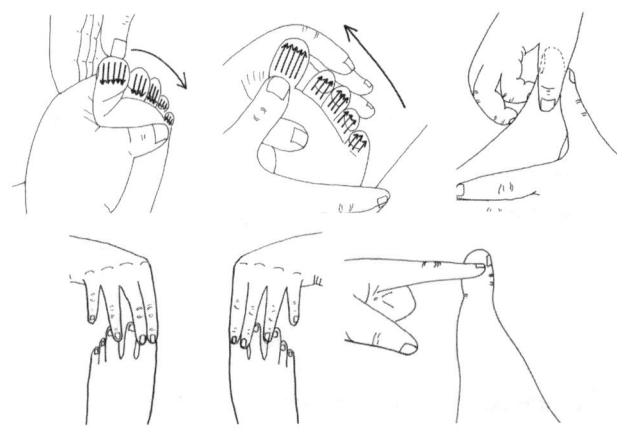

3. NECK/SHOULDERS: LEFT FOOT THEN RIGHT:
3.1, 3.2., 3.3, and 3.4

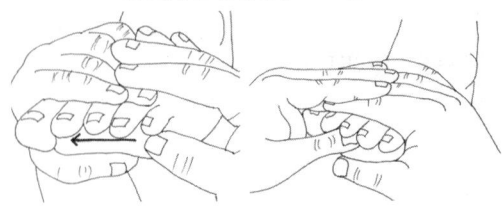

OPTIONAL/ALTERNATIVE

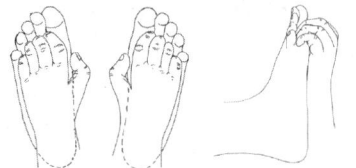

4. CHEST: *LEFT FOOT THEN RIGHT: 4.1, 4.2,* AND *4.3*

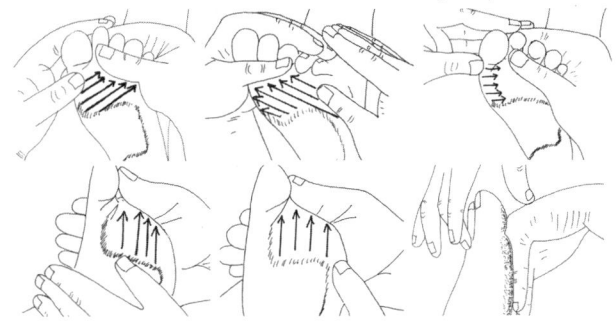

ALTERNATIVE   EXTRA

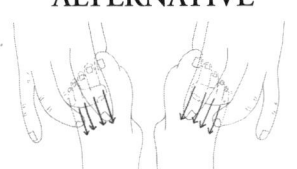
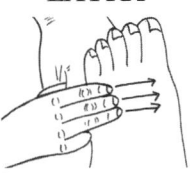

5. ABDOMEN/DIAPHRAGM TO BUTTOCKS: *LEFT FOOT THEN RIGHT*

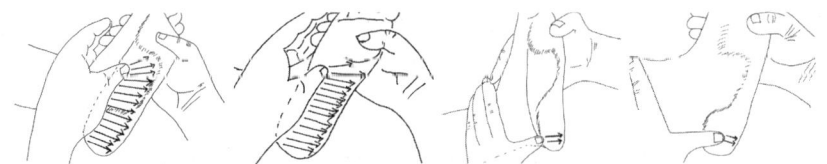

6. LARGE INTESTINES (*BOTH FEET TOGETHER*)

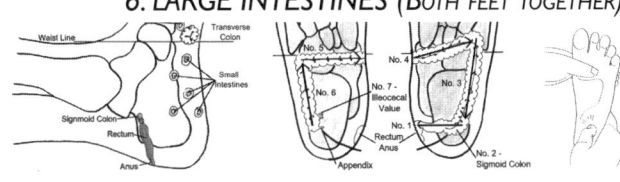

7. REPRODUCTIVE REFLEXES (INSIDE AND OUT): BOTH FEET TOGETHER:
7.1, 7.2, 7.3, 7.4, 7.5, 7.6, 7.7, 7.8 and 7.9

FEMALE & MALE – inner pelvis

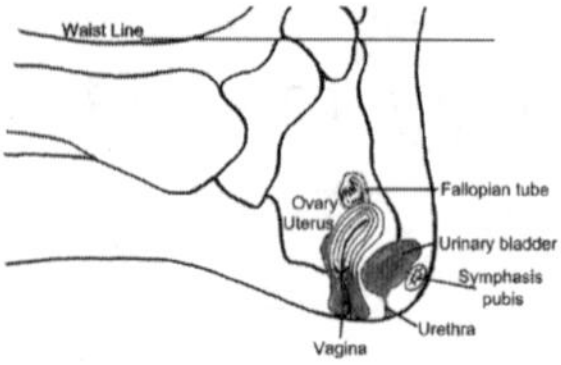

FEMALE & MALE – pelvis (Sole)

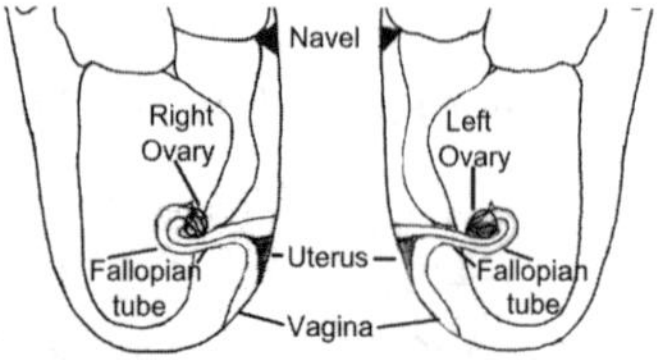

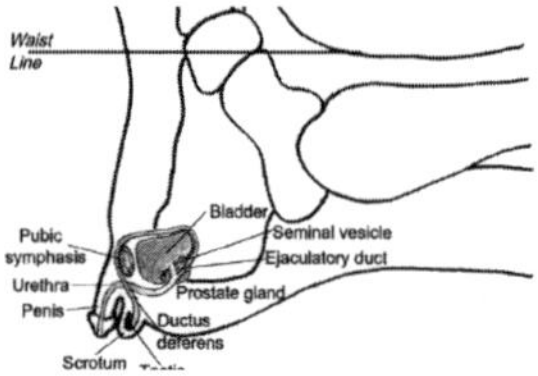

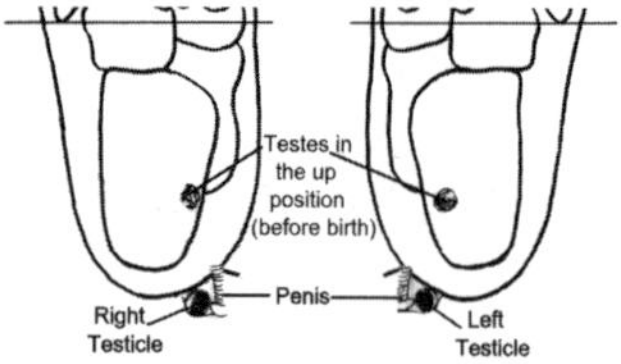

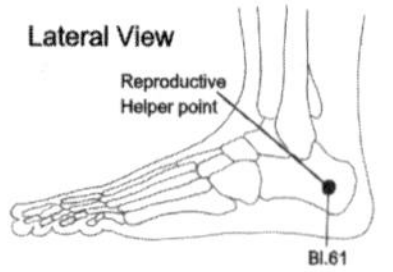

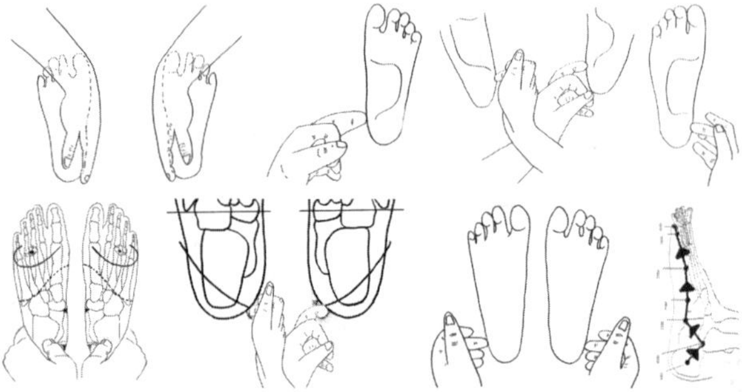

8. INNER AND OUTER PELVIS: LEFT THEN RIGHT FOOT:

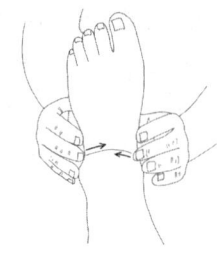

9. MEDIAL: INSIDE THE BODY: RIGHT THEN LEFT FOOT:
9.1 & 9.2: CNS/Spine + other three lines (back, inner organs & abdomen)

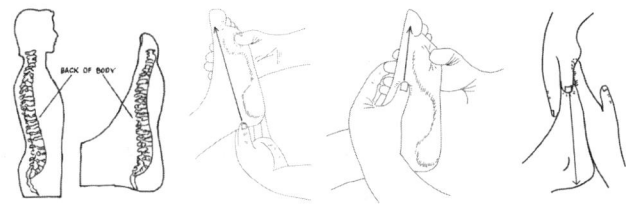

10. SHOULDER AND UPPER ARM: LEFT THEN RIGHT FOOT:

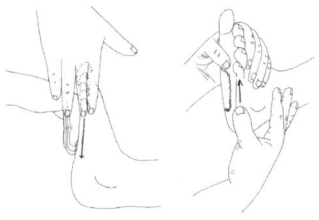

11. KNEE. LEG, HIP AND LOWER BACK:
RIGHT THEN LEFT FOOT:

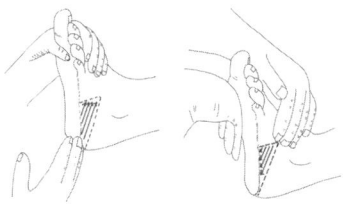

12. OUTER HIP: LEFT THEN RIGHT FOOT:

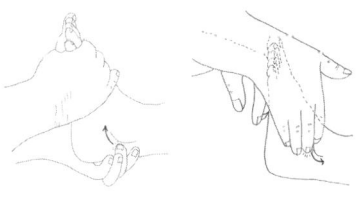

**ALTERNATIVE/Opening–
Inner/Outer Hip**

13. KIDNEYS AND ADRENALS: BOTH FEET TOGETHER:

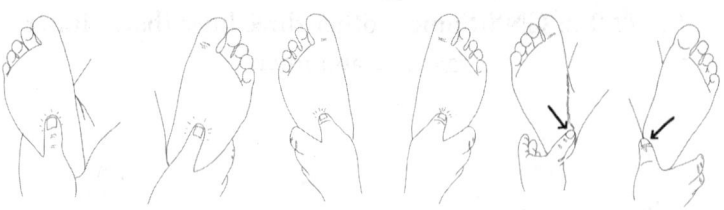

14. FIGURE EIGHT/INFINITY: FINISH WITH BOTH FEET TOGETHER.
Tai Chi on Feet

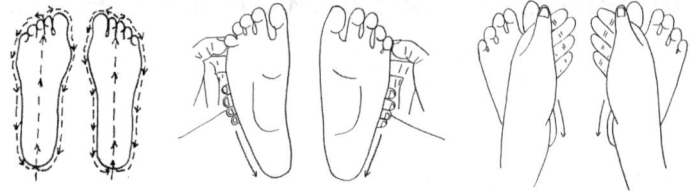

SECTION 3
SYSTEMATIC APPROACH
to REFLEXOLOGY

"Medicine is Science,
as Reflexology is Medicine"

CHAPTER 25
Anatomy and Physiology of the Foot and Leg

As an introduction to Anatomy and Physiology (abbreviated as A & P) of the foot and leg, the major structures of the foot and leg are outlined briefly below because as professional Reflexologists need to understand the instrument being used.

So, for the Reflexologist it is important to realise that there are many structures found in the feet including skin, muscles, fascia, tendons and ligaments, bones, arches of the foot, blood vessels and nerves.

As A & P is heavily jargon based, at the end of this Chapter you will find a Table of jargon used in this Chapter to help you understand these terms. NOTE: The Table of Jargon at the end of this Chapter will also be included in Appendix A: Glossary.

BONES OF THE FOOT AND LEG

There are 26 bones in the foot, and the foot is broken up into the Fore foot and the Rear foot. The Forefoot is composed of the five metatarsals (numbered one to five inside to outside) and the toes bones or phalange (Two phalange of the Big toe, and three phalange of each of the other four toes). The Rear foot is the rest of the bones of the foot behind the metatarsals, that is, the three Cuneiform bones, the Navicular, the Cuboid, Calcaneus and Talus. See Illustration 102 below.

Starting from the toes, the Big toe has two phalange (singular Phalanx) bones and the first one is called the Distal phalanx of the Big toe (Hallux or Great toe) and the second bone is called the Proximal phalanx of the Big toe. The other four toes have three bones in each toe and they are called (from tip of toe):

- The Distal phalanx of the 2nd, 3rd, 4th and 5th toes;
- The Intermediate (or Middle) phalanx of the 2nd, 3rd, 4th and 5th toes; and
- The Proximal phalanx of the 2nd, 3rd, 4th and 5th toes.

ILLUSTRATION 102: Bones of the Foot and Leg

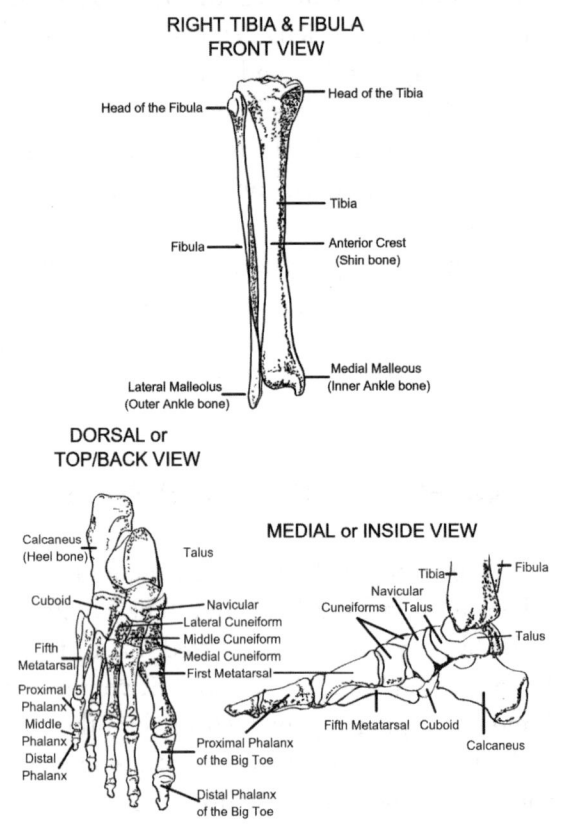

NOTE: On the inside (medial) view of the bones of the foot above, you can see BOTH the 5th Metatarsal and Cuboid bones, but these are outside bones.

The heads of these distal phalange of the five toes articulate with the distal heads of the 5 metatarsal bones, which together comprise the Fore Foot.

Before going on, a comment on heads of bones is necessary. Most, if not all, bones have two heads, and so the method of distinguishing one from the other is the use of the terms: distal and proximal. Distal simply means further away from the mid-line of the body or middle of the body (torso) and proximal means closer.

The rest of the bones of the foot, working backwards from the metatarsals, are firstly the three Cuneiform bones:
• Medial (inside) Cuneiform
• Intermediate or Middle Cuneiform and
• Lateral (outside) Cuneiform

Behind the three cuneiforms is the Navicular bone and beside the Lateral cuneiform and the Navicular is the Cuboid, which is on the outside of the foot. Then there is the Calcaneus (commonly called the Heel bone) and above it, articulating with the Calcaneus and Navicular, is the Talus. These then are the bones of the foot.

The inside leg bone is the Tibia, which is the bigger of the two leg bones and its distal head is called the Medial Malleolus, which is commonly known as the inner anklebone. On the outer leg is the Fibula, and its distal head is called the Lateral Malleolus, which is commonly known as the outer anklebone. So it is important to realise that the inner and outer anklebones are actually not bones of the feet, but are in fact the two distal heads of the leg bones.

There are two other bones (called Sesamoid bones, which are bones within a tendon) in the feet that everyone has, but are not included in A & P. These two sesamoid bones are located on the ball of the foot under the Big toe and are there to help in the ability to walk (push off the ground, which is part of what in medicine is called gait). See Chapter 26. So there are actually a total of 28 bones in the foot. Reflexologists need to know about these two extra bones as they may while working the chest, encounter them and be misled as to what they are.

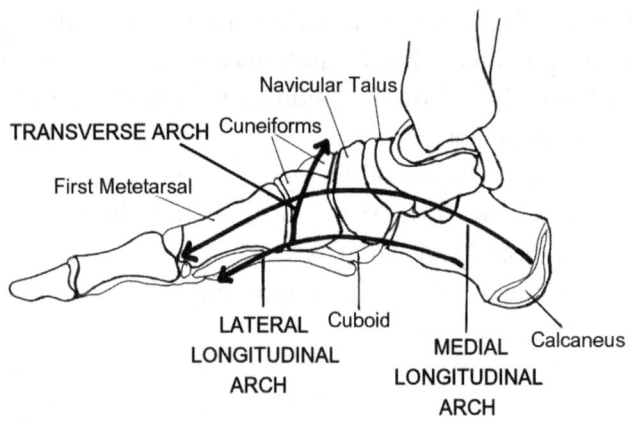

ARCHES OF THE FOOT

ILLUSTRATION 103: Arches of the Foot

There are three arches of the foot, with two longitudinal (length of the foot) arches, one inside and one outside, as well as one transverse (across the foot) arch. The medial longitudinal arch is formed by the Calcaneus, Talus, Navicular, the three Cuneiform bones and the first three Metatarsals (Metatarsal 1, 2 and 3). This is the arch that determines high or low arches.

ILLUSTRATION 104: Sole Arch Structures

The Lateral (outside) Longitudinal Arch is formed by the Calcaneus, Cuboid and the 4th and 5th Metatarsal bones. The third arch of the foot is the Transverse Arch, which runs across the front of the rear foot. It is formed by the three Cuneiforms and the Cuboid. (See Dorsal View Illustration 102: Bones of the Foot and leg, above).

MUSCLES OF THE FOOT AND LEG

It is worth noting that there are actually muscles in the sole of the feet and these are illustrated below. These muscles move the toes and the Table (Illustration 106) below outlines the name, origin, insertion, function and innervation of these muscles.

ILLUSTRATION 105: Muscles on the sole of the foot

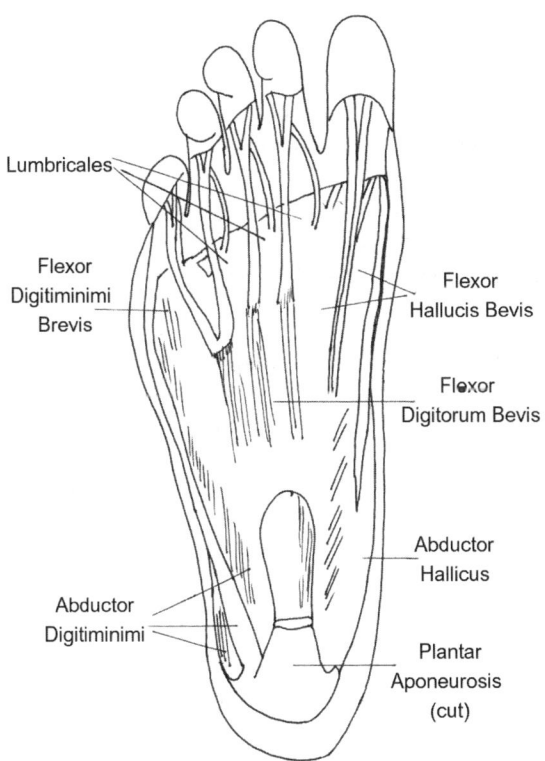

Lumbricales

Flexor Digitiminimi Brevis

Flexor Hallucis Bevis

Flexor Digitorum Bevis

Abductor Hallicus

Abductor Digitiminimi

Plantar Aponeurosis (cut)

ILLUSTRATION 106: Table: Muscles Moving the Toes

Muscle	Origin	Insertion	Function	Innervation
Flexor hallucis Brevis	Cuboid, 3rd cuneiform	Base of proximal phalanx of great toe	Flexes great toe	Lateral and medial Plantar
Flexor hallucis Longus	Posterior surface of Fibula	Base of distal phalanx of great toe	Flexes great toe	Posterior Tibial
Extensor hallucis Longus	Fibula & interosseous Membrane	Dorsal surface of distal phalanx of great toe	Dorsi flexes ankle, extend great toe	Deep peroneal
Interossei Dorsales	Surfaces of adjacent metatarsal bones	Extensor tendons 3rd, 4th toes	Abduct, flex toes	Lateral plantar
Flexor Digitorum Longus	Posterior surface of shaft of tibia	Distal phalanges of lateral toes	Flex toes, extend foot	Posterior tibial
Extensor digitorum longus	Anterior surface fibula, lateral condyle tibia, interosseous membrane	Common extensor tendon of four lateral toes	Extends toes	Deep peroneal
Flexor digitorum osseus brevis	Medial tuberosity of calcaneus, plantar fascia	Middle phalanges of four lateral toes	Flexes toes	Medial plantar
Abductor Hallucis	Medial tuberosity of calcaneus, plantar fascia	Medial surface of base of proximal phalanx of great toe	Abducts, flexes great toe	Medial plantar
Abductor digiti Minimi	Medial & lateral tubercles of calcaneus; plantar fascia	Lateral surface of base of proximal phalanx of 5th toe	Abducts little toe	Lateral plantar

There are a few terms used in this table that need explaining:
• **The Origin:** is the attachment point to the bone of the fixed end of the muscle.

- **The Insertion:** is the attachment point to the bone of the more flexible end of the muscle.
- **The Function:** is what type of movement the muscle does; and
- **The Innervation:** is the nerve that sends the message of movement to the muscle.

The majority of the movements of the feet actually come from the muscles of the leg rather than the muscles of the feet. So it is the lower leg muscles or calf muscles that do this.

ILLUSTRATION 107: Muscles of the Leg

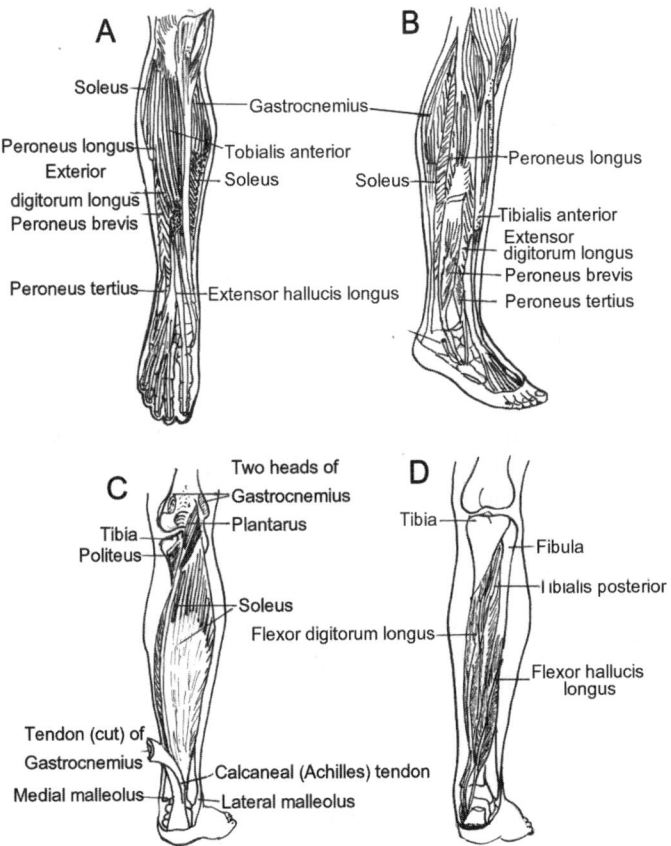

The following Table outlines the movements of the feet and toes, by the leg muscles.

ILLUSTRATION 108: Table:
Muscles Moving the Foot & Leg

Muscle	Origin	Insertion	Function	Innervation
Gastrocnemius	Two heads from lateral and medial condyles of femur, beside knee	Tendo calcaneus	Plantar flexes foot (points toes); flexes leg; supinates foot	Tibial
Soleus	Posterior aspect head of fibula and medial border of tibia	Tendo calcaneus	Plantar flexes foot	Tibial
Tibialis posterior	Interosseus membrane between tibia and fibula	Three cunei-form; cuboid, navicular bone; 2nd, 3rd, 4th metatarsals	Plantar flexes foot	Tibial
Tibialis anterior	Lateral condyle and upper por-tion of lateral surface of body of tibia	Under surface of medial cuneiform and base of 1st metatarsal	Dorsally flexes foot	Deep peroneal
Peroneus tertius	Lower 3rd of anterior surface of fibula and lateral tuberos-ity of tibia	Dorsal surface of base of 5th metatarsal bone	Everts; plantar flexes foot	Deep peroneal
Peroneus longus	Head and lat-eral surface of body of fibula	Lateral side of 1st metatarsal and medial cuneiform	Everts foot	Peroneal
Peroneus brevis	Lower 2/3rd of lateral surface of body of fibula	Tuberosity at base of 5th metatarsal Calcaneus	Plantar flexes foot	Peroneal
Plantaris	Lateral condyle of femur		Plantar flexes foot	Tibial

FASCIA

Fascia is the semi-elastic (much like string) connective tissue that encloses and separates muscles and is an important structure of the foot (as well as of the body). The fascia of the foot holds the muscles of the feet in place and helps to promote various movements of the foot and toes. It also helps create the illusion of the two (medial and lateral) longitudinal arches of the foot. The most important point about the fascia of the foot is that a thick band of it runs between the Big and 2nd toes (between zones 1 & 2) of the arch of the foot. Remember in Reflexology jargon this is called the Tendon Line. It is important to make sure that the Tendon Line (the thick band of fascia) is not damaged during Reflexology. If the fascia is tight, the Reflexologist should be careful not to use strong, deep pressure on or over the fascia as it can be damaged.

CALCANEAL SPUR

Commonly called a Heel spur which is the growth of bone from the heel or calcaneus bone. It is the result of pressure, not on the bone, but on the fascia, especially the thick band of fascia (Tendon Line). As the fascia is, for various reasons, put under pressure, it sometimes becomes over-stretched and is damaged.

Once fascia is grown, the body loses the ability to grow more: fascia does not have its own blood supply and it is blood that heals damaged tissue or cells. Fascia receives blood through what is called osmosis (seeping in), which makes fascia very slow to heal, especially in the feet where the fascia, if damaged, is basically re-damaged every time weight is put on the feet.

So, as the body cannot grow more fascia, the alternative is for it to grow bone. Thus, a calcaneal or heel spur results. Rarely does the actual heel spur (bone) cause pain, unless it grows downwards rather than in line with the fascia, which does not often happen as the bone growth is for the purpose of taking the pressure off the fascia. Remember, the outside of bones is dead cells and has no nerve supply, and therefore cannot cause pain. However, if the spur does grow downwards (towards the floor), then every step would be painful as the spur would be pushing into the tissues of the foot. Therefore, in this case the person is in constant pain with every step taken.

What is called heel spur pain is usually the result of re-damaging the fascia. It is a simple matter to determine if the pain is actually the result of the fascia, and that is if it is painful when the person first puts weight on their feet in the morning, and/or, after being off the feet for some time. If this is the case, it indicates that the pain is most likely not the result of the spur (bone growth) but of the fascia being re-damaged, so it is worse of a morning or after resting for a period of time, and then the pain decreases (it is not constant).

One of the myths of Reflexology is that with regular treatments it can break down the spur. Even if this was possible, it is not desirable, as the spur is decreasing the stress on the fascia. Reflexology, however, can help speed up the healing process of the fascia. But the underlying cause has not been dealt with and this is best done by a podiatrist, who can access the reasons behind the bone growth, which usually relates to the person's gait (method of walking).

OTHER STRUCTURES IN THE FOOT

The other structures of the foot are skin, tendons, ligaments, blood vessels (arteries and veins) and nerves. A tendon is a band of connective tissue that connects a muscle to a bone, while a ligament is a band of connective tissue that holds two or more bones together. There are both tendons and ligaments in the feet. The foot, of course, to function needs blood supply and nerves. The blood flows to the leg and foot through arteries and veins take de-oxygenated blood and toxins away from the foot and leg.

Finally, nerve supply is also needed by the foot and this occurs through a number of nerves called as a group lumbosacral nerves, or commonly sciatic nerve.

JARGON USED IN THIS CHAPTER
ILLUSTRATION 109: List: Glossary of Terms

Arteries — Blood vessels that travel from the heart with oxygenated blood to every organ and cell in the body.

Articulate — A place where two bones come together, commonly called a joint.

Calcaneal Spur — Heel Spur: See Spur

Calcaneus — Commonly called heel bone.

Cuneiform — Three wedge-shaped bones of the front of the Rear Foot.

Distal — Means further away from the mid-line or middle of the body (torso).

Dorsal — Top or back of the foot.

Fascia — A semi-elastic (string-like) connective tissue that encloses and separates muscles.

Fore Foot — All the structures of the foot in front of and including the proximal heads of the metatarsal bones, i.e. the metatarsal and phalange bones.

Frontal — Front of the body.

Hallux — Big toe or Great toe (First toe).

Insertion — The attachment point to the bone of the more flexible end of the muscle.

Innervation — The nerve that sends the message of movement to the muscle.

Intermediate — Middle, that is the bones between the distal and the proximal bones, in this case the middle phalanx of each of the 2nd to 5th toes and the middle cuneiform, between the lateral and medial cuneiform bones.

Lateral — Outside.

Ligament — A band of connective tissue that holds two or more bones together

Longitudinal — Long ways or length-wise.

Malleoli — Plural (Singular: Malleolus). Head or end of leg bones. Commonly called the inner and outer ankle bones.

Medial — Inside.

Metatarsals — "Meta" means middle, and "tarsus" means foot, i.e. middle foot bones. The long middle bones of the foot. There are five in total, numbered from the inside to the outside.

Origin — The attachment point to the bone of the fixed end of the muscle.

Osmosis — Diffusion of solvent (fluid or blood) through a membrane (barrier).

Phalange — (Singular Phalanx) Toe bones (also finger bones).

Plantar — Sole or bottom of the foot.

Proximal — Closer to the mid-line/middle of the body (torso).

Rear Foot — All the structures of the foot behind the proximal heads of the metatarsal bones, i.e. the three Cuneiforms, Navicular, Cuboid, Talus and Calcaneus bones and structures around these bones.

Spur — Calcaneal or Heel Spur.

Tendon — A band of connective tissue that connects a muscle to a bone

Tendon Line — The thick band of fascia that runs between the Big and 2nd toes (zones 1 & 2) of the arch of the foot.

Transverse — Going across the body (or foot).

Veins — Blood vessels which travel away from cells towards the heart with de-oxygenated blood and waste products.

CHAPTER 26
Biomechanics: An Introduction

Biomechanics is the science of how we walk, run, jump, etc. via analysis of the process of each action, and the relevant lower limb joint movements which accomplish this. Biomechanics explains how and why deformities of the foot develop over time as a result of improper movement of the foot, ankle, leg, knee and hip, and results in problems developing in other parts of the body, especially the lower limbs, pelvic region, lower and even upper back. Therefore, it is largely postural, skeletal and muscular problems which develop. This can be the result of bone, or tissue (muscular) imbalances. The study of Biomechanics has concluded there is a direct relationship between the feet and the body, so that foot problems can cause problems in other parts of the body and vice versa.

One of the results of Biomechanics as a science is the development of orthoses, (commonly called orthotics, which is actually an adjective) designed to adjust an individual's gait to alleviate problems which have developed in other parts of the body. So orthoses are not a cure but are preventative as they prevent the repetitive injuries from occurring. The reason for this is that once an individual has developed their gait by actually using their body, the body does not have the ability to change its gait.

Thus, Biomechanics can be found in Sports Medicine and Podiatry (formerly called and in some parts of the world is still known as Chiropody) and as a result of its findings has relevance to the science and art of Reflexology. Reflexologists are now trained to assess the need for Biomechanical intervention and therefore referral to a Podiatrist.

This investigation into how and why athletes kept breaking down with the same injury led Sports Medicine to analyse the gait of the athlete. To do this, video was used as the actual movement and process of taking a step cannot be seen with the naked eye. The result was an analysis of the process of gait: gait can be defined as the process of taking a step, the lifting of one foot and placing it on the ground, which is then repeated, step after step.

This analysis led to the discovery of an array of information on a process of gait that had, up until this time, not been analysed. The key finding was that to take a single step there is a whole process of movements which take place.

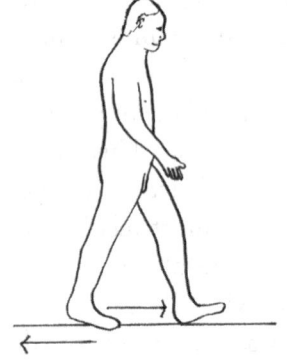

ILLUSTRATION 110:
Gait or Walking

Thus, to take a step, one does not merely pick up one leg and foot and place it down and then pick up the other leg and foot and put it down. Briefly what actually happens is:
• The foot goes through a whole range of movements or motions too subtle for the naked eye
• The knee joint moves and especially rotates
• The hip joint likewise moves and rotates.

What was also discovered was that no human being moves biomechanically correctly and this imperfection in everyone's gait can not only cause foot problems, but problems with the lower limb (calf, leg and thigh); the pelvis, including the hips; the lower back; and even the mid and upper back right up to the neck.

ILLUSTRATION 111: Axes of Gait

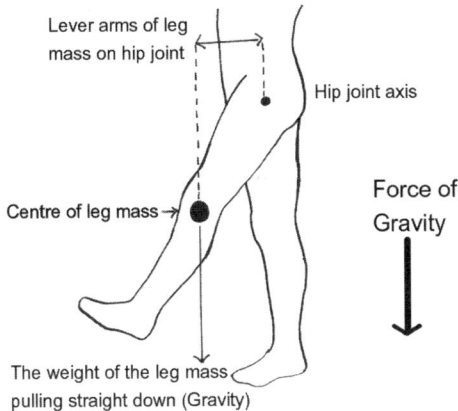

The result of this investigation into the gait of human beings is that we now know that the feet actually have the greatest number of motions of any joint in the body. The shoulder joint has the greater range of movement, but the foot actually goes through more types of movement. A further discovery was that the sub-talar joint, the joint below the Talus bone and above the Calcaneus (heel) bone, is the axes of motion of all these movements of the foot. It is this joint which creates the various movements the foot can do: Adduction and Abduction; Inversion and Eversion; and Plantarflexion, and Dorsiflexion.

ADDUCTION AND ABDUCTION

To understand adduction and abduction, one needs to visualise a 360-degree circle drawn on the ground or floor around the feet. **Adduction** is movement of the foot towards the mid-line or centre of the body, which increases the circle towards 360 degrees. **Abduction** is moving the foot away from the mid-line of the body and therefore decreasing the 360-degree circle.

ILLUSTRATION 112: Adduction and Abduction
ABDUCTION   ADDUCTION

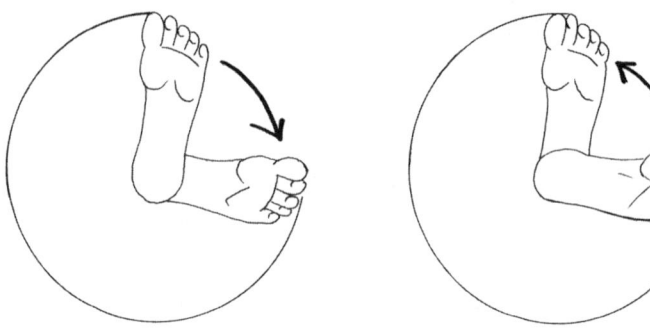

INVERSION AND EVERSION

Inversion is simply moving the sole of the foot towards the midline of the body, that is pointing the sole inwards; **eversion** is the opposite, moving the sole of the foot away from the midline of the body, or pointing the sole outwards.

ILLUSTRATION 113: Inversion and Eversion
INVERSION   EVERSION

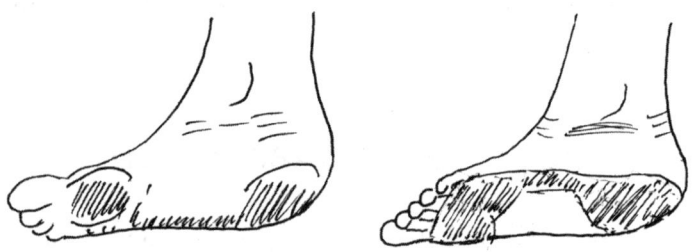

PLANTARFLEXION AND DORSIFLEXION

Plantarflexion is pointing the toes to the ground, or moving the sole of the foot downward towards the ground. **Dorsiflexion** is the opposite, that is moving the top of the foot upwards away from the ground, or pulling the toes upwards.

ILLUSTRATION 114: Plantarflexion and Dorsiflexion
PLANTARFLEXION   DORSIFLEXION

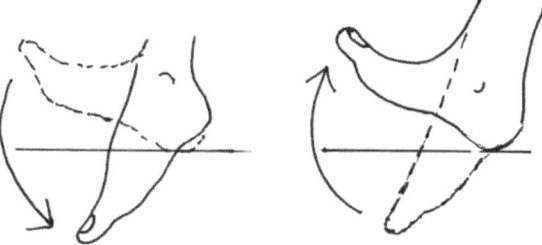

Each of these motions: Adduction and Abduction, Inversion and Eversion, and Plantarflexion and Dorsiflexion cannot be performed by the foot in isolation or on its own. The foot cannot, for example, adduct without inverting and plantar flexing at the same time. Conversely, the foot cannot abduct without also everting and dorsi flexing at the same time.

SUPINATION AND PRONATION

Given that the foot cannot actually do any of the abovementioned motions in isolation, what the foot does is supination and pronation, which is the combination of the three motions together. Therefore, **supination** is a combination of adduction, inversion and plantarflexion, while **pronation** is a combination of abduction, eversion and dorsiflexion.

ILLUSTRATION 115: Supination and Pronation
SUPINATION   PRONATION

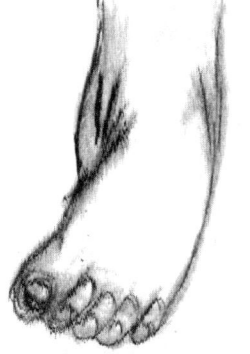 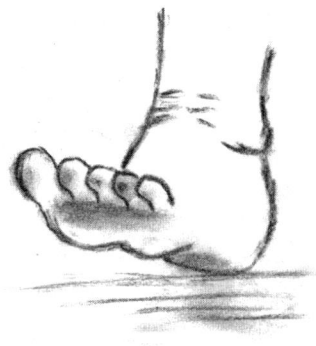

Supination then is where the sole of the foot is swept up and towards the midline, turning the sole inwards and the toes upward; while **pronation** is where the sole of the foot moves away from the midline, turns the sole outwards and the toes downward.

These then are the actions the foot actually does and the reason for this is that the foot, when it first strikes the ground, needs to be locked to take the impact like a shock absorber. It then needs to be loose to adjust to the uneven surface of the ground, and finally to push off the ground, the foot joints need to be locked so that we have a solid level with which to push off. This is the reason that the foot goes through **locked**, **unlocked** and **locked** again with each step. This is also the reason for the pattern on the sole of the foot. The pressure starts at the heel, with contact to the surface, and then rolls outward along the outside of the sole and then across the ball of the foot up the Big toe (the solid lever).

The problem that arises with the foot is not so much doing these motions or not, but the timing of each and the change from one to another: either being too early or too late causes problems.

EXERCISE AND THE FEET

As far as the foot is concerned the best form of exercise is in water (swimming) and walking on natural surfaces. Especially good is walking on wet sand, or any surface that gives and yet at the same time supports. The worse scenario for the feet is walking on hard surfaces, and sports which lock the foot either in one position or an abnormal position, or both.

FOOTWEAR

There are many opinions on this matter, however the best thing you can do for your feet is to walk bare footed on natural surfaces.

But when exercising on hard and unnatural surfaces such as cement, asphalt and bitumen, it is vital that well-designed supportive shoes are worn to decrease the impact of this activity on the feet as well as the whole body. In both Biomechanics and Reflexology (Anatomical Reflection Theory), this potential negative impact is damage to the feet and thus to the body as well.

CHAPTER 27
Reflexology and the Systems of the Body

Reflexology training includes a systematic (Anatomy and Physiology) approach to the science of Reflexology. It is vital to understand how the body functions, but one of the problems with the systematic approach to the human being is that it cuts the body up into separate and isolated bits, and as a result promotes the proposition that the body is a mechanical device and therefore needs a mechanical approach to problems or imbalances of the body. The systems of the body do not function in isolation, but are part of a whole, and again, are we but the systems of the body? Are we more than the sum of our parts?

Before proceeding with an analysis of the systems of the body and their reflections in Reflexology, it is worth noting that this systematic approach is only one way of cutting the body up into its bits, which has now taken on the mantle of a tradition.

This systematic (A & P) approach to the human being is not by any stretch of the imagination wholistic, which is why on a purely physical level Reflexology uses helper areas to help the Reflexologist put the body back together. The tendency is to see the trees rather than the forest.

It is important that Reflexologist begin with this approach for many reasons, but it is absolutely vital that afterwards the body is put back together and dealt with as a whole. However there are times when a systematic approach is useful, such as balancing the Endocrine system or the glands, which is the second major communication system (through blood) of the body.

The systematic (A & P) approach to the human being is a beginning and learning tool, but should not remain the major approach. The purpose of this chapter is to, as accurately as possible reflect the systems of the body onto the feet for the benefit of Reflexologist's understanding of Reflexology rather than A & P. Therefore, what follows is a brief outline of each system, an illustration of said system and then the reflection of each system onto the feet.

i. CARDIOVASCULAR SYSTEM

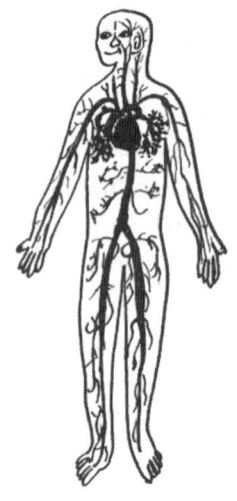

ILLUSTRATION 116:
Cardiovascular System

Major Components: The Heart is the major organ and pump of the system, plus blood vessels (circulatory system of arteries and veins) and blood.

Functions: The circulatory system transports nutrients, waste products, gases (oxygen and carbon dioxide) and hormones throughout the body. It also plays a part in the immune response and the regulation of body temperature. The Heart is the body's most powerful muscle as it pumps 7 570 litres of blood throughout about 112 630 kilometres of blood vessels every 24 hours.

CARDIOVASCULAR SYSTEM THROUGH THE FEET:

The major organ of the Cardiovascular system is the heart, which is located in the chest area below both 1st toes (longitudinal zone 1 on both feet) and under the 2nd toe longitudinal zone 2) on the left foot, as the heart is in the mid-line (mid-sagittal plane) of the body but larger on the left side.

ILLUSTRATION 117: Heart through the Feet

5432
2345
5 4 3 2 1
1 2 3 4 5

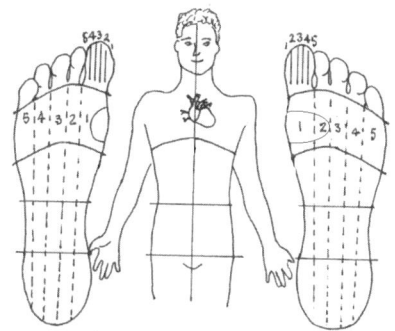

ILLUSTRATION 118: Heart and Major Arteries, Sole View

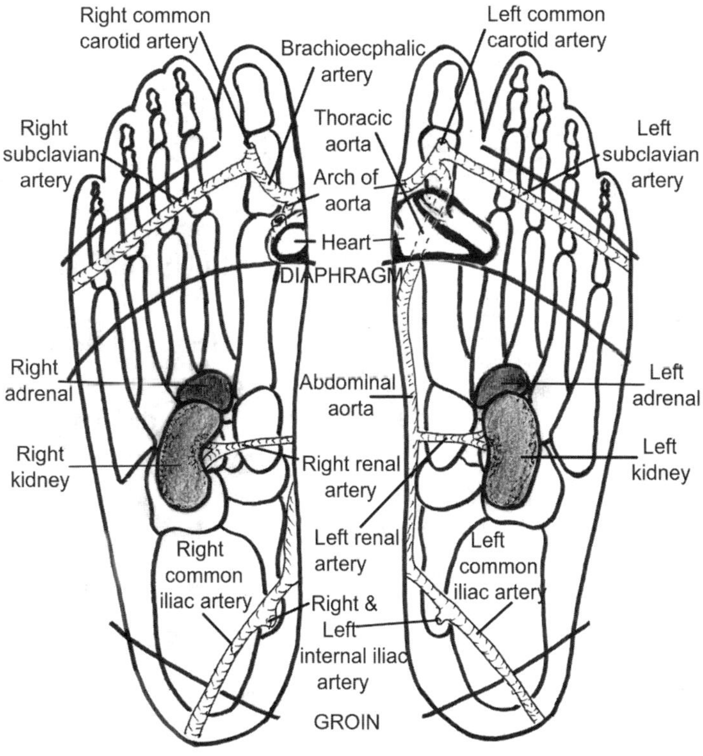

Right common carotid artery
Brachioecphalic artery
Left common carotid artery
Right subclavian artery
Thoracic aorta
Left subclavian artery
Arch of aorta
Heart
DIAPHRAGM
Right adrenal
Abdominal aorta
Left adrenal
Right kidney
Right renal artery
Left kidney
Left renal artery
Right common iliac artery
Left common iliac artery
Right & Left internal iliac artery
GROIN

ILLUSTRATION 119: Heart and Major Veins, Sole View

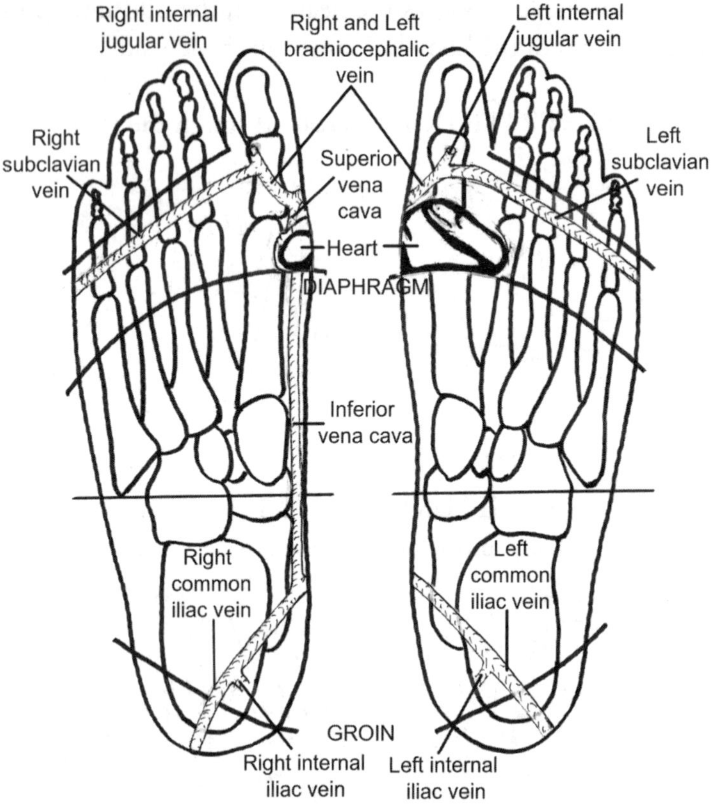

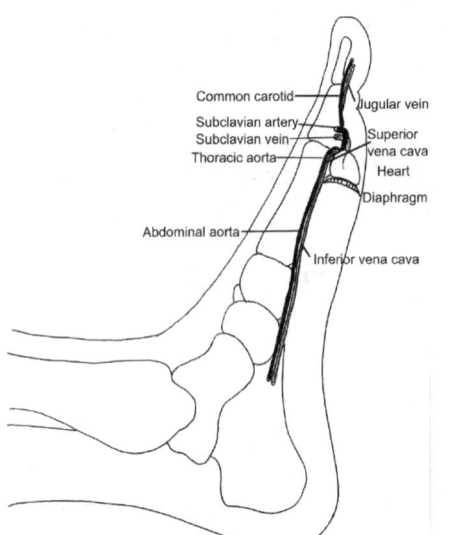

Right internal jugular vein

Right and Left brachiocephalic vein

Left internal jugular vein

Right subclavian vein

Superior vena cava

Left subclavian vein

Heart

DIAPHRAGM

Inferior vena cava

Right common iliac vein

Left common iliac vein

GROIN

Right internal iliac vein

Left internal iliac vein

Common carotid

Jugular vein

Subclavian artery

Subclavian vein

Superior vena cava

Thoracic aorta

Heart

Diaphragm

Abdominal aorta

Inferior vena cava

ILLUSTRATION 120: Heart and Major Arteries and Veins, Inside View

ILLUSTRATION 121: Arteries and Veins through the Head and Neck (Outside Big & 5th Toes)

Arteries   Veins

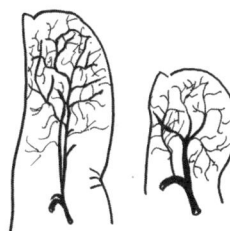 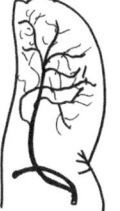 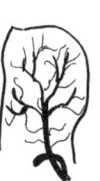

As arteries and veins go everywhere, right down to the cellular level, they cover the whole feet. So, using the Anatomical Reflection Theory, to locate a cardiovascular or circulatory problem simply find the appropriate reflex area/s. For example, leg circulatory problems are the lower limb or leg reflex.

ILLUSTRATION 122: Arteries and Veins through the Feet

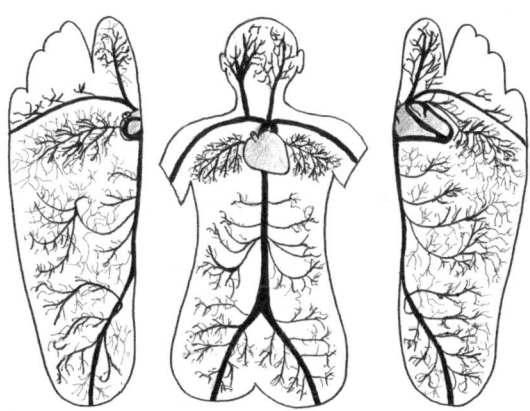

ii. DIGESTIVE SYSTEM

Major Components: The Digestive system runs from the mouth (and tongue) through the whole body to the rectum and anus. From the mouth (tongue), food travels through the

Oesophageus into the Stomach and from here into the tube from the Stomach (called the Duodenum, in which the Pancreas sits and excretes pancreatic juices and the Gall Bladder, which excretes bile) to the Small Intestines. The Liver produces bile and the Gall Bladder stores concentrated bile. Absorption (taking in of nutrients) occurs in the Duodenum, Jejunum and Ileum, and the Small Intestines. From here, what is left after absorption travels into the Large Intestine and Sigmoid colon to the rectum and finally the anus.

ILLUSTRATION 123: The Digestive System

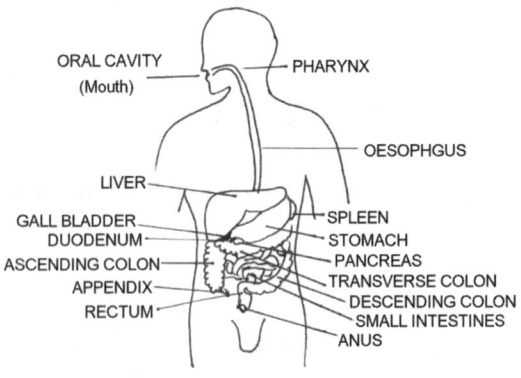

ORAL CAVITY (Mouth)
PHARYNX
OESOPHGUS
LIVER
GALL BLADDER
DUODENUM
ASCENDING COLON
APPENDIX
RECTUM
SPLEEN
STOMACH
PANCREAS
TRANSVERSE COLON
DESCENDING COLON
SMALL INTESTINES
ANUS

Functions: The digestive system performs the mechanical and chemical processes of digestion (breaking down of food into simple molecules that the body can absorb and utilise), absorption of nutrients and elimination of waste. The **Ileocecal Valve** is the valve that controls the passage of the contents of the Small Intestine into the Large Intestine. The **Appendix**, although part of the Lymphatic system as it is full of lymph nodes, is at the bottom and beginning of the Ascending Colon of the Large Intestine.

NOTE: The Large Intestine is composed of the Ileocecal Value, Appendix, Ascending Colon, Hepatic Flexure (Liver corner), the Transverse (across the body) Colon, the Splenic Flexure (Spleen corner), the Descending Colon, Sigmoid Colon, Rectum and Anus.

THE DIGESTIVE SYSTEM THROUGH THE FEET:

ILLUSTRATION 124: Digestive System, Sole View

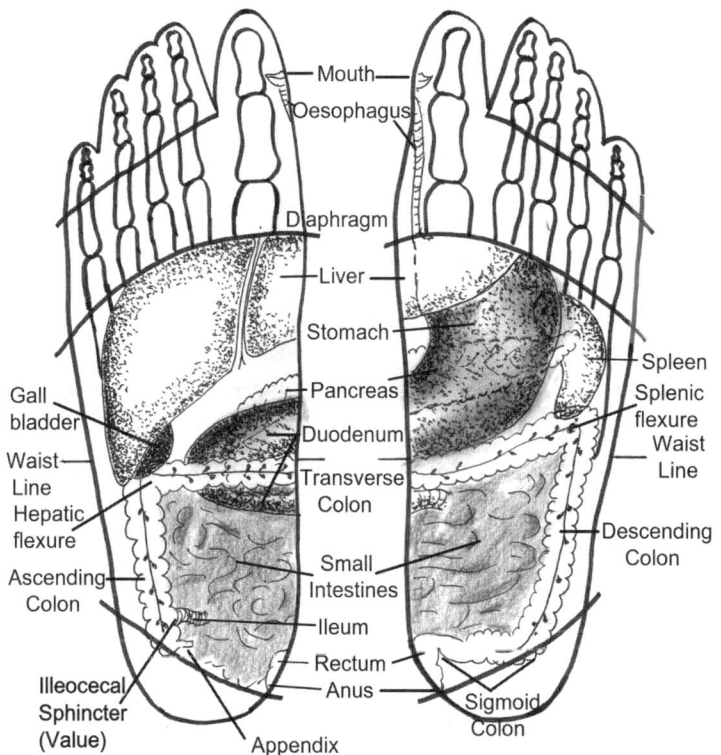

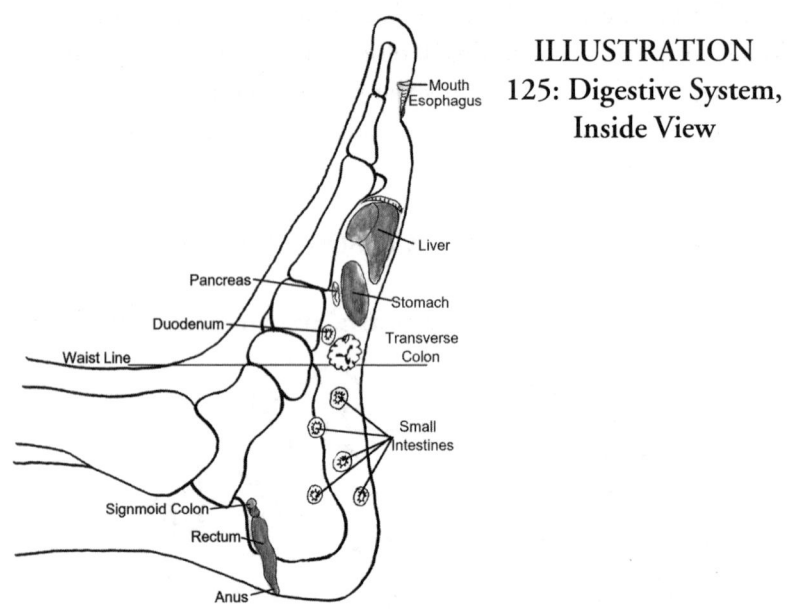

ILLUSTRATION 125: Digestive System, Inside View

iii. ENDOCRINE SYSTEM

Major Components: The major glands of the body are the Pineal, Pituitary, Thyroid and Parathyroid, Thymus, Adrenal glands, Islets of Langerhans (on the Pancreas), and the gonads (ovaries in females and Testes in males).

ILLUSTRATION 126: The Endocrine System

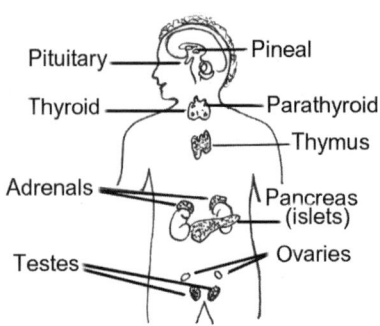

Functions: The secondary communication system (the Nervous system is the first and major communication system) and a major regulatory system as it participates in the regulation of metabolism, reproduction and most functions of the body. It activates and deactivates the Digestive and Reproductive systems, as well as regulates growth and development.

THE ENDOCRINE SYSTEM THROUGH THE FEET:
ILLUSTRATION 127: Endocrine System, Sole View

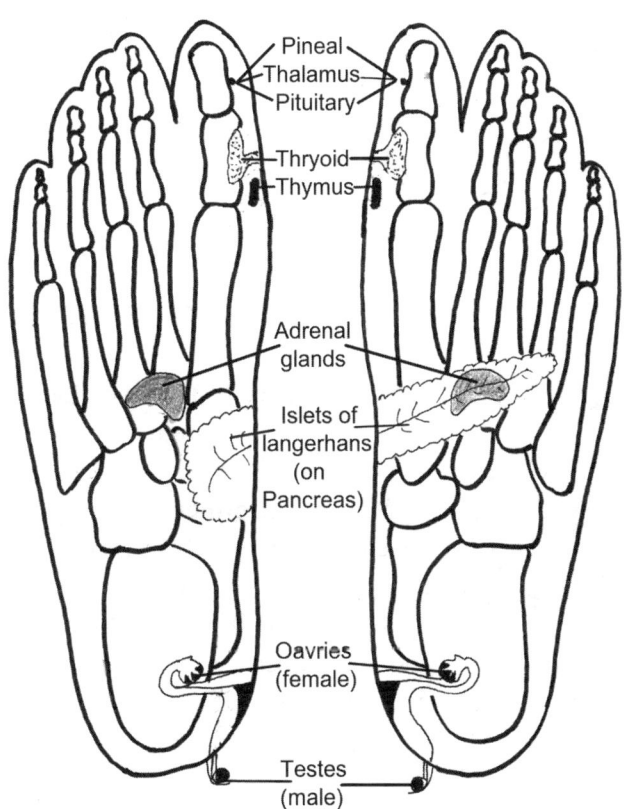

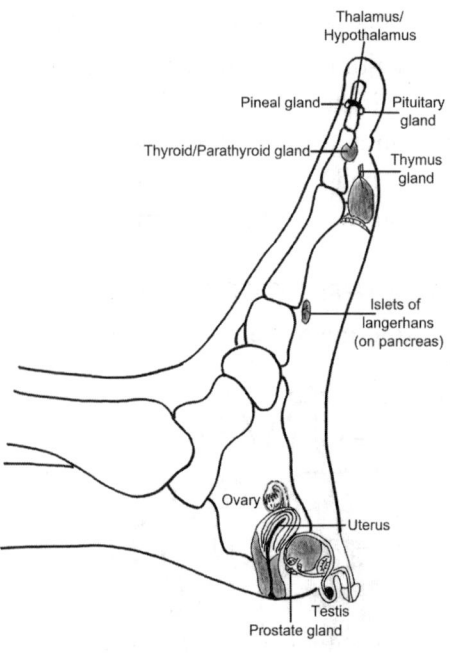

Thalamus/
Hypothalamus

Pineal gland

Pituitary
gland

Thyroid/Parathyroid gland

Thymus
gland

Islets of
langerhans
(on pancreas)

Ovary

Uterus

Testis

Prostate gland

ILLUSTRATION 128:
Endocrine
System, Inside View

iv. LYMPHATIC SYSTEM

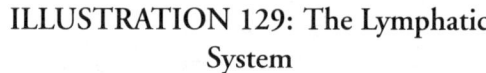

ILLUSTRATION 129: The Lymphatic
System

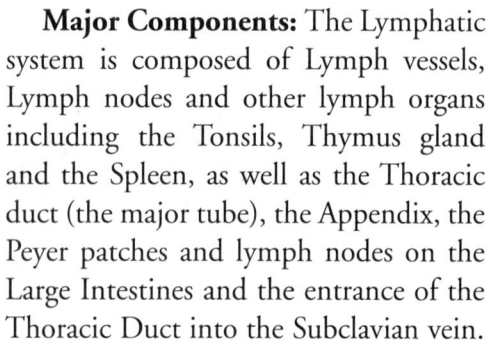

Major Components: The Lymphatic system is composed of Lymph vessels, Lymph nodes and other lymph organs including the Tonsils, Thymus gland and the Spleen, as well as the Thoracic duct (the major tube), the Appendix, the Peyer patches and lymph nodes on the Large Intestines and the entrance of the Thoracic Duct into the Subclavian vein. Lymph nodes are concentrated in the neck region, the Axilla (arm pit or underarm) and the groin (Inguinal nodes), although there are nodes in the elbow and back of the knee. The majority of the lymph system is superficial (close to the surface) and in muscles. Unlike the heart in the Cardiovascular system, there is no pump for the Lymphatic system and so the muscles and body movements do the pump work.

Functions: The Lymphatic system removes foreign substances and complex molecules from the blood and breaks them down into their chemical constituents, combats disease (and is therefore part of the immune system), maintains tissue fluid balance and absorbs fats.

THE LYMPHATIC SYSTEM THROUGH THE FEET:

As the lymphatic system is largely frontal (on the front of the body) and superficial it is mostly on the sole of the feet, although some is located on the inside and outside of the feet (body).

ILLUSTRATION 130: Lymphatic System, Sole View

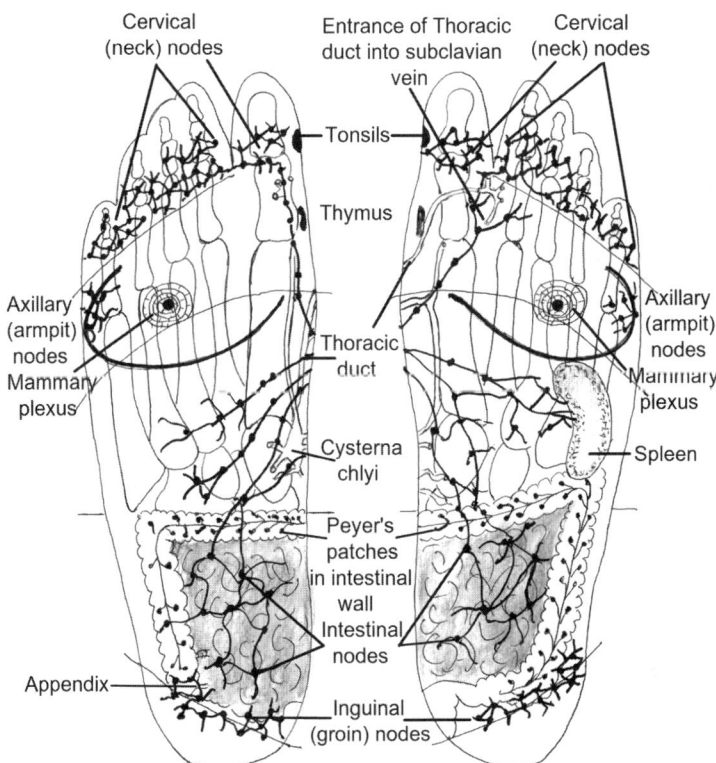

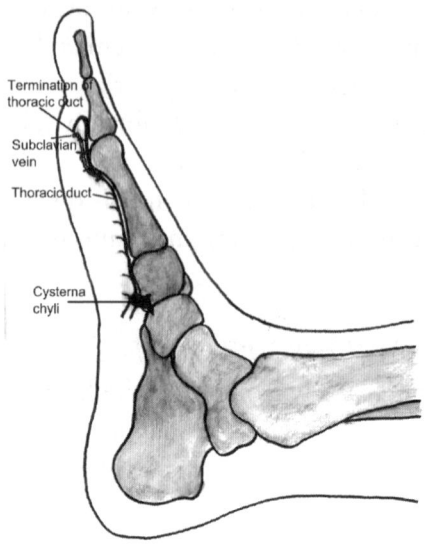

ILLUSTRATION 131: Lymphatic System, Inside View

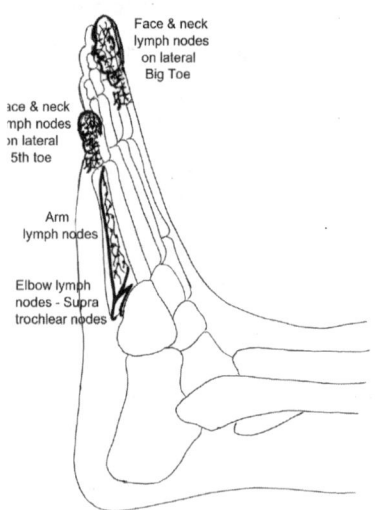

ILLUSTRATION 132: Lymphatic System, Outside View

NOTE: There are certain points on the Back/top of the feet that most Reflexologists have been taught are Lymph. These points are helper areas for Lymph as they are actually energy points that have an effect on the Lymphatic system, and so they will be included as Helper areas on the chart below.

ILLUSTRATION 133: Lymph Helper areas on Back of the Feet

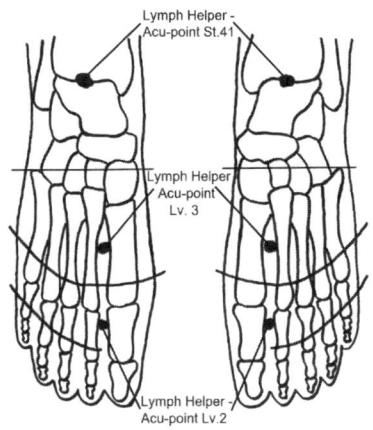

Lymph Helper -
Acu-point St.41

Lymph Helper
Acu-point
Lv. 3

Lymph Helper -
Acu-point Lv.2

v. MUSCULAR SYSTEM

Major Components: There are gross muscles, which are superficial and are attached to the skeleton or bones, and there are internal muscles of the inner organs (NOTE: the inner organs are actually smooth muscle).

Functions: Gross muscles allow the body to move and maintain the posture of the body (in conjunction with bones, or the skeleton) as well as produce body heat and work other systems of the body.

ILLUSTRATION 134: Muscular System

THE MUSCULAR SYSTEM THROUGH THE FEET:

As the muscular system is largely superficial, other than the limbs (arms and legs) the muscles are on the torso and the back. As to the limbs, the muscles of the limbs reflect in the same place as the limbs reflect. In the diagrams below, the muscular system is stylized as the reflexes of the parts of the body also reflect the muscle structure of that part of the body. For example, chest muscles reflect in the chest while upper back muscles reflect in the upper back, and so on.

ILLUSTRATION 135: Muscular System, Sole and Back of Foot Views

Sole/Front   **Back**

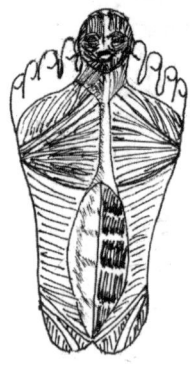 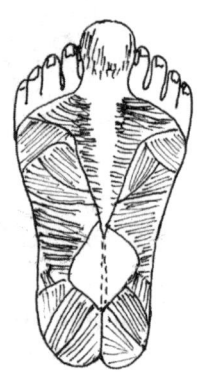

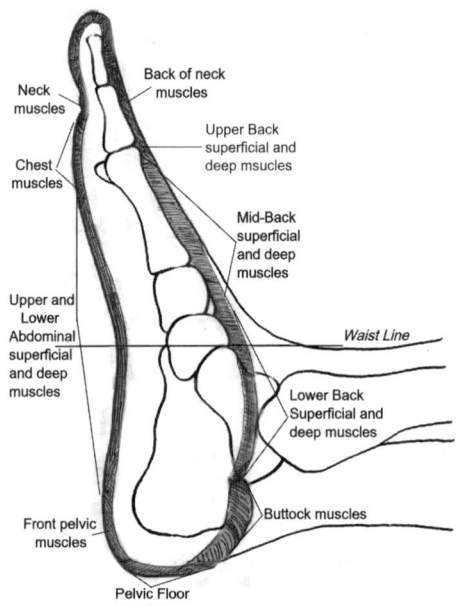

Neck muscles

Back of neck muscles

Upper Back superficial and deep msucles

Chest muscles

Mid-Back superficial and deep muscles

Upper and Lower Abdominal superficial and deep muscles

Waist Line

Lower Back Superficial and deep muscles

Buttock muscles

Front pelvic muscles

Pelvic Floor muscles

ILLUSTRATION 136: Muscular System, Inside View

vi. NERVOUS SYSTEM

Major Components: The Nervous system is broken up into the Central Nervous system (CNS), which is composed of the brain and spinal cord; and the Peripheral Nervous system (PNS), which is composed of the nerves and sensory receptors, which link all systems of the body to the Central Nervous system.

Functions: Together the Nervous system is the major communication system and therefore major regulatory system of the body, as it detects sensations, controls movements and controls physiological and intellectual functions.

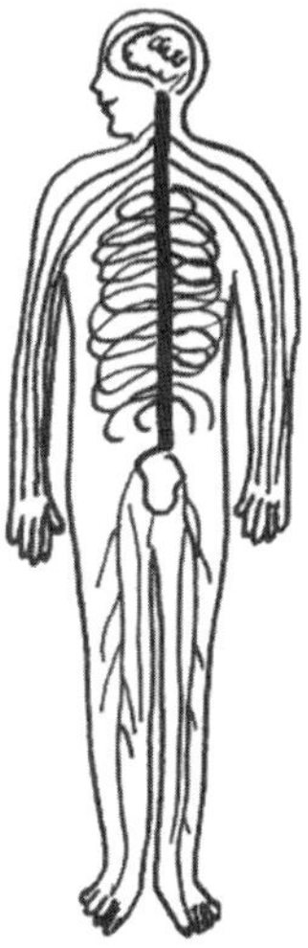

ILLUSTRATION 137:
Nervous System

NOTE: It is worth consulting an A & P textbook to learn about each individual nerve of the spine, the parts of the body that each nerve sends messages to (innervation) and the related conditions or imbalances that can be associated with said nerve. These individual nerves can be accessed down the inner aspect of the foot/feet (as illustrated below), and so these individual nerves become Helper areas for particular conditions and imbalances. For example, the coccyx nerve innervates the rectum and anus and is a useful Helper area for haemorrhoids and pain at the end of the spine.

THE NERVOUS SYSTEM THROUGH THE FEET:
a) Central Nervous System (CNS) through the feet:

ILLUSTRATION 138: Central Nervous System (CNS), Inside View

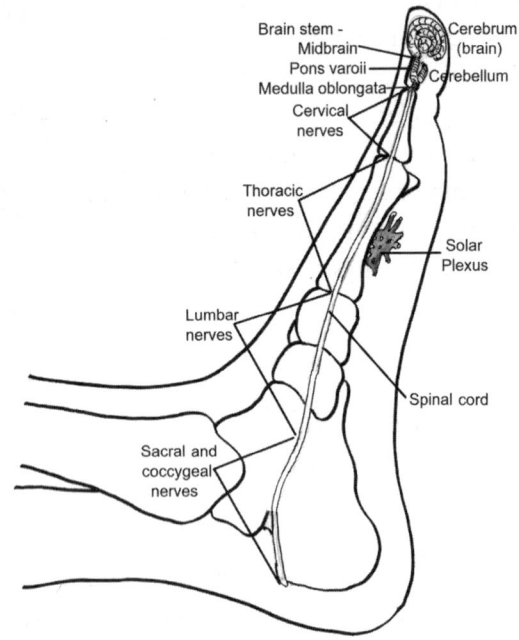

ILLUSTRATION 139: Brain, Outside Big Toe

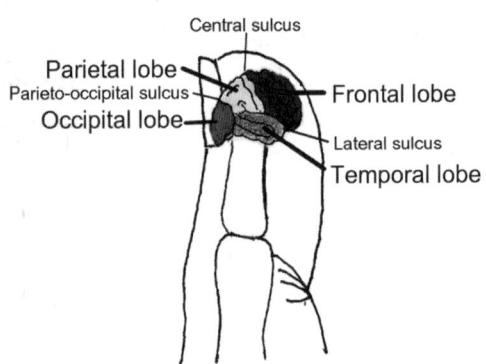

ILLUSTRATION 140: Nervous System: Brain, Sole of Toes

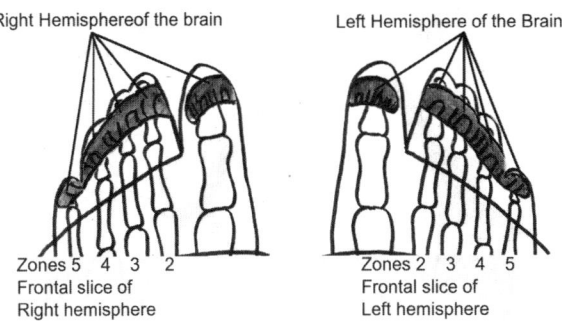

Right Hemisphereof the brain

Left Hemisphere of the Brain

Zones 5 4 3 2
Frontal slice of
Right hemisphere

Zones 2 3 4 5
Frontal slice of
Left hemisphere

ILLUSTRATION 141: Brain, inside & outside of Toes:
2nd Toe   3rd Toe

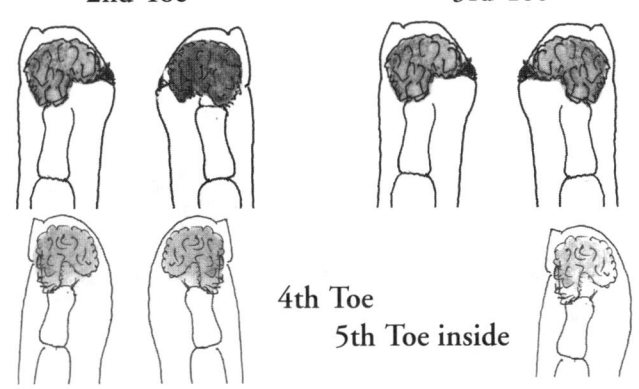

4th Toe
5th Toe inside

b)Peripheral Nervous System through the feet:

As the peripheral nervous system goes down to the cellular level, the nerves of the body are everywhere in the body and therefore in the feet. Thus, when there is a nerve innervation (sending of a message to and fro) problem with a part of the body, outside of the Central Nervous system, then it is simply a matter of using the Anatomical Reflection Theory to locate the problem in the feet.

ILLUSTRATION 142: Peripheral Nervous System, Sole View

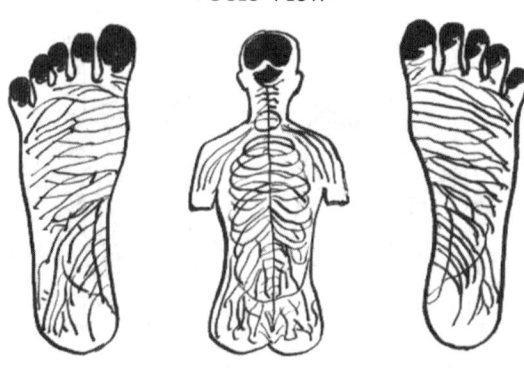

ILLUSTRATION 143: Peripheral Nervous System, Back View

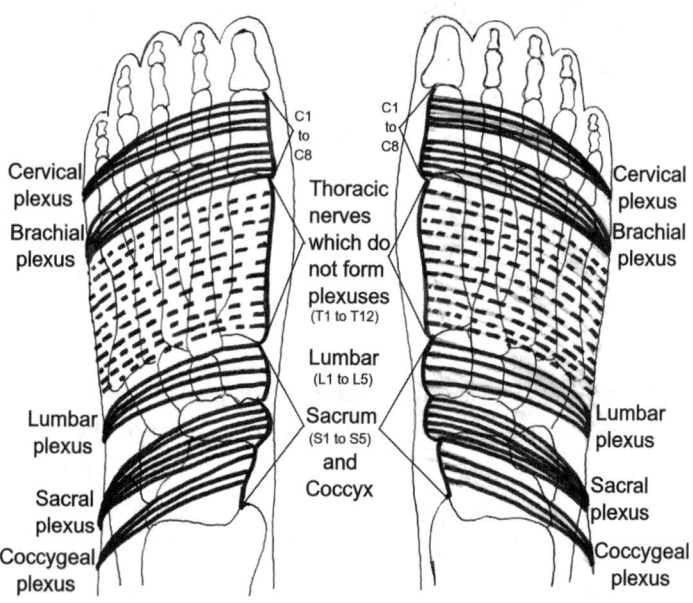

ILLUSTRATION 144: Peripheral Nervous System, Outside View

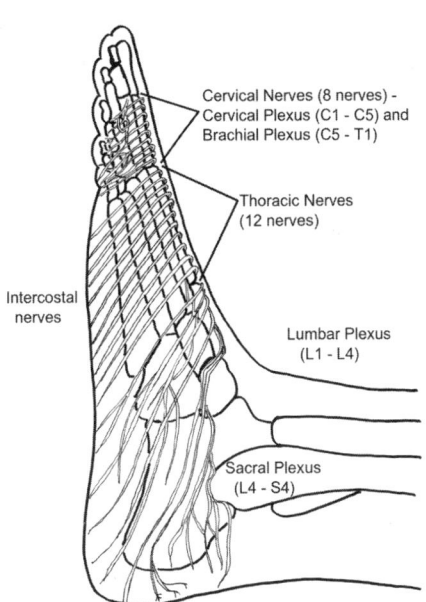

Cervical Nerves (8 nerves) - Cervical Plexus (C1 - C5) and Brachial Plexus (C5 - T1)

Thoracic Nerves (12 nerves)

Intercostal nerves

Lumbar Plexus (L1 - L4)

Sacral Plexus (L4 - S4)

vii. REPRODUCTIVE SYSTEM

Major Components: The Gonads, the organ of sex cells production: in females the ovaries and in the male the testes. The sexual organs of the female are the Vagina, the Uterus (or womb), the Ovaries and the Fallopian tubes. The sexual organs of the male are the Penis, the Testes, the Prostate Gland, the Epididymis (structure that holds and matures sperm), the Ductus Deferens (Duct of the testicle) and the Seminal Vesicle (a glandular structure that excretes components of semen).

ILLUSTRATION 145: The Reproductive System
Male   Female

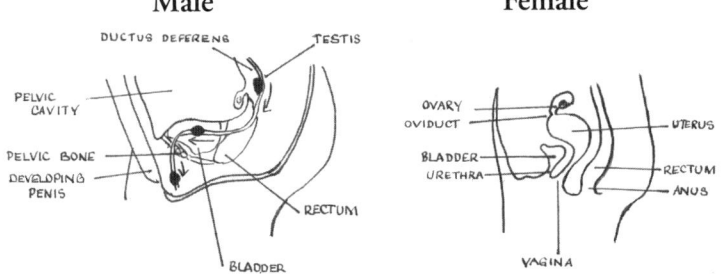

DUCTUS DEFERENS   TESTIS

PELVIC CAVITY

PELVIC BONE

DEVELOPING PENIS

RECTUM

BLADDER

OVARY
OVIDUCT

BLADDER
URETHRA

UTERUS

RECTUM

ANUS

VAGINA

Functions: Performs the process of reproduction and controls sexual functions and behaviour.

THE REPRODUCTIVE SYSTEM THROUGH THE FEET:

Other than the breasts, all the structures of the Reproductive system in both males and females are located in the pelvic region. Also NOTE that both the male and female reproductive systems (as illustrated above) begin in the same location before birth, and they are reflected in this position in the feet, which indicates that the feet reflect not only anatomically accurately but also in the foetal position. However, as the male testes move downwards usually towards the end of the gestation period, they also reflect in the down position in the feet.

ILLUSTRATION 146: Female Reproductive System, Sole View

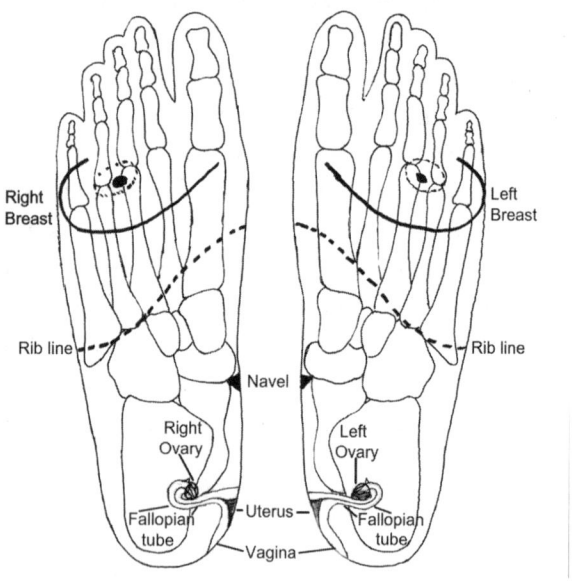

ILLUSTRATION 147: Female Reproductive System, Inside View

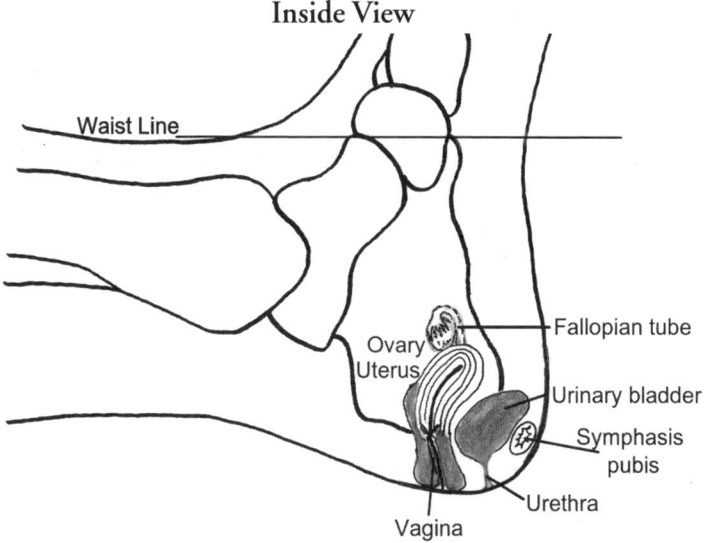

ILLUSTRATION 148: Male Reproductive System, Sole View (Pelvis/Heel area)

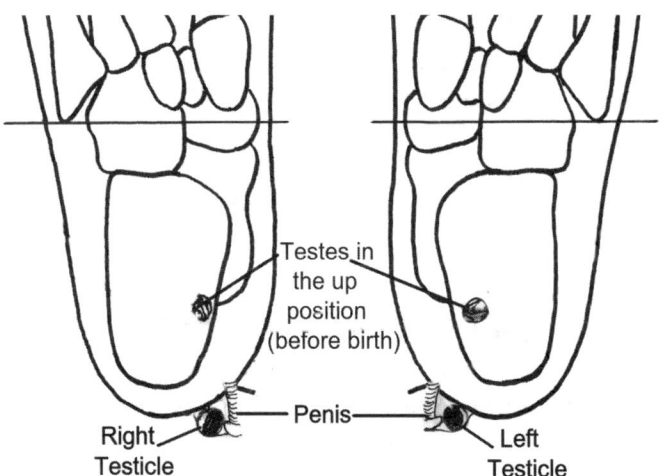

ILLUSTRATION 149: Male Reproductive System, Inside View

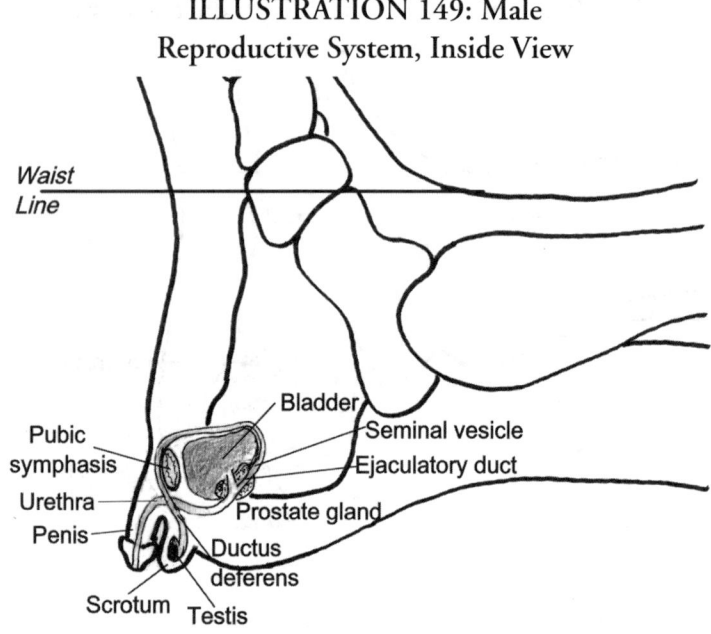

ILLUSTRATION 150:
Reproductive Helper
point (Outside)

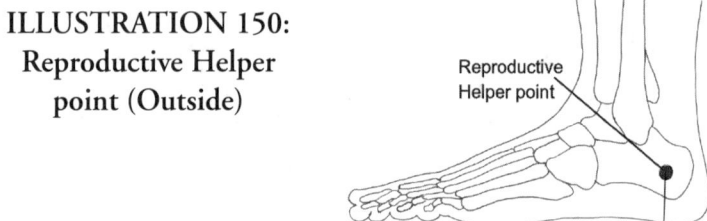

viii. RESPIRATORY SYSTEM

Major Components: The Lungs and Respiratory passages, i.e. the nose and nasal cavity, Pharynx (throat), Larynx (speaking), Trachea (windpipe), and the Bronchi (plural for bronchus or commonly bronchials) and the Diaphragm (muscle of breathing)

ILLUSTRATION 151: The Respiratory System

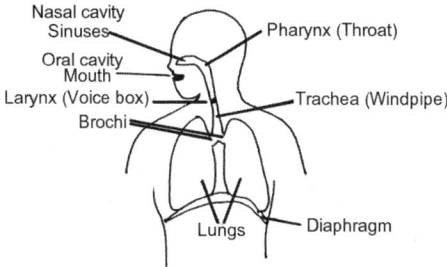

Function: Breathing is the process by which gases (oxygen and carbon dioxide) are exchanged between the blood and the air. It also regulates blood pH (i.e. acid alkaline balance of the body).

THE RESPIRATORY SYSTEM THROUGH THE FEET:

ILLUSTRATION 152: Respiratory System, Sole View

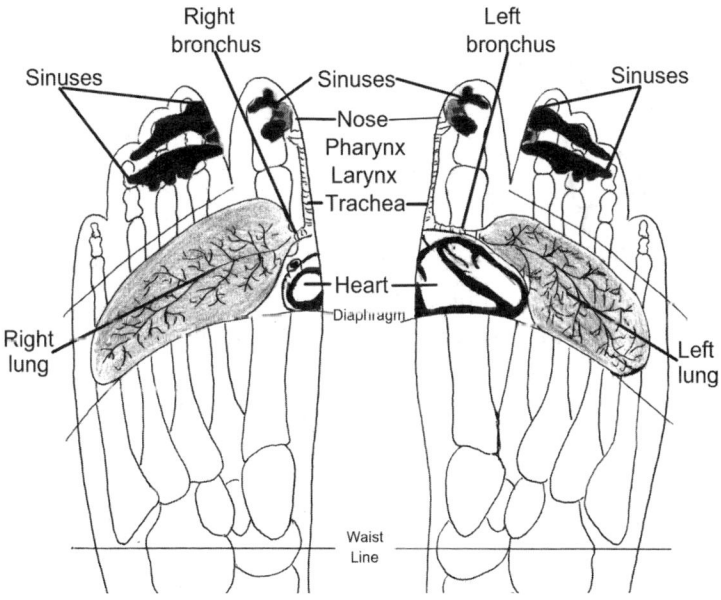

Reflexology

ILLUSTRATION 153: Respiratory System, Back View

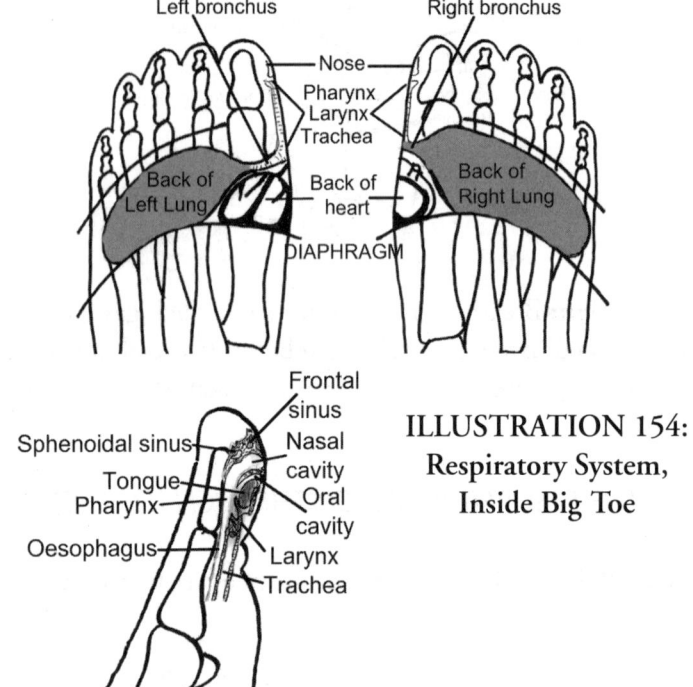

ILLUSTRATION 154: Respiratory System, Inside Big Toe

ILLUSTRATION 155: Sinuses, Outside Big Toe and inside and outside toes:

Outside Big Toe   Inside and out 2rd toe

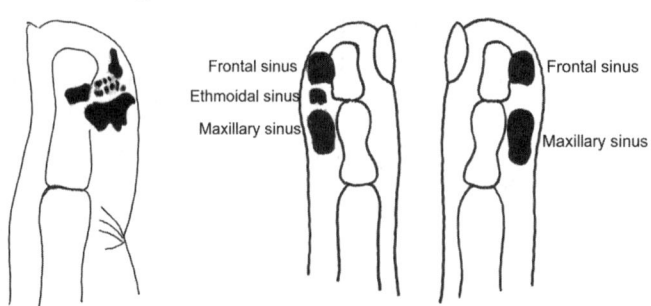

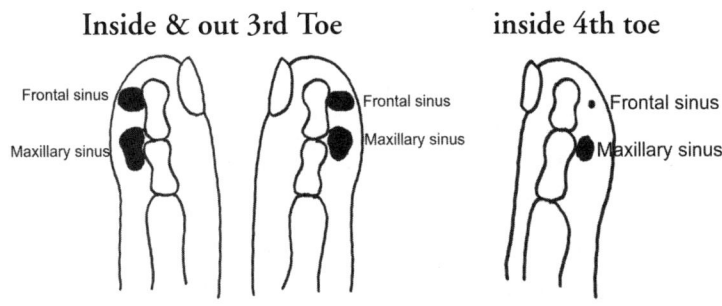

Inside & out 3rd Toe

Frontal sinus
Maxillary sinus

Frontal sinus
Maxillary sinus

inside 4th toe

Frontal sinus
Maxillary sinus

ix. SKELETAL SYSTEM

ILLUSTRATION 156: Skeletal System

Major components: The Skeletal system consists of 206 bones and associated cartilage and joints.

Functions: It protects and supports the body, and is a major component in the body being able to move. It also produces blood cells and stores minerals.

The skeletal system is the full collection of the bones of the body: the major bones are the spinal column, the skull, the ribs, the pelvic bones and the bones of the upper and lower limbs.

THE SKELETAL SYSTEM THROUGH THE FEET:
ILLUSTRATION 157: Skeletal System, Outside Views
Big Toe   **5th Toe**

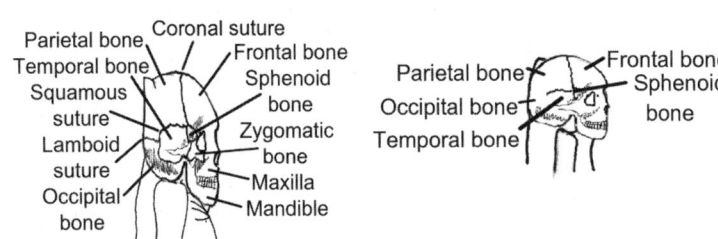

Parietal bone
Temporal bone
Squamous suture
Lamboid suture
Occipital bone

Coronal suture
Frontal bone
Sphenoid bone
Zygomatic bone
Maxilla
Mandible

Parietal bone
Occipital bone
Temporal bone

Frontal bone
Sphenoid bone

ILLUSTRATION 158: Skeletal System, Sole View

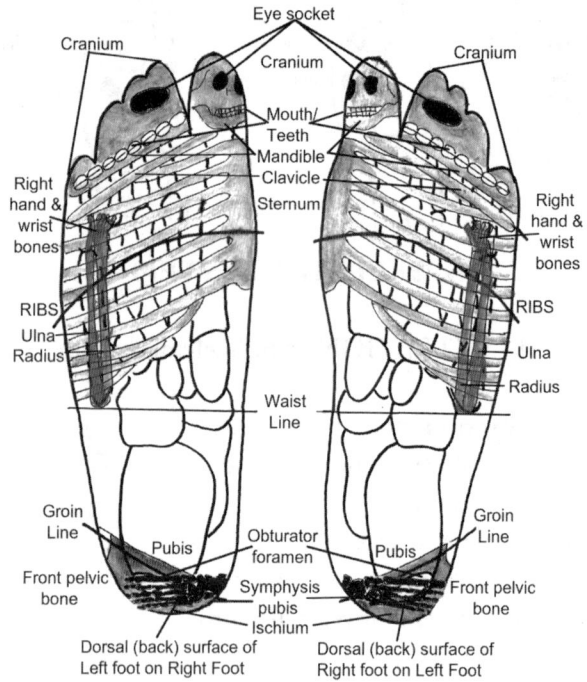

Eye socket

Cranium

Cranium

Cranium

Mouth/ Teeth

Mandible

Clavicle

Sternum

Right hand & wrist bones

Right hand & wrist bones

RIBS

Ulna

Radius

RIBS

Ulna

Radius

Waist Line

Groin Line

Pubis

Obturator foramen

Pubis

Groin Line

Front pelvic bone

Symphysis pubis

Ischium

Front pelvic bone

Dorsal (back) surface of Left foot on Right Foot

Dorsal (back) surface of Right foot on Left Foot

ILLUSTRATION 159: Skeletal System, Back View

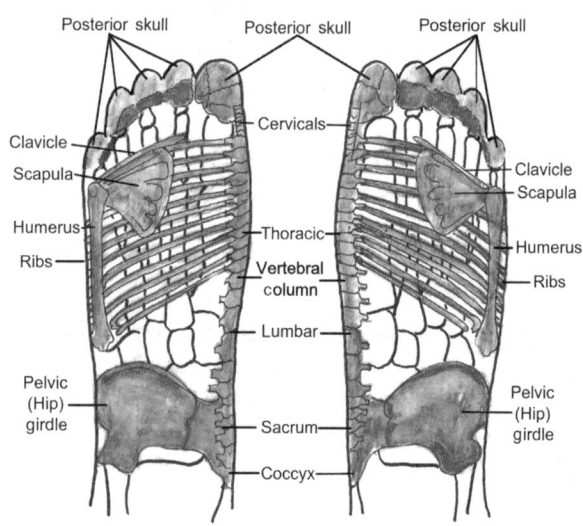

Posterior skull

Posterior skull

Posterior skull

Clavicle

Scapula

Cervicals

Clavicle

Scapula

Humerus

Ribs

Thoracic

Vertebral column

Humerus

Ribs

Lumbar

Pelvic (Hip) girdle

Sacrum

Coccyx

Pelvic (Hip) girdle

ILLUSTRATION 160: Skeletal System, Skull, Back View

Parietal bone
Parietal bone
Parietal bone
Sagittal suture
Lamboid suture
Occipital bone
Foramen magnum
Temporal bone
Lambdoid suture
Lambdoid suture
Temporal bone
Temporal bone
Occipital bone
Occipital bone

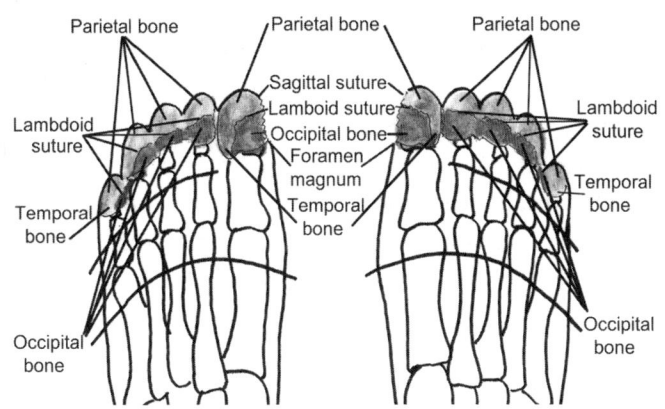

ILLUSTRATION 161: Skeletal System, Inside View

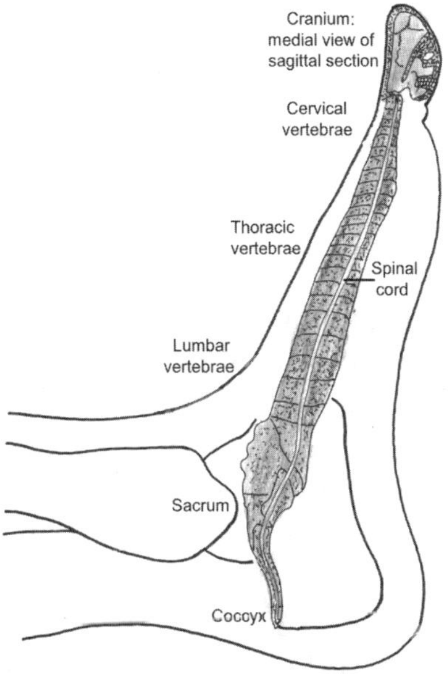

Cranium: medial view of sagittal section
Cervical vertebrae
Thoracic vertebrae
Spinal cord
Lumbar vertebrae
Sacrum
Coccyx

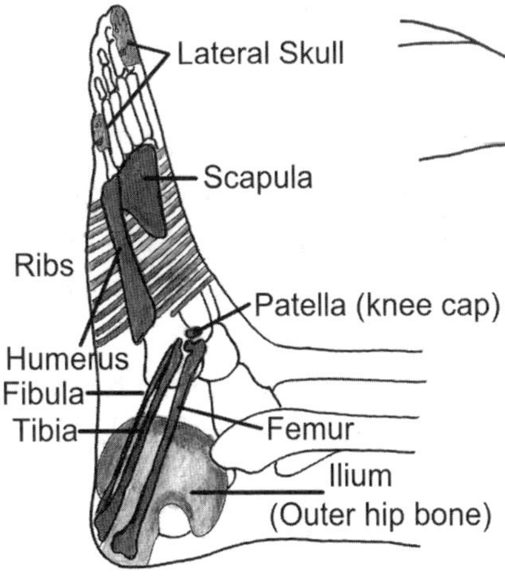

Lateral Skull
Scapula
Ribs
Patella (knee cap)
Humerus
Fibula
Tibia
Femur
Ilium
(Outer hip bone)

ILLUSTRATION 162: Skeletal System, Outside View

x. SPECIAL SENSES: SENSE ORGANS

Skin: is called the Integumentary system. It consists of the dermis, epidermis, body hairs, nails and sweat glands. It function is to protect the internal and prevent water loss and to help regulate the body's internal temperature; it produces Vitamin D, contains excretory glands (release waste through the skin), and has nerve receptors for touch, pain, cold and heat.

Olfactory Sense (Smell): The nose can recognize 4 000 different aromas and is used to clean and moisten the air before it enters the lungs.

Gustatory Sense (Taste): The tongue has receptors, or taste buds, which recognise four groups of tastes: sour, salty, bitter and sweet. Sweet taste buds are located mainly on the tip of the tongue; bitter at the back; salty at the sides and tip; and sour at the sides. The tongue is also essential for speech and aids in swallowing.

Visual Sense (Eyes): The eyes are one of the most complex organs of the body. All impulses are carried to the brain through the optical nerve.

Hearing and Balance (Equilibrium), The Ear: Three parts: external, middle and inner ear. The semi-circular ducts achieve equilibrium/balance: one of the canals reads up and down motion, one reads forward motion and the third one lateral or side motion.

THE SENSORY ORGANS THROUGH THE FEET:

Skin is located all over the outer body as it is in the feet. So the specific area of skin of the body reflects in the reflexes of appropriate area in the feet. For example, lower limb or leg skin problems reflect in the lower limb/leg reflex.

Also, other than the skin, all the senses are in the head and are related to the brain, and therefore are located in the toes.

ILLUSTRATION 163: Sense Organs, Sole View

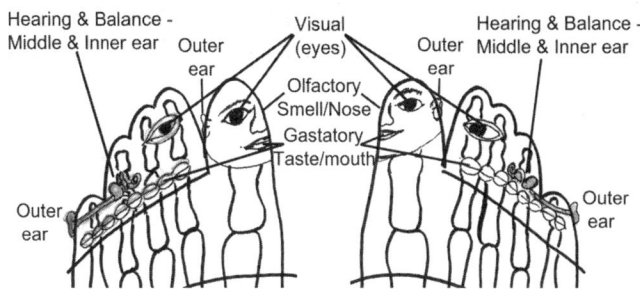

ILLUSTRATION 164: Sense Organs, Olfactory (Smell): Inside View, Big Toe

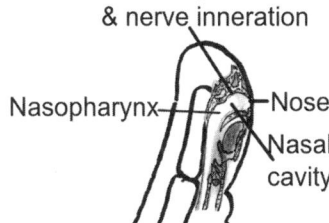

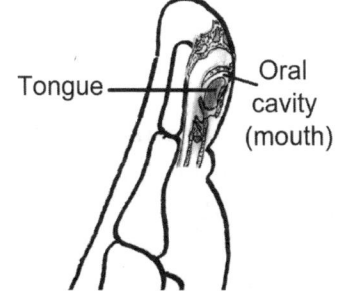

ILLUSTRATION 165: Sense Organs, Gustatory (Taste): Inside View, Big Toe

ILLUSTRATION 166: Sense Organs, Visual (Eyes): Inside: Lateral 2nd Toe / Medial 3rd Toe

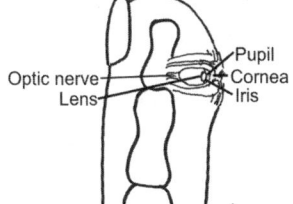
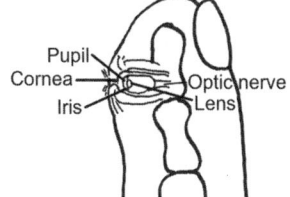

ILLUSTRATION 167: Sense Organs, Hearing and Balance
a) Outside View– Auricle of the Ear or Ear Lobe

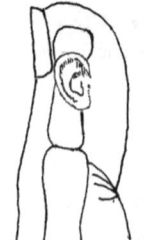

Big Toe

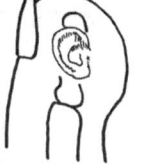

5th Toe

b) Inside View

Lateral 4th

Medial 5th Toes

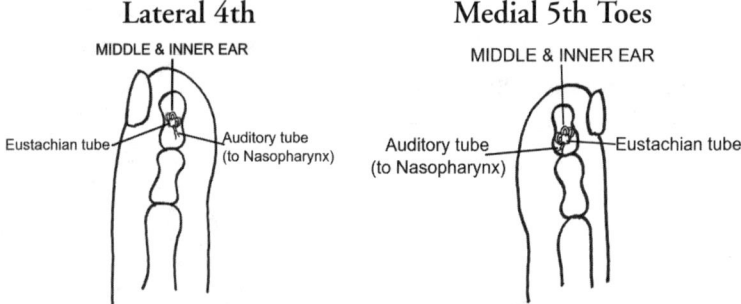

MIDDLE & INNER EAR

Eustachian tube

Auditory tube (to Nasopharynx)

MIDDLE & INNER EAR

Auditory tube (to Nasopharynx)

Eustachian tube

xi. URINARY SYSTEM

Major components: Kidneys, Ureter tubes (tube from the kidney to the bladder), the bladder and the urethra (duct that carries urine from the Bladder to the outside world).

ILLUSTRATION 168: Urinary System

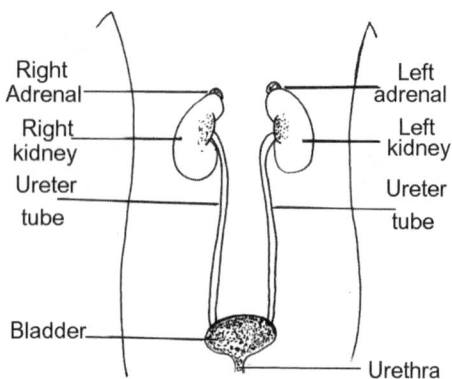

Right Adrenal

Right kidney

Ureter tube

Left adrenal

Left kidney

Ureter tube

Bladder

Urethra

Functions: It removes waste products from the circulatory system (blood), regulates blood pH (Acid/Alkaline balance), ion balance and water balance.

THE URINARY SYSTEM THROUGH THE FEET:

As the kidneys and the ureter tubes are bi-lateral, that is there are two and they are on both sides of the body, they do not reflect on the inner aspect of the feet. However, as the Bladder and urethra are in the mid-line of the body they reflect both on the inside and sole views of the feet.

ILLUSTRATION 169: Urinary System, Sole View

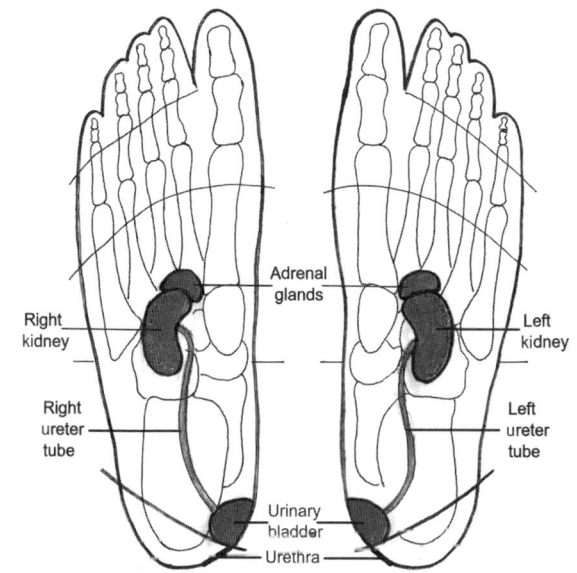

ILLUSTRATION 170: Urinary System, Inside View
Female   Male

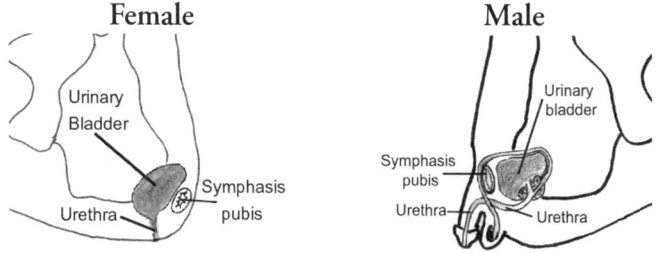

SECTION 4
Receivers of Reflexology

"As ye receive, so shall ye give.
As ye give, so shall ye receive."

CHAPTER 28
Reflexology Session

One of the major advantages of Reflexology is that all you need is knowledge, practical skills, experience, and your hands to practice it. So, as long as you can get to the feet, a Reflexology session can be done anywhere and at any time, and the receiver can gain benefit. The flexibility of a Reflexology session is one of its strengths.

However, for professional Reflexology and a complete treatment more is needed. The first question that arises here is: Is Reflexology performed in your own space or someone else's? If it is in someone else's space, such as a clinic, then you have little control over the setting. If it is in your own space, there are many questions that need answering.

The two most common methods of working as a Reflexologist are either with or for someone else, or in your own clinic. Each has their advantages and disadvantages. If working with or for someone else, most, if not all, of the decisions discussed below are out of your control. Initially, for experience, both are worth doing, but ultimately you have to decide which suits you best. So with this in mind, here, what will be dealt with is in your own clinic: preparing for a session and the session structure.

PREPARING FOR A SESSION

The first thing a Reflexologist needs to do is to work out what services they offer and how they are going to work. It is highly recommended that you draw up a portfolio of your clinic (a resume or CV of the clinic) from the beginning as this will provide the structure and motivation to make practice decisions. This portfolio can then be left in the reception area. It should also be edited and updated regularly for as you grow, so will your clinical experience. Most new Reflexologists, especially initially, attempt to be everything to everyone, and try to please their potential receivers rather than working out these questions for themselves first.

A) WHAT DO YOU DO? WHAT ARE YOU OFFERING?

The first and most important question is: What do you do? To some extent this decision comes from experience. There is no right and wrong. It is simply a matter of decision-making. Most when they begin do not even ask themselves these questions. Part of the answer comes from your training and your definition of Reflexology. Your Reflexology session will be structured by your own beliefs and, initially, what you have been taught Reflexology to be.

There are other questions which arise here as well that have an influence on your decision such as:
• Business vs. Practice
• Clinic and/or mobile.

If the business side of your clinic is a weakness, then small business training is vital, but this is only half the story. It is a fine line between them, but as a suggestion:
• While working in your clinic, you are a therapist and there for the receiver and their needs ONLY.
• Once outside your Clinic, it is your livelihood and business.

This is a very important distinction that many do not make, and so these two issues become blurred.

One of the common problems that arise is selling things within the clinical setting. Usually the reason is for business and money making rather than the receiver's needs (Unto thyself be true.). The resultant danger is the tendency to sell and promote these products rather than be the Reflexologist and therapist.

Another difficulty which arises is the question of marketing strategies. These should occur outside the clinical setting rather than within. Firstly, offering specials or discounts to different groups of people and first-time discounts, etc. are strategies better suited to other industries rather than health care.

Discounts are a major issue and I recommend offering no discounts for two reasons:

1. The health care industry does not do this as it cheapens the profession (if it is a profession)
2. Receivers have to value what is offered. This initially comes from you (Do you value what you do?), your pricing (which reflects your valuation in your market place) and your decision-making concerning marketing and especially discounts.

Pricing is another major issue that needs to be dealt with. Getting an idea of the current pricing in your area is important and needs to be taken into consideration, but ultimately your pricing reflects your valuation of what you do. Too cheap or too expensive.

Finally a word, excuse the pun, on word of mouth. Ultimately your clinic will prosper or not on the basis of word of mouth and reputation. The more decisions are consciously made about all these issues the better. Word of mouth comes from what you do and how you do it: your decisions.

There are so many decisions that are best made at the beginning rather than later, and so the more you can make these decisions consciously and deliberately the better. Once you have defined what you are offering and how you are offering it, you can then begin to structure the session accordingly.

B) THE SPACE TO WORK

(See Chapter 18 for more details)

Next it is important to look at the issue of the space you work in, first and foremost for yourself. This is paramount as you are the one who will have to spend your working day in this space.

The second question to ask is what sort of space do you want for your receivers?

The possible responses are: medical, clinical, professional, friendly, warm and inviting, but always reflective of you. Ultimately a combination of these is probably the best: professional and friendly, clinical and inviting, but always reflective of you.

A minimum of two rooms are recommended, one as an office and reception area and the other as a treatment area, and the treatment area should be a quiet, isolated and individual space separate from anything else and used for this purpose only.

C) EQUIPMENT NEEDED

(See Chapter 18)

The first item required is either a massage table or a reclining reflexology chair, plus a stool or seat for the Reflexologist to sit on while working. See Chapter 18 for a discussion of the advantages and disadvantages to each of these options. Next the question arises: Are you going to work from your own space or will you be mobile? This will clearly have an influence upon your choice of equipment.

Also desirable is a massage table that can be raised at the head end so that the receiver can sit up. This was chosen as some receivers for various reasons cannot, or prefer not to, lay supine, such as pregnant women, children and the elderly. For these receivers there needs to be plenty of pillows available so that they can sit up comfortably.

Lastly a stool or some other type of seating for working

at the end of the massage table or reclining chair is needed. There are again a number of options here and again the decision is yours.

As record keeping is an important aspect of the profession of Reflexology, paperwork needs to be designed and used. This includes Initial and Subsequent visit consultation sheets as well as a method of storing them. Also one needs an appointment book (diary) and promotional material such as business cards and flyers.

You will also need a desk and at least two chairs (one for the receiver and the other for you). As towels are used, a storage space for the towels is required, as well as a good supply of towels. It is wise, for the cooler months, to have heating and a light blanket to place over the receiver if necessary. In the warmer months, cooling may be needed.

D) THE ENVIRONMENT

(See Chapter 18)

The environment or atmosphere created is important for both you and the receiver. Again, this links with all that was said above concerning the space, as everything done within this space and what it contains help create the environment.

As much as is possible decrease and hopefully eliminate noise and interference from the outside world. Work in a peaceful, quiet environment. If this is not possible, the alternative is to decrease the negative impact of outside noise and interference.

The telephone ideally should be in the reception area and not the treatment room. However, if this is not possible, take the telephone off the hook or put the telephone on silent (e.g. mobile/cell phone) when actually treating.

E) THERAPEUTIC RELATIONSHIP

This is such as important issue involving two people: the giver (Reflexologist) and the receiver. There are so many aspects which contribute to the therapeutic relationship that they cannot adequately be covered here. In fact the majority of the therapeutic relationship is outside the control of the giver, and so it is difficult to qualify and yet is easier to damage than it is to build.

Essentially it is the process of building a relationship of trust and confidentiality, of shared values and professional intimacy. It does not happen immediately but is something that grows and develops over time and although the Reflexologist is involved, as are their ethics, morality and belief system, the majority of this lies outside the control of the Reflexologist as it is largely in the hands of the receiver.

Aspects of the therapeutic relationship include communications, questioning, discussion and counselling skills, although this does not mean counselling professionally. Listening and questioning skills are vital, as are a non-judgemental and non-discriminatory approach, which is why it is important to examine your own belief system as it plays a major role in developing and maintaining a therapeutic relationship. Vital is a desire to truly listen to the receiver, not only to what they are saying, but also to how they are saying it. This is again another aspect of being a professional that cannot be taught, but comes from experience.

F) PROFESSIONALISM: MEMBERSHIP AND CODE OF ETHICS AND/OR CODE OF PRACTICE

It is a requirement of most professional organisations that you display your qualifications, professional membership certificate and Code of Ethics and/or Code of Practice in a place where receivers can easily and readily see and read them. It is important for the sake of the receiver that you are qualified, recognised and professional, rather than important to and for you, the Reflexologist.

TREATMENT STRUCTURE

1. FIRST CONTACT: Telephone Checklist

Usually the first contact with a prospective receiver is actually over the telephone. So telephone communication skills are extremely important and a much ignored aspect of the Treatment Structure. First impressions are so important and as this is the first contact, it is doubly important. It is recommended that a Telephone Check List be drawn up and pasted in the front of the appointment book for reference when speaking to a prospective client by you or your secretary, to avoid problems at the Initial Consultation.

Also it is important to answer the enquirer's questions but it is just as important to give a good impression of you as a person as well as a professional. Just as important is structuring the treatment situation over the telephone while educating the caller on Reflexology, what you do, how you do it, etc. Being prepared, structured and organised is vital to the impression of the caller, as is being courteous and informative. Avoid being vague and general. Be specific and to the point; friendly and professional. Know what you are doing, and let them know you know what you are doing.

One suggested method for drawing up a Telephone Checklist is to role-play a scenario. For example, get a friend to ring you and record the conversation. It is amazing how revealing this can be. A Telephone Checklist could be the difference between getting receivers or not.

2. INITIAL CONSULTATION

Always be punctual and prepared. Be ready to work when you say you will be. Never keep receiver's waiting. This is an ethical and moral question. So many health care professionals keep people waiting and this is unprofessional and disrespectful to the receiver. If you make an appointment time, keep it.

Time structure is important as this will determine the structure of the session. The most common structure is a one-hour appointment. This will be discussed in more detail in Chapter 30.

Another Information sheet worth drawing up is an Initial Consultation Sheet, and the one I drew up when I first began is below (See Illustration 172). The reason for this is to make sure I covered everything I wanted to at the beginning of the First Consultation.

ILLUSTRATION 171: List: Initial Consultation Options
Reflexology Treatment: Here there are two options:
While studying and early in development:
1. Openings
2. Examining the feet: visual and touch
3. Full treatment Sequence
4. Balance and Figure Eight to finish
Later on: Be specific
1. Openings
2. Examining the feet: visual and touch
3. What they are coming for (What are they paying you for?)
4. Related reflexes, regions. sections, helper areas, systems, etc.
5. Balance and Figure Eight to finish.

NOTE: In the second option above I have "What are they paying me for?" The receiver is coming for a specific reason. It may be for a specific problem, or simply to experience what I do, or hopefully preventative wellbeing management. However, as this is what they are parting with their hard-earned money, I feel obliged to put this as a priority, which is why I have as one of the first questions I ask: Reason for the treatment, and in fact I ask this over the telephone and write it in my appointment book beside their name and telephone number, and Initial Consultation sheet, so that this becomes my priority even before they arrive.

Initial Consultation: Information
ILLUSTRATION 172: List

1. Please take off your shoes and socks.
2. What is your reason for having the treatment?
3. If you get COLD or HOT, **please let me know**.
4. Once on the massage Table:
   * Lay down, on your back.
   * I'm going to place a pillow under head (more if needed) and under your knees for support
   * I'm going to place BOTH feet on foot rest / cushion / baluster.
5. During the treatment, you may get a reaction. Please let me know if you do have any reaction whatsoever. You may feel like releasing something: a sigh, groan, laugh, cry, etc. **Feel free to do so.**
6. You may fall asleep. If so, that's fine.
7. Some points/areas/reflexes of the feet may be tender or sore. I may ask you about these or you may let me know if you feel anything. DO NOT WORRY if areas/points/reflexes are tender/sore. It does not mean that anything is necessarily wrong. Most, if not all people have tender/sore reflexes/points somewhere. It indicates an imbalance in the energy/chi of that region or reflex, which is NOT NECESSARILY physical.
8. If any points are sore, please let me know, and let me know the type of pain: sharp or dull. I may ask you to compare points/reflexes. If so, I am looking for the difference, not the similarity.
9. Close your eyes, but keep your attention on the experience and stay alert throughout. Keep you mind focused on the present NOW and on what's happening for you and your body. **Avoid thoughts** wandering to future concerns or dwelling on the past. If this happens draw yourself gently back to the NOW.

10. At the end, I will ask for feedback. Please feel free to express anything that you wish.

11. The treatment is done in **active silence**. Verbal communications will be kept to a minimum. BUT if you wish to speak, feel free to do so.

12. At the end, I will leave you on the table for a few minutes. Just lie there and be conscious of what has and is happening for you.

13. The energies take up to **twenty four to thirty six hours** to completely penetrate all of you and to balance your system. Any reactions within this time indicate the energy received and balanced. It is a good sign rather than a bad one. Please take note of what happens, and the time that it occurs.

During the treatment many things may happen, as mentioned in the list above, and as I work I record down on my consultation sheets any feedback from the receiver as well as my observations and information received from working the feet. So although the Reflexology treatment is performed in silence, it is an active, listening and observing silence.

After the Reflexology treatment of approximately 35 to 45 minutes, I leave the receiver for a few minutes on the massage table while I return to my desk and record anything else that I was unable to during the treatment. This time is also when I record anything I picked up but did not have time to include in this treatment in the section: To Do Next Time (SEE Appendix B: Consultation Sheets), which is actually planning future treatments as this will be transferred to the To Do of the next Client Information sheet. Leaving the receiver on the table gives me time to do this and gives the receiver a few minutes to absorb the effects of the treatment.

3. SUBSEQUENT VISITS

Subsequent Visits are basically the same as above except the time structure is one to one and a quarter hours. The Initial and Subsequent Visits will be looked at in detail in Chapter 30.

CHANGE

Lastly a comment on change: It is another of the foundation aspects of any therapy and needs mentioning here. Our whole ethos is anti-change and so most of us find ourselves resistant to change to some degree or another. This is understandable.

Over time and treatments changes occur and often as they are subtle, the receiver is unaware of these, which is why I always ask at the beginning of each subsequent visit the reason why the receiver initially sought my help. Often the receiver does not even realise that changes have occurred. These I call the side effects of the treatment. The reality of the situation is that we are constantly changing. Change is the most natural of the processes of life and death. Therefore:

"You do not have to change. You are changing."

Allow change to happen. Do not try and make change happen. If and when something is meant to happen it will, naturally, quickly and easily.

CHAPTER 29
Receiver's Responses and Reactions, and the Myth of the Healing Crisis

There are two situations in which reactions can occur and they are during the treatment and afterwards.

RESPONSES AND REACTIONS DURING A TREATMENT

During a treatment the range of responses varies from receiver to receiver. So the first and most important point about responses is that they are unique to each individual receiver and so there are as many responses as there are receivers.

The most common response is an extremely deep meditative level of relaxation, but for others who do not meditate the tendency is to go to sleep. Generally males will fall asleep, some the moment you begin.

The other common responses receivers experience during a treatment, include:

- Verbalisation and sounds: sighing, laughing, a few tears, memories (the past), etc. and some receivers will talk about all sorts of aspects of their life. This is more common down the track once the therapeutic relationship has been established but can happen during the initial consultation. The Reflexologist can also actually trigger past memories and emotions, but my experience is that this is more as amazement than

disquieting or painful.
- Sensations in their body, quite often related to the reflex/region of the body currently being worked or just worked.
- Pain or discomfort.
- Body responses (sounds), commonly stomach and bowel sounds, again quite often related to the reflexes/region of the body currently being worked or just worked.
- Usually immediately after the treatment comments such as 'It feels like I have had a full night's sleep.' or comments regarding feelings of wellness or being balanced, grounded and centred.
- Other common comments to do with their feet and how light they are and/or how much they can feel them, are conscious of their feet, etc.
- A feeling of being spaced out and not really fully back.

TWO TYPES/GROUPS OF RESPONSES FROM INITIAL TREATMENT:

Experience has indicated that there are two groups or types of responses to the initial treatment. These are:

1. FEEL EVERYTHING: The Open receiver: Those receiver's who feel everything, including pain during the treatment. Throughout the treatment they are mentioning 'Oo', 'ouch', 'arh' etc.
2. FEEL NOTHING: the Closed receiver: Those receiver's who feel nothing, even when you pick things up who will respond in the negative.

NOTE: These two groups or types are caricatures and no one receiver is completely one or the other as most people are a combination of both.

What is important to know about these two types is that the first group who feel everything and are therefore open will find that pain and discomfort decrease quite quickly over time and that they generally gain results and improvements from their symptoms and imbalances quite quickly. So the process is quicker for these receivers.

However, for the second group this is not the case. What tends to happen here is that over time with each treatment they will feel more, often saying things like 'What's that! That wasn't sore before." when in fact this has been noted by the Reflexologist during earlier treatments. These receivers are for whatever reason closed, that is they have turned themselves off from their own body. Therefore, the Reflexologist must turn them back on before seeing improvement in their symptoms and imbalances. This type also tends to be mental beings, which does not necessarily mean they have mental imbalances but rather that they tend to be mental and intellectual, and have used this ability to ignore their body in some way or another. Furthermore, the tendency with this group is for things to get worse before they get better (Perhaps as a result of the belief structure of these receivers?). Therefore the process takes longer. This group should be warned that this may be the case.

But always remember the response is unique to each individual receiver. The range is actually limitless.

RESPONSES AND REACTION AFTER THE TREATMENT

The variety of responses and reactions after a treatment, is endless, limited only by the number of receivers. Rarely, if ever, is there an increase in the receiver's symptoms, such as pain, after a treatment. However, there are sometimes strange physical reactions (out of the ordinary). They may get no benefit, but they do not get worse. The worst that happens is nothing happens.

However, many actually gain improvement in their presenting symptoms to the extent that they do not even realise. Quite often their response when quizzed is along the lines of 'Oh, I forgot. That hasn't been a problem.' And they themselves are quite surprised. The most common phrase that receivers use is something like: 'Better able to cope' and 'No longer a problem'. Receivers repeat these types of phrases often. The most likely time for a person to have a reaction is after the first treatment.

There are two reasons for this. Firstly the treatment continues to work through the receiver's whole system for 24 to 36 hours, that is, it is a minimum of 24 hours and is usually one full day. If the receiver does have a reaction, it is very important to note down the reaction and especially the time that it happens.

The other reason for the 24 to 36 hours for a reaction after the first treatment is the fact that most bodies have been out of balance for many years, and so it is a mild shock to the system. Generally it is a short-term (five to ten minutes) reaction ranging from very subtle that they themselves do not even notice (and those around them tend to see the reaction) through to strange physical reaction, which is usually the case when there are physical imbalances and long-term problems.

Recommend that receivers do nothing mentally or physically active for an hour or two after the treatment, and to be over-cautious when driving. If the receiver is driving a long distance, suggest stopping locally for a cupper or a meal for a while (an hour or two) before driving home.

Not everyone says that they have a reaction, but they usually do. Quite often those around them notice something different rather than the receiver. This is quite common. Sometimes the side effects are more significant and powerful than the actual reaction.

At times, receivers have unexpected and unforeseen responses and outcomes, which I call side effects as they have not specifically been worked on during the treatment process. Often these side effects are the most important and significant aspect of the treatment. They are always gentle, quite rapid and easy and include physical, emotional, mental, and/or spiritual changes and shifts. There have been so many varieties of these side effects and often other problems that the receiver has not consciously come to treatment for occur.

I am not an Astrologer, but one last observation from experience is that receivers with either a strong Pisces, or Neptune (the planet that rules Pisces) influence in their Natal Astrology chart will either love or hate Reflexology. There is no in-between. The reason for this is that Pisces and Neptune rule the feet astrologically. Reflexology will be extremely effective on these people, or they will absolutely hate it.

THE MYTH OF THE HEALING CRISIS

The Healing Crisis has been previously mentioned. It is extremely rare but there is the very odd occasion when it occurs. The Healing Crisis means that it takes a few days to recover from the treatment as the symptoms increase before decreasing, so pain and discomfort increase before improvement. However, this does not mean that strange, weird and wonderful things do not happen after a treatment. What it means is that there is literally never an increase in symptoms, especially pain after a treatment. Most of the time the symptoms decrease easily, quickly and naturally; or not at all.

Think about it: If the body is designed to heal itself, why would it be hard and difficult for the body to do this? The only explanation I have come up with for this is the belief system of the person concerned and that most significantly the Healing Crisis is in fact a response of the body to the actual treatment.

Reflexology and most therapies, especially body therapies, have latched onto this concept to explain what happens immediately after the treatment. It has become an excuse and in fact most of what is called the Healing Crisis is the result of the treatment itself. It is the body's attempt to re-balance itself as a result of the treatment. It is the treatment actually making it harder on the body to do what it is trying to do, as it must first deal with the abuse (I do not use this word lightly.) caused by the treatment. So the treatment actually makes it harder for the body to do what it is trying to do, that is, the treatment is not working with the body but rather against it.

CHAPTER 30
Receiver's Management and Care

As a professional the Reflexologist needs to manage the receiver and their care, as well as the clinic. There are many aspects to this that need to be taken into consideration.

One question worth asking yourself is: What is the aim with each receiver and for each treatment session? Is it:

- To help?
- To balance the whole person on all levels?
- To aid the body to heal itself?
- To travel with the receiver on their journey?
- To counsel?
- To dictate?
- To heal?
- To do what you think is best?
- To take over the receiver's journey or to make the receiver's journey yours?
- To fix everything up?
- To do what the receiver asks you to do?
- To take responsibility for the receiver and their imbalances?
- To treat specific physical, emotional, mental and/or spiritual imbalances?
- To do something else altogether?

The answer to these and similar questions will determine what you do and how you do it, so this is the basis of your clinical treatment sessions. Once again this comes from your belief system. Honesty is the best policy, and unto thyself be true.

You will realise that there are so many aspects to managing receivers and their care that it cannot all be covered adequately here. The issues will briefly be raised once more for you as a professional Reflexologist to consciously decide.

SESSION STRUCTURE: TIME MANGEMENT

Firstly, the issue of time is an important one. Many Reflexologists and health care providers do not keep appointment times. This is unprofessional and no receiver should wait more than a few minutes for an appointment. So time management is an extremely important aspect.

Earlier the first and subsequent Consultations have been outlined and discussed. Here the question is more about time organisation. One of the first and most important organisational matters, for yourself and the receiver, is structuring the times of the day you will work. There are many options.

The one-hour appointment time structure is the most common organisation of a Reflexologist's day and the most likely structure that you will encounter, especially if working for someone else.

ILLUSTRATION 173: Time Structure: One-Hour Option
8.00am to 9.00am
9.00am to 10.00am
10.00am to 11.00am
11.00am to 12.00 noon
12.00 noon to 1.00pm (or Lunch)
1pm to 2pm: Lunch (or appointment)
2.00pm to 3.00pm
3.00pm to 4.00pm
4.00pm to 5.00pm
5.00pm to 6.00pm (or Evening meal)

6.00 to 7.00pm: Evening Meal (or appointment)
7.00pm to 8.00pm
8.00pm to 9.00pm
9.00pm FINISH or extra appointment time if needed

There are advantages and disadvantages to this structure. One of the major advantages is the number of treatments that can be done in a working day, an advantage of this structure surrounds income. Therefore this structure is more of a business and income-based choice. This structure is also more stressful on the Reflexologist as the pressure is to make sure you manage the time accurately, otherwise receivers have to wait. This is one of the disadvantages of this structure as it is difficult not to keep people waiting. This structure is more mechanical and suits a production-line type approach to Reflexology. However, for the therapist and the treatment, this structure gives less flexibility, and more pressure. This then is a therapist-centred approach. It suits the manager, the business-person and the mechanic rather than the Reflexologist as therapist.

Under this time structure, the one-hour would be broken up into something like:

1. **5 to 10 minutes:** Record taking (Not a great deal of time for this.)
2. **35 to 45 minutes:** treatment
3. **5 to 10 minutes:** conclusion
4. **5 minutes maximum:** preparation of next receiver.

It leaves very little room for error or flexibility. There is no time to spare, perhaps a maximum of 5 minutes. There is little time to finish with the previous receiver, change towels and such, and to get ready for the next receiver.

Also, there is no extra time for the First Consultation under this structure, or the alternative is for First or Initial visit to book a double appointment (two-hour time period) but most do not do this and therefore medical and personal history note-taking and questioning is sacrificed. Alternatively, the receiver could fill in the paperwork beforehand or while waiting. These are the options available, and the tendency is to limit it to the one-hour and therefore sacrifice something of the Initial Consultation, especially questioning, discussing and record keeping. Also, there would be no change in fee of course, between Initial and Subsequent visits. An advantage or a disadvantage?

Finally under the above style of time management, record keeping which is so necessary and important (and will be discussed below), is far more difficult as there is very little time available for this.

An alternative structure for the Initial Consultations is approximately one and a half hours and subsequent visits are an hour to an hour and a quarter, as outlined below.

ILLUSTRATION 174: Time Structure: One-& a Quarter Hours Option

1 to 1.15 Hour Structure (Mine)

9.00am to 10.15am

10.15am to 11.30am

11.30am to 12.45pm

12.45pm to 2.00pm: LUNCH

2.00pm to 3.15pm

3.15pm to 4.30pm

4.30pm to 5.45pm

5.45 to 7.00pm: TEA

7.00pm to 8.15pm

8.15pm to 9.30pm

9.30pm – FINISH or extra appointment time if needed

NOTE: Under this structure, the Initial Consultation appointment takes two time periods, that is up to two and a half hours, which allows for greater flexibility in the delivery of the Initial Consultation, but the disadvantage is two time periods are used.

It is obvious that this time management structure also has advantages and disadvantages. Firstly, as the appointment time is longer fewer appointments can occur in one day, which means less income, but hopefully more therapy. Also, rarely is the next receiver kept waiting for any time at all.

This structure gives greater flexibility and less stress in the delivery of the service of Reflexology as there is more time for both the giver and the receiver, and is a much more receiver-centred approach and less a business one.

Under this time structure the Initial Consultation would be something like this:

1. **20 to 30 minutes:** Me asking questions and filling in consultation sheet and explaining what I do and how.
2. **35 to 45 minutes:** Treatment
3. **10 to 15 minutes:** Conclusion, feedback, discussion, suggestions, payment, etc.
4. **5 to 10 minutes:** Prepare for next receiver.

TOTAL – 1.5 hours and up to two and a half hours, if necessary.

And Subsequent Visits of a maximum of an hour and a quarter would be:

1. **5 to 10 minutes:** Initial contact, discussion, feedback, current state of health, etc. (longer if needed).
2. **35 to 45 minutes:** Treatment.
3. **5 to 10 minutes:** Conclusion, feedback, discussion, suggestions, payment, next appointment, etc., and
4. **5 to 10 minutes:** preparation of next receiver.

TOTAL – 1.15 hours.

One of the most important factors, once in practice, is to make sure you keep control of the time factor. It is so important to learn simple techniques to keep track of time. For example, simply mentioning what is left to do or next draws the attention of the receiver back to the situation at hand. These techniques courteously done are important for you, the Reflexologist, the current and the next receiver.

INITIAL CONSULTATION INFORMATION SHEET AND TELEPHONE CHECKLIST

As mentioned earlier, an Initial Consultation Information sheet is a good idea for you to draw up so that initially when first in practice, you make sure you cover everything that you want to cover, it helps you to be better organised and more professional. Also, as a suggestion, a Telephone Checklist is a good idea. See Chapter 28 for more details.

RECORD KEEPING

Another extremely important issue is Record Keeping. See Appendix B: Consultation sheets. **NOTE:** The first Initial Consultation sheets in the appendix are actually the ones I designed when I began to practice, and following these are my current three-page consultations sheets. Over the years my Consultation sheets have grown and evolved along with me as a professional Reflexologist and therapist.

Your consultation sheets are vitally important for many reasons. I highly recommended you draw up your own consultation sheets as they reflect your own biases, prejudices, belief system and strengths and weaknesses, and most importantly where you are currently at. No one draws up the perfect consultation sheets as you can only assess their value or otherwise by using them and the tendency is to simply use the Consultation sheets provided whereas they should evolve over time. Use a system of boxes for ticking and crossing as much as possible and develop an abbreviation and notation system as well, which allows for speed of record keeping. This will make the task of keeping receiver records up-to-date much easier.

Another suggestion to help be well prepared before each treatment is to put aside time at the beginning (or end) of each week and prepare all paperwork for the following week. Review what you have written and plan what you are going to do. This way, when your receiver arrives you are prepared, ready and professional. It has a further advantage which is that it is as a learning process for yourself and ultimately for the benefit of your receivers.

Detailed records must be kept for a variety of reasons, including:

1. It is difficult to keep everything in your head.
2. Professionalism: you will need to refer back to previous records for a variety of reasons. If they are not detailed enough, you will not know what to do, and yet they need to be brief enough that this process is quick and easy.
3. If there are any problems with receivers, your records will be vital. It is amazing how often, if a problem arises, simply looking back on your records can eliminate so many potentially difficult situations.
4. There may also be legal requirements concerning your records, that is, it is a legal obligation to keep records, and they may, under certain circumstances, be required or subpoenaed.

CONFIDENTIALITY AND DUTY OF CARE

Confidentiality and Duty of Care are also very important aspect of being a professional Reflexologist, and they are an important component in the development and maintenance of the therapeutic relationship as well as a moral and legal requirement. All Professional organizations' Codes of Ethics or Codes of Practice stress this.

As many receivers are often in a vulnerable position and the Reflexologist is in a position of trust, receivers often open up and reveal information that is meant to be between the Reflexologist and the receiver only. As you are in a privileged position, you will hear information about the receiver that you are morally, ethically and legally obliged to keep to yourself. Revealing these details is a breach of trust.

Because of this privileged position it is paramount that the professional reflexologist realise he/her duty of care for the receiver. Like all health care providers, Reflexologists also need to realise their legal and moral obligations of care while performing a Reflexology session.

FEEDBACK

This is extremely important and should be encouraged at every opportunity. It is also a component of the therapeutic relationship. As a therapist you learn so much from feedback, about what you do and how, as well as about the therapeutic situation, health and wellbeing, and so on. Both positive and negative feedback is worthwhile, as both will teach you something, so encourage such.

You learn so much about so many things by encouraging feedback and initially for learning and early professional development it is such a great tool. Another reason to ask for feedback is that it helps build trust and interest between yourself and the receiver.

One final point to remember is that if you do not ask, you will not know, and it is amazing how often a simple question related to feedback can provide you with so much information.

I cannot stress enough the importance of feedback.

RECOMMENDATIONS/SUGGESTIONS

On your consultation sheets you should have a section (usually at the bottom) for recommendations. There are many reasons for this, but the most important is that you cannot remember everything you recommend to a receiver, such as self-help, and it is important to keep a record of these. It is also important, as misunderstanding can so easily arise, especially at the end of a treatment when the receiver is so relaxed.

TO DO

This is a section I would highly recommend you have on your consultation sheets so that you can plan ahead and be prepared before the arrival of the receiver. This links to what I said earlier about being prepared, planning ahead and if you are serious about this process you need to put time and effort into it. This is an example of that. It is a brief way of doing a Treatment Plan for the receiver.

NEXT TIME

Also suggested for your consultation sheets is a section, usually at the bottom, for things that you did not get time to do this time and therefore wish to do next time you see this receiver. So, at the end of the consultation by recording this you are already beginning to plan and structure the next session and as such this will be transferred to 'To Do' mentioned above.

BE PREPARED

This is again an important aspect of professionalism. Make sure you are set up and everything is done, such as cleaning and disinfecting the room, heating/cooling, towels, table, consultation sheets, etc. and that everything is clean, neat and tidy, well before the receiver arrives. These are all little details, but important ones that help to provide you with a more professional appearance and allow you to work from a centred space rather than from a rushed one.

APPEARANCE

This is another of the issues you need to make a decision

about. For example, medical standards commonly include dressing in suits or at least a collar and tie and wearing a white overcoat. How will you present yourself professionally either in a clinic or health care setting?

When working in someone else's clinic or within the health care system you will need to take your lead from their standards and requirements. Some may have requirements and you will need to find these out and work within them.

In your own clinic you will need to decide your professional presentation. Think about what you want to wear. What do you think is appropriate? Should you wear some sort of uniform? These are questions you need to ask yourself.

I have always worked in white clothes, bare feet and sandals (with a white sleeveless jumper and white socks in winter) to perform Reflexology.

CONCLUSION

A conclusion is an ending and I find it difficult to write a conclusion as Reflexology is alive; it is a living, growing part of me and a journey that I have not as yet reached its end. I am still learning, developing and discovering, and I am excited about the future as there is so much yet to discover and understand; the journey has just begun. Reflexology as we have it today is no more than a third developed; there is at least two-thirds yet to discover. Reflexology chronologically is a young child that needs to grow up and mature, and so the future should be bright, but the path ahead is a challenging one: the rocky road that Reflexology is currently taking is recognition and promotions at any cost and perhaps the price is too high and the risk is that we could be lost along the way without a strong and solid road base, to continue the analogy, upon which to stand. We stand upon the earth but we reach for the heavens.

Reflexology, like all natural therapies is going through a transition period where it is increasingly being recognised within the health care system. What we do today will determine the future of Reflexology's tomorrow. This is the responsibility we now face. It is past time that the theoretical and practical foundations of Reflexology were examined. It is time to stop and reflect upon these foundations, so that we can move ahead as professional Reflexologists with knowledge, intuition and compassion, confident in the foundations upon which we stand, rather than the shifting sands of poor theoretical and practical knowledge.

Any structure is only as good as it foundations. If the foundations are poorly constructed and weak then the structure is doomed. This has been the aim of this current work: to begin the process of creating a solid foundation upon which the profession of Reflexology can stand and prosper. Does this work finish this process? Not by a long shot. It is a beginning, perhaps a good one, but that is for others to judge.

There are so many contradictions in the basic theory and practice of Reflexology that need to be aired, analysed and critically assessed; another reason for writing this book. It is both controversial and challenging, for that is its purpose. I have proposed a consistent perspective of the feet, and followed it. It is now up to each and every one of you to make your own decisions. If you have thought, assessed and made decisions about Reflexology, then I have achieved what I set out to do. If the Reflexology profession begins to look at its theoretical and practical foundations, then again I have achieved my aim.

The main reason for this work is to answer the questions of Reflexologists, by presenting a consistent perspective of the feet in theory and practice; to provide Refleoxlogist with a detailed analysis of the basic premises upon which Reflexology is based so that each and every one can make their own conscious decisions about what they do, how they do it and why they do it. It is only with knowledge that these decisions can be made, for in knowledge lies the power. So many either do not have the knowledge or have failed to share that knowledge and I find this surprising, for in sharing it grows.

In Section One, there is much theory and critical analysis which is new:

- The sacred art of working the feet
- The reassessment of the theories of Reflexology and a consistent perspective proposed and consistently applied
- The Anatomical Reflection Theory and the resultant new more detailed physical charts of the systems of the body through

the feet
- The critical analysis and explanation of the Solar Plexus reflex, which is actually K.1/TB acu-point.
- Diagnosing through the feet and how Reflexologists diagnose
- A re-examination of the ancient and modern history and evolution of Reflexology

In Section Two the practical applications of these theoretical foundations are explained including:
- Preparing to work the feet
- How to hold the feet and why
- My basic rules and why I consider these important
- The treatment options and techniques available to Refleoxlogist; the choices as therapist we always have
- The Openings (rather than relaxers) which open up the area of the body before working.
- The Basic Procedure for a full Reflexology treatment: head to tail, reproductive, inside and out.

Then in Section Three the physicality of Reflexology is examined including and especially the reflection of each medical system of the body accurately through the feet and the detail of the complexity of the human anatomy reflected in the detailed reflexes of the feet. Knowledge that is vital for the foundations of Reflexology and at the same time to establish Reflexology as a credible therapy. Ironically the very thing that so many crave. If we could but get our house in order and our foundations established, then we could take it to the world of medicine, not as subordinates but as professional collaborators. A dream and a vision.

In the last section you have learnt about carrying out reflexology treatments, running a clinic and managing clients and a practice. I have explained what and how I work so that you can make your own decisions about these issues: to work out what you do and don't do and why. Conscious decisions once again. And finally there is the Appendices of the glossary, my consultation sheets, numbers and Reflexology: Wholistic

(Soul-Growth) Numerology, recommended reading and Reflexology resources and concluding with Reflexology around the world, all of which follows this conclusion.

So much currently available in Reflexology neglect so much of what has been covered in this work and concentrates on perpetuating the myths of the past. This work is the beginning of the process where I have explained what I have discovered through my Reflexology journey, why I do what I do, how I do what I do. Is it right? It is for me. For you now I pass on the responsibility to make your own decisions, consciously and with knowledge and wisdom.

There are so many contradictions within current Reflexology theory and practice that have been exposed in this book; brought out into the light of day and critically analysed, with a consistent perspective espoused. Is it right? I think so, but unless these questions are asked, and then the answers cannot be found.

For the first time Reflexology theory has been explained in detail. Perhaps the reason I am one of the few to have taken this journey is that I started again, and attempted to understand through experience and through working intuitively on the feet while at the same time attempting to understand what I was doing and why. Knowledge (yang) and intuition (yin) working together in harmony. The artist rather than the mechanic at work.

The Reflexology journey shared in this book is both radical and revolutionary. I accept both, for both are quite true. Unless these issues are brought out, how can we make decisions about them for yourselves as individual Reflexologists but perhaps more importantly as a profession. How can we ever be a profession until this process has at least begun. It is an on-going, never-ending process and as we learn more, understand more, develop more; so will our understanding of this most beautiful of therapies.

"JUDGE THE MESSAGE, NOT THE MESSENGER."

I hope you have gained insight into this fantastic therapy called Reflexology and at the same time have made conscious decisions about Reflexology and about the profession you are part of; that you have learned along the way and have stronger foundations in the theory and practice of Reflexology. This is what it is all about. Unless knowledge is shared it dies, and therefore it cannot grow least of all be questioned and challenged. I have made my decisions and it is now time for you to make yours.

The longest journey begins with the first step. May my sharing have added a step or two to your Reflexology journey.

APPENDICES

APPENDIX A:
GLOSSARY

Abduction: Is moving the foot away from the mid-line of the body.

Adduction: Is moving the foot towards the mid-line of the body.

Acu-points: Chinese energy points of the body and feet, which are each individual and unique energy centres or vortexes of energy.

Anatomical Position: Is the person standing with legs apart facing forward, with their palms forward. It is the position in which everything to do with the body is described.

Anatomical Reflection Theory: (See Chapter 7) Major premise upon which Reflexology is based: that the two feet reflect your body anatomically accurately.

Anatomy & Physiology (A & P): Scientific study of the structures and vital processes or functions of the body, via a systematic approach to the body.

Arteries: Blood vessels that travel from the heart with oxygenated blood to every organ and cell in the body.

Articulates: A place where two bones come together, commonly called a joint.

Balance: Chinese concept: we strive for balance, which is a yin state of inactivity but we do not really want balance, as firstly nothing can exist unless it has two aspects or qualities (yin &

yang), and secondly, we need movement, which is provided by activity, which is yang. Therefore, the key is not so much Balance, but avoidance of extremes (i.e. Extreme yin and extreme yang). In other words, Moderation in all things and on all levels.

Biomechanics: The science of gait, that is how we move, walk and run.

Calcaneal Spur: Heel Spur: See Spur

Calcaneus: Commonly called heel bone.

Cardiovascular System: The systems of blood flow around the body via arteries and veins and include the heart, which is the pump of the system.

Central Nervous system (CNS): The brain, brain stem and spinal chord.

Change: Basic premise of life. It is the natural law of the universe. Everything is in a state of movement, flux and change.

Chakras: Energy vortexes which are the major aspect of the Indian energy system. There are seven chakras, from Crown, Brow (Third Eye), Throat, Heart, Solar Plexus, Sacral and Base (Root) chakras.

Cuboid: One of the bones of the rear foot. It is located on the outside behind the fifth and fourth metatarsal bones and in front of the calcaneus or heel bone.

Cuneiform: Wedge-shaped bones of the front of the Rear Foot, located behind the first, second and third metatarsals and in front of the navicular.

Chi: Is the energy within everything that exists in the universe. It is the building blocks of everything in the universe. It is energy just before it becomes physical.

Chi (Life-force) creation and Distribution: Chinese process of how the body creates and distributes energy through out the body.

Chi: Deficient energy: Low or not enough energy. It is characterised by emptiness, dull pain, bruised feeling, softness, a good pain, cold; etc.

Chi: Excess energy: High or too much energy. It is characterised by hardness, fullness, heat, inflammation, strong pain, ouch pain that makes you sit up and take notice; etc.

Chi-Reflexology: Advanced Reflexology approach developed by Moss Arnold. It is a combination of a philosophical approach, including the Chinese philosophy, with the science of Reflexology.

Clinical Reflexology: or Professional Therapeutic Reflexology: Therapeutic approach to the science and art of Reflexology, i.e. Reflexology as a therapy.

Contraindications: Any condition that may be harmful for the receiver and therefore something Reflexologist should not work.

Criss-cross Motion: Is obtained by working an area in two directions, first in one direction diagonally upwards and then stop, reverse hands and work back in the opposite upwards direction. Usually, worked on an angle across the foot from inside to the outside and then back again.

Crystal Deposits Theory: Are found in the feet. They feel like grains of sand. They are toxins gathered in the feet. By working these you are helping the body eliminate toxins from the body.

Diaphragm (Diaphragm Line): Is a thick muscle forming the floor of the chest or upper cavity of the body at the base of the lungs (base of the metatarsal pad/ ball of the foot, where the skin changes colour).

Digestive System: The system of absorption of nutrients and elimination of waste, running from the mouth to anus, and including the majority of the organs of the abdomen and pelvis.

Dis-ease: Dis = Not; ease = balance (homeostasis) i.e. out of balance.

Distal: Means further away from the mid-line of the body or middle of the body (torso).

Dorsal: Top or back of the foot.

Dorsiflexion: Is moving the dorsi surface (back/top of the foot) upwards from the ground, or pulling the toes upwards. Its opposite movement is Plantarflexion.

Endocrine System: The major glands of the body, which communicate via hormones, which travel to various parts of the body through the blood.

Energy: See Chi. In Indian Chakra energy system it is called prana.

Eversion: Is moving the sole or plantar surface of the foot away from the mid-line of the body. It is pointing the sole outwards. Its opposite movement is inversion.

Extremes: Good or bad taken to its extreme results in greater degree of imbalance, and thus is to be avoided.

Fascia: Medical term for semi-elastic (much like string) connective tissue, which encloses and separates muscles. In the arch of the foot the fascia runs from the Calcaneus (Heel) bone to the ball of the foot, with a thick band of fascia between zones 1 and 2.

Fibula: The lateral or outside smaller and thinner bone of the lower leg.

Figure Eight technique: See Infinity technique; concluding or finishing technique.

Finger Walking: Basic Reflexology technique designed to cover the whole reflex.

Fore Foot: All the structures of the foot in front of and including the proximal heads of the metatarsal bones, i.e. the metatarsal and phalange bones and structures of the foot.

Four Levels of Existence: *Physical, emotional, mental* and *spiritual.* Physical and mental are yang (masculine/active) in nature, while emotional and spiritual are yin (feminine/passive) in nature = balanced; i.e. Father, Mother, Son and Daughter. The four seasons, four elements, etc.

Frontal: Front of the body

Gait: Medical term for all the movements needed in the action of walking, or taking a step.

Gonads: The sexual organs that produce sex cells: in females the ovary and in males the testes.

Groin (Groin Line): Is found at the end of the soft arch area just below where the heel starts. The heel itself is darker in colour and of a heavier texture. The line is a curve upward from medial (inside) to lateral (outside), and below the colour change.

Hallux: Big toe or Great toe (First toe)

Hand Reflexology: The older form of Reflexology. It is working the reflexes of the hands.

Healing Crisis: The healing crisis occurs after a treatment and it takes a few days to recover from the treatment as the symptoms increase before decreasing. Therefore it means an increase in symptoms, pain and discomfort immediately after a treatment.

Heel Spur: See Calcaneal or Heel Spur.

Helper Areas: Reflexology's attempt at putting the systems of the body back together and dealing with any imbalance or problem wholistically. They are other reflexes not the direct reflex and outside the system of the imbalance, that may help a particular imbalance.

Hippocratic Oath: *I shall do no harm.* It is the basis of the health care system.

Holding Techniques: Methods of holding the feet (the person) while working.

Homeostasis: Medical term for equilibrium/balance/harmony of the internal environment of the body.

Imbalance: Moving away from a balanced state, either yin (too little or deficiency) or yang (too much or excess).

Industrial Medicine: Term used for western allopathic medicine, as distinct from wholistic, alternative, complimentary and traditional medicine.

Infinity Technique: Finishing technique where the feet are closed down using a figure eight movement over each foot at the same time, and disconnecting from the energies of the receiver.

Innervation: Is the nerve that sends the message of movement to the muscle

Insertion: Is the attachment point to the bone of the more flexible end of the muscle.

Inside of the Foot: Is the Big toe or medial side of the foot.

Intention: The reason you are doing what you are doing, in this case Reflexology.

Intermediate: Middle, that is the bones between the distal and the proximal bones.

Intuition: A yin quality as opposed to the logical, knowledge based approach which is a yang quality. It is the artist at work. It is flexible, adaptable and fluid.

Inversion: Is moving the sole or plantar surface of the foot towards the mid-line of the body. It is pointing the sole inwards. Its opposite movement is eversion.

Lateral: Outside of the body or feet

Lateral Longitudinal Arch: Is the outer arch of the foot which is formed by the calcaneus, cuboid, and fourth and fifth metatarsal bones.

Ligament: Is a band of connective tissue that holds two or more bones together.

Longitudinal: Means longways or length-wise.

Lymphatic System: System that removes foreign substances and complex molecules from the blood and breaks them down. Part of the immune system.

Malleoli: Plural (Singular: malleolus) Distal heads of the leg bones (tibia and fibula) commonly called anklebones.

Medial: Closer to the mid-line of the body or feet. The inside.

Medial Longitudinal Arch: Is the inner arch of the foot formed by the calcaneus, talus, navicular, the three cuneiform bones and the first three metatarsal bones.

Metatarsal Pad: Or the Ball of the foot or chest area, between the *Shoulder Line* and the *Diaphragm.*

Metatarsals: Meta means middle, and tarsus means foot, i.e. middle foot bones. The long middle bones of the foot that run the length of the foot. There are five in total, numbered from the inside to the outside.

Mid-sagittal plane: Mid-line of the body, that is cutting the body right down the middle.

Muscular System: Gross muscles, which allow the body to move and maintain posture as well as producing body heat.

Navicular: Is a rear foot bone, behind the three cuneiform bones and in front of the calcaneus bone.

Nervous System: The major communication system of the body, including the brain and spinal chord (Central Nervous system) and the nerves and sensory receptors (Peripheral Nervous system).

Nervous System Theory: Major theory of Reflexology used for medical and general public. By working the feet you are working all the nerve endings in the feet and therefore working through the nervous system to all parts of the body.

Numbers/Numerology: *Numbers* are a system by which one can count and is applicable to Reflexology in relation to the number of times a technique is performed. *Numerology* is an ancient science of numbers which explains why certain numbers are used in performing the practical techniques of Reflexology.

Origin: Is the attachment point to the bone of the fixed end of the muscle.

Osmosis: Diffusion of solvent (fluid or blood) through a membrane (barrier).

Outside of the Foot: Is the little toe or *lateral* side of the foot.

Pain: One of the major message systems employed by the body.

Phalange: Singular phalanx. Toe (and finger) bones.

Plantar: Sole or bottom of the foot.

Plantarflexion: Is pointing the toes to the ground, or moving the plantar surface (sole) of the foot downward towards the ground. Its opposite is dorsiflexion.

Pronation: Is the combination of abduction, eversion and dorsiflexion that is where the sole of the foot moves away from the mid-line, turns the sole outwards and the toes downward. Its opposite movement is supination

Proximal: Means closer to the mid-line or middle of the body (torso).

Rear Foot: All the structures of the foot behind the proximal heads of the metatarsal bones, that is the three Cuneiforms, Navicular, Cuboid, Talus and Calcaneus bones and structures around these bones.

Reflection: The physical aspects of the body reflected in the feet and vice verse.

Referral Areas: Is an anatomically related area which can be worked instead of, or in addition to, the area of imbalance. This is true for all referral areas. The basic reason these areas are called *referrals* is simply because of the anatomical relationship existing between them.

Reflex: Is the term used to represent an area of the foot that relates to a particular part or area of the body.

Reflexion: The energy aspects of the body reflecting in the feet and vice versa.

Reflexology: Is the science that deals with the principle that there are reflex areas in the feet and hands, which correspond to all the structures of the body anatomically accurately and proportionally. Reflexology is a unique method of using the thumb and fingers on these reflex areas.

Reflex Zone Therapy: Original name of Reflexology, based on Zone Theory which is where the name came from.

Reproductive system: The system that performs the process of reproduction and controls sexual functions and behaviour via the gonads (male and female reproductive organs).

Respiratory system: Breathing, which is the process of exchanging gases between the air and blood, as well as regulating blood pH (i.e. acid/alkaline balance of the body)

Safety Precautions: Safety Precautions are conditions and/or situations which the Reflexologist needs to be conscious of in the therapeutic situation.

Sedation: A yin technique for decreasing excess imbalances, bringing the body back towards a more balanced state of existence.

Sense Organs: System of the body to do with the five senses: touch (skin), smell (nose), taste (mouth), sight (eyes), and hearing and balance (ears).

Shoulder Line: Is the line formed at the base of the second, third, fourth and fifth toes. It is the division between the toes (head/neck) and the ball of the foot (chest). *NOTE*: Not the Big toe.

Skeletal System: Protects and supports the body and is a major component of body movement. It also produces blood cells and stores minerals.

Solar Plexus: A chakra of the Indian energy system, located just below the end of the sternum (breastbone) and in the mid-line of the body, which penetrates the body to a point in the mid-thoracic of the spine.

Spur: Calcaneal or heel spur: bone growth as a result of fascia of the foot/feet being under pressure and/or damaged. The bone growth is the body's response to take the pressure off the damaged fascia.

Stimulation: A yang technique for increasing deficient imbalances, bringing the body back towards a more balanced state of existence.

Sub-talar joint: Is the joint below the talus bone and above the calcaneus bone. It is the location of the axes of motion for all the foot movements.

Supination: Is the combination of adduction, inversion and plantarflexion, that is where the sole of the foot is swept up and towards the mid-line, turning the sole inwards and the toes upward. Its opposite movement is pronation.

Talus: Is a strange shaped bone located between the distal heads of the tibial and fibula and above the calcaneus bone.

Tendon: Is a band of connective tissue that connects a muscle to a bone.

Tendon Line: Reflexology jargon for the thick band of longitudinal fascia in the arch of the foot (*between the diaphragm line and the Groin Line between Zones 1 and 2 i.e. between the Big toe and the second toe*). When you flex the Big Toe it will protrude and feel like a taut band of tissue.

Thrombosis: Also known as economy class syndrome: blood clotting.

Thumb Walking: The major technique of Reflexology designed to cover the whole reflex.

Tibia: The medial or inside larger bone of the lower leg.

Transverse: Going across the body (or foot), i.e. from inside to out or outside to in.

Transverse Arch: The arch of the foot that runs across the front of the rear foot and is formed by the three cuneiform and the cuboid bones.

Urinary System: Excretory system that removes waste product from blood, regulates pH (acid/alkaline balance), ion balance and water balance.

Veins: Blood vessels that travel away from cells towards the heart with de-oxygenated blood.

Waist (Waist Line): Is an imaginary line around the body found with the arm by the side in a relaxed position, and is drawn across the body just under the bottom of the elbow. On the foot it is found by locating the high spot or *bump* (Fifth metatarsal bone) on the outside of the foot about half-way down. After finding this high spot, draw an imaginary line across the foot, just below the *bump*; this will be the waistline.

Walking the Ridge: Is a technique where you use either your thumb or finger, and walk along the top of the Metatarsal pad (ball of the foot) or the Shoulder Line and then the necks of the toes.

Western Industrial Medicine: See Industrial Medicine

Wellbeing: The complete health of a human being on all levels: physical, emotional, mental and spiritual.

Wholistic/Wholism: Or Holistic/Holism: concept of the whole. In health care it is dealing with the whole person and all aspects: physical, emotional, mental and spiritual or the four levels of existence.

Yang: Yang is the active principle associated with expansion and intangibility. (Cannot exist in isolation)

Yang Imbalance: Characterized by *Excessive Chi.*

Yang Techniques: See Stimulation. Treats yin (deficiency) imbalance by strong pressure with fast clockwise action.

Yin: Yin is the passive principle associated with contraction and is tangible. (Cannot exist in isolation)

Yin Imbalance: Characterized by *Deficient Chi.*

Yin Techniques: See Sedation. Treats yang (excess) imbalance by light pressure (but still under the skin), with slow anti-clockwise action.

Zone Theory: Is the original theory that connects the feet to all parts of the body. It runs along a series of imaginary longitudinal lines, each encompassing a zone. There are TEN lines or zones (FIVE *either side of the body/foot*), one for each toe/finger, and they run the entire length of the body from the top of the head to the tips of toes, and from the toes to the base of the heel on the foot.

APPENDIX B:
CONSULTATION SHEETS

As far as consultation sheets are concerned, you need to draw up your own and to use them and allow them to evolve and grow through experience. There are no perfect consultation sheets. Collecting a variety of consultation sheets is a wise course of action as you will learn a great deal about the person who designed them, their biases and prejudices, and therefore, assist you to make decisions about what you ask, how you ask it, and what is important and therefore worth including and what is not, and even how you record information.

You will see a huge difference between the two sets of consultation sheets provided below. This is not by accident and is actually quite deliberate. The other point worth making is that many consultation sheets appear to be quite thorough and record down a great deal of information, such as the first example provided below, but with experience and the time constraints placed on the professional Reflexologist it becomes vital to develop consultation sheets that allow you to record information as briefly, succinctly and accurately as possible, without lengthy written records.

What follows are two examples of consultation sheets, both Initial and Future visits. The first two are the first consultation sheets (two pages) I drew up and used, and the second set is my current consultation sheets (4 pages). They are provided for two reasons: to show that consultation sheets evolve and grow as you do as a professional Reflexologist, and secondly to show that all consultation sheets reflect the designer's biases and prejudices.

CONSULTATION SHEET 1: First Initial Consultation (1 page)

REFLEXOLOGY: CLIENT INFORMATION AND ASSESSMENT
INITIAL VISIT: CONFIDENTIAL

NAME: . . . . D.O.B.: . . . . . / . . . . . /
DAY: . . . . DATE: . . . . / . . . . . TIME: . . . . am / pm
ADDRESS: . . . . Ph.: (H) . . . . (W) . . . . :
. . . . HEALTH FUND . . . .
Referred by: Word of Mouth / Advert. / Yellow Pages / Flyer / Other: . . . .
PRESENT OCCUPATION: . . . . SEX: Male / Female AGE: . . . .
REASON FOR CONSULTATION: . . . .

PRESENTING SYMPTOMS OR CONDITION
Principal diagnosis: . . . . Diagnosed by: GP / Specialist / Other . . . .
When diagnosed: . . . . Symptoms: . . . .
Current treatment / medication / vitamins: . . . .
Other therapies tried previously: . . . .

MEDICAL HISTORY
History of blood clotting ☐ Thrombophlebitis ☐ Pregnant / problems with pregnancy ☐ IDDM ☐ Epilepsy ☐ Cancer ☐ Unstable BP ☐
Allergies: . . . .
. . . .
. . . .
. . . .
. . . .

HEADACHE: ☐ Forehead (St. or LI) ☐ Top of Head (Lv & P) ☐ Both sides of Head (GB & TH) ☐ Back of Head (B & SI)
OPERATIONS / ACCIDENTS: (Broken bones, sprains, back problems)
. . . .
. . . .
PERSONALITY: Yang Tendency: Agitated, Outward, Talkative, Aggressive & Irritable   Yin Tendency: Passive, Inward & Quiet manner

LIFESTYLE
EXERCISE: Occasional / 1-4 days per week / 5-7 days per week.   Type of exercise: . . . .
DIET: No special diet / Vegan / Vegetarian / Low fat / Other: . . . .
WEIGHT: Average / under / over   Coffee / day: . . . . Tea / day: . . . . Cigarettes / day: . . . . Water / day: . . . . Alcohol / day: . . .
STRESS LEVELS: Work (L) 1 2 3 4 5 (H); Home (L) 1 2 3 4 5 (H)
LEISURE ACTIVITIES: . . . .
SLEEPS WELL: Every night / Mostly / Sporadically / Wakes regularly at: . . . .
EMOTIONAL STATE (How client feels): . . . .

PULSE: (40-60 beats / minute): . . . . (beats / min.)

TOUCH EVALUATION	Right	Left
Temperature	cool all over / warm all over / cool toes / cold	cool all over / warm all over / cool toes / cold
Moisture	very moist / moist / dry / scaly	very moist / moist / dry / scaly
Colour (overall)		
Joint mobility		
Odour		
Injuries		
Operations		

Biomedical observations: . . . .
Orthotic Podiatrist Recommended   ☐ Yes   ☐ No

Comments: . . . .

Blemishes / moles
Tinea
Planter warts
Prominent veins
Creases
Dry patches

R plantar L plantar   R lateral L lateral   R med L med   R dorsal L dorsal

Corns
Spurs
Callouses
Bunion
Hammer toes
Enlarged toe joints
Arch

CONSULTATION SHEET: First: Each Reflexology
Treatment (1 page)

REFLEXOLOGY: CLIENT INFORMATION

CONFIDENTIAL

NAME: . . . . Visit No.: . . . .

Day: . . . . Date: / / Time: . . . . am / pm

Feedback from previous massage:

Changes since last massage (e.g. illnesses, emotional state, mental state, treatments, medications, pregnancy, periods etc.)

REPORT

RECOMMENDATIONS / SUGGESTIONS:

CONSULTATION SHEET: Current Initial Consultation
(2 pages)

CHI-REFLEXOLOGY - Initial Consultation
CLIENT INFORMATION AND ASSESSMENT: **CONFIDENTIAL**

NAME: .... D.O.B.: / /   SINGLE / MARRIED / SEPARATED

DAY: .... DATE: / /   TIME: .... am / pm

ADDRESS: .... Ph.: (H) .... (W) ....

.... HEALTH FUND ....

Referred by: Word of Mouth / Advert. / Yellow Pages / Flyer / Other: ....

PRESENT OCCUPATION: .... SEX: Male / Female   AGE: ....

REASON FOR CONSULTATION: ....

PRESENTING SYMPTOMS OR CONDITION

Principal diagnosis: .... Diagnosed by: GP / Specialist / Other

When diagnosed: .... Symptoms: ....

Current treatment / medication / vitamins: ....

Other therapies tried previously: ....

MEDICAL HISTORY Thrombophlebitis ☐ IDDM ☐ Epilepsy ☐ Cancer ☐ Unstable BP ☐ Pregnant /pregnancy problems ☐

OPERATIONS / ACCIDENTS: (Broken bones, sprains, back problems, allergies)

LIFESTYLE

EXERCISE: Occasional / 1-4 days per week / 5-7 days per week.   Type of exercise: ....

DIET: No special diet / Vegan / Vegetarian / Low fat / Other: ....

Coffee / day .... Tea / day: .... Water / day: ....

Cigarettes / day: .... Alcohol / day: ....

WEIGHT: Average / under / over

WEIGHT: ☐ Obesity + dull, pale complexion, shortness of breath and weak muscles – Yang Chi Deficiency

☐ Emaciation + yellow/grey, lustreless complexion, delicate muscles and dry skin – Deficiency of Yin – Blood.

APPETITE: ☐ POOR (deficient or Dampness in ST or SP) ☐ EXCESSIVE (Excess ST Fire; too Yang, too dry) ☐ NORMAL

STRESS LEVELS: Work (L) 1 2 3 4 5 (H);   Home (L) 1 2 3 4 5 (H)

LEISURE ACTIVITIES: ....

SLEEPS WELL: Every night / Mostly / Sporadically / Wakes regularly at: ....

EMOTIONAL STATE (How client feels): ....

COMMON SYMPTOMS: ☐ COLD – Yin / Deficiency   ☐ HEAT – Yang / Excess

---

PERSONALITY: Yang Tendency: Agitated, Outward, Talkative, Aggressive & Irritable

               Yin Tendency: Passive, Inward & Quiet manner

TIME OF DAY

Like			Dislike		
☐ 11-1pm (H)	☐ 1-3pm (SI)	☐ 3-5pm (B)	☐ 11-1pm (GB)	☐ 1-3pm (Lv)	☐ 3-5pm (Lu)
☐ 5-7pm (K)	☐ 7-9pm (P)	☐ 9-11pm (TH)	☐ 5-7pm (LI)	☐ 7-9pm (ST)	☐ 9-11pm (SP)
☐ 11-1am (GB)	☐ 1-3am (Lv)	☐ 3-5am (Lu)	☐ 11-1am (H)	☐ 1-3am (SI)	☐ 3-5am (B)
☐ 5-7am (LI)	☐ 7-9am (ST)	☐ 9-11am (SP)	☐ 5-7am (K)	☐ 7-9am (P)	☐ 9-11am (TH)

HEADACHE: ☐ Forehead (St. or LI) ☐ Top of Head (Lv & P) ☐ Both sides of Head (GB & TH) ☐ Back of Head (B & SI)

PAIN: Related to –	PERSPIRATION:
Location ☐ Chest (H or Lu disharmony)	☐ Normal
☐ Flank (Lv or GB)	☐ Spontaneous (Deficient Defensive Chi)
☐ Abdomen (ST, SP, SI)	☐ Night Sweats (Deficient Yin; H & L)
☐ Lower Abdomen (B, LI, Uterus, Genital area)	☐ No Perspiration (Cold; Deficient Yin / Blood)
☐ Lower Back (K disharmony)	☐ Profuse Sweating (H)

TASTE IN MOUTH:	BOWEL MOVEMENT:
☐ Bitter (Lv or GB Heat; Excess)	☐ Regular (Once a day). WHEN: . . . .
☐ Sweet (Damp-Heat in SP & ST)	☐ Irregular. HOW OFTEN: . . . .
☐ Salty (Cold in K)	**Stool:** ☐ Hard & Dry (Yang excess)
☐ Sour (Overacting or Heat in LV & ST)	☐ Normal
☐ Tasteless (Deficient St & SP Chi)	☐ Loose and Wet (Dampness + Earth / Water
☐ Metallic (Lu)	Sp/St and/or K/Bl)

URINE: ☐ Clear (Yin) ☐ Dark or Scanty (Yang) ☐ Normal

TONGUE:
☐ Heart and lungs – Front of tongue
☐ Liver & Gall Bladder – Sides of tongue
☐ Stomach and Spleen – Middle of tongue
☐ Kidneys – Back of tongue
☐ Red and moist – Sufficient Chi and blood
☐ Pale – Deficiency of Chi and blood
☐ Thin white and moist coating – Sufficient stomach Chi

☐ Yellow coating – Exhaustion of stomach Chi
☐ Red and black or grey coating – Extreme heat
☐ Pale and black or grey coating – Extreme cold
☐ Deep red / purple – Heat in blood system
☐ White coating – Cold syndrome
☐ Yellow coating – Heat syndrome
☐ Bluish – Blood stagnation (Liver problems)

PULSE: (40-60 beats / minute): . . . . (beats / min.)

LEFT WRIST	HEART (Ex / Def)	LIVER (Ex / Def)	KIDNEY YIN (Material) (Ex / Def)
SUPERFICIAL			
MIDDLE			
DEEP (Internal)			
RIGHT WRIST	LUNGS (Ex / Def)	SPLEEN (Ex / Def)	KIDNEY YANG (Function) (Ex / Def)
SUPERFICIAL			
MIDDLE			
DEEP (Internal)			

TOUCH EVALUATION	Right	Left
Temperature	cool all over / warm all over / cool toes / cold	cool all over / warm all over / cool toes / cold
Moisture	very moist / moist / dry / scaly	very moist / moist / dry / scaly
Colour (overall)		
Joint mobility		
Odour		
Injuries		
Operations		

Biomechanical observations: . . . .
Orthotic Podiatrist Recommended   ☐ Yes   ☐ No

Comments: . . . .

Blemishes / moles
Tinea
Planter warts
Prominent veins
Creases
Dry patches

R plantar   L plantar   R lateral   L lateral   R med   L med   R dorsal   L dorsal

Corns
Spurs
Callouses
Bunion
Hammer toes
Enlarged toe joints
Arch

GENERAL OBSERVATIONS: . . . .
. . . .

CONSULTATION SHEET: Current: Each Reflexology
Treatment, including diagnostic (2 pages)

REFLEXOLOGY: CLIENT INFORMATION
CONFIDENTIAL

NAME: . . . . Visit No.: . . . .

Day: . . . . Date: / / Time: . . . . am / pm

Feedback from & changes since last massage (e.g. illnesses, emotional state, mental state, treatments, medications, pregnancy, periods etc.)

TO DO: . . . .

REPORT
Lv – Ex/Def . . . .
GB – Ex/Def . . . .
P – Ex/Def . . . .
TB – Ex/Def . . . .
H – Ex/Def . . . .
SI – Ex/Def . . . .
Sp – Ex/Def . . . .
St – Ex/Def . . . .
Lu – Ex/Def . . . .
LI – Ex/Def . . . .
K – Ex/Def . . . .
B – Ex/Def. . . . .

BALANCE USED – Standard   Yes [ ]   No [ ]
                Integration Yes [ ]   No [ ]
                Mu/Shu   Yes [ ]   No [ ]
                Toe Balance Yes [ ]   No [ ]

Crystal: [ ] Yes [ ] No
Lymphatic Drainage: [ ] Yes [ ] No
Oil used: . . . .

Spiritual Healing: [ ] Yes [ ] No
Balance Organ: [ ] Yes [ ] No
P. C. . . . .

RECOMMENDATIONS / SUGGESTIONS:

NEXT TIME:

CHI-REFLEXOLOGY - Diagnostic
Client Information
CONFIDENTIAL

	Pulse
FIRE: Heart	
Pericardium	
EARTH: Spleen	
METAL: Lung	
WATER: Kidney	
WOOD: Liver	

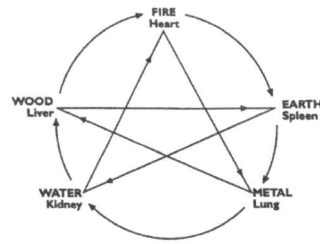

DIAGNOSTIC:

HEART EX	Spleen (Ex)	Lung (Def)
HEART DEF	Spleen (Def)	Lung (Ex)
SPLEEN EX	Lung (Ex)	Kidney (Def)
SPLEEN DEF	Lung (Def)	Kidney (Ex)
LUNG EX	Kidney (Ex)	Liver (Def)
LUNG DEF	Kidney (Def)	Liver (Ex)
KIDNEY EX	Liver (Ex)	Heart (Def)
KIDNEY DEF	Liver (Def)	Heart (Ex)
LIVER EX	Heart (Ex)	Spleen (Def)
LIVER DEF	Heart (Def)	Spleen (Ex)

APPENDIX C:
NUMBERS AND REFLEXOLOGY

It amazes me how complete a system of thought and knowledge, intuition and experience I have developed. It was not a conscious thing but a process that evolved and grew. It was not until I had to explain what I did and why, initially to share it and later to put pen to paper that I began to realise this. My approach is actually a complete one and everything is interrelated. Therefore, nothing is done by accident or without a reason. This includes the number of times techniques are done.

Wholistic (Soul-Growth) Numerology is part of what I have developed. It is a complete Numerological approach, with twelve numbers, like Astrology has twelve houses and twelve signs. It is based on the Four Levels of Existence: physical (in this case practical as well), emotional, mental and spiritual, and like Astrology there are three numbers (Signs and Houses) for each of the four levels of existence.

What follows is an introduction to Wholistic (Soul-Growth) Numerology and its applications to any therapy, including Reflexology.

ILLUSTRATION 175: Numbers of the Four Planes

SPIRITUAL	11	12	22	AIR
MENTAL	3	5	9	FIRE
EMOTIONAL	2	6	7	WATER
PRACTICAL/PHYSICAL	1	4	8	EARTH

The relevance of numbers and their vibrational influence on any therapy, including Reflexology is summarised in the following table.

ILLUSTRATION 176: Numbers and Their Effects

2   Emotional Balance

3   Mental Balance

4   Physical and wholistic balance – due to the FOUR levels of existence (Physical, emotional, mental and spiritual)

12 Spiritual and wholistic balance (4 X 3 or four groups of three)

6   Treatment Number

I do not generally use the numbers **two** or **three** as they are specific levels rather than wholistic. However, for specific purposes, such as emotional and mental balance, they may be useful.

You can see why **four** and **twelve** are extensively used, as is the number **six** for treatment. Why six for treatment? Initially it is because it is the Chinese number of treatment, but there are other reasons. Six is ruled by the planet Venus, the planet of Love: concern, compassion and nurturing, and is yin. Thus when you are treating repeat the technique six times or for six out-breaths of the receiver (breath is our rhythm of life) not only for treatment but to treat with concern and to nurture the receiver. And finally as six is a yin number, it is treating through yin energies and the feet are our yin instrument of movement and our connection to Mother Earth, our connection to yin energies, which flow up into the human being through and from the feet. (See Chapter 2 for a more detailed explanation) So there are a multitude of reasons for using six for treatment.

These are all of relevance of Wholistic (Soul-Growth) Numerology to Reflexology. However, there is much more to this system of numerology and the following Table outlines the content of Wholistic (Soul-Growth) Numerology as there are so many aspects that complete the numerological vibrations.

Wholistic (Soul-Growth) Numerology Contents
ILLUSTRATION 177

INTRODUCTION:
a) Numbers and the Four Levels of Existence
b) Numbers, Planets, Yin (Masculine)/Yang (Feminine)
c) The Purpose of Life
d) Number Quality, Attainment and Spiritual Lesson/Task

NUMEROLOGICAL ENERGY PATTERNS

HOW TO CALCULATE NUMBERS:
• 11, 12 & 22 what to do?
• Number Combinations

NUMEROLOGY CHART:
a) Governing Factor and Birthday Synopsis
b) Personality Factor
c) Maturity Factor
d) Secondary Vibrations
e) Destiny Factor
f) Pyramids
g) Danger Signals in Birth chart

VIBRATIONS IN YOUR BIRTH NAME:
a) Spiritual Purpose (Vowels)
b) Egoic Desire (Consonants)
c) Overall Self-Expression
d) Other Lessons in your Name
e) Karmic Patterns
f) Other names used

ARROWS IN THE BIRTH CHART:
Twenty-two Arrows: their calculation and explanation.

NUMEROLOGY: FUTURE INFLUENCES
a) Year Vibration
b) Monthly Vibration

NUMEROLOGY CHART: CALCULATION SHEETS

APPENDIX D
RECOMMENDED READING AND REFLEXOLOGY RESOURCES

RECOMMENDED READING

There are so many reflexology books that they cannot all be listed below. And most reflexology books are not significantly different. What are listed below are the author and title and comments about the text where applicable.

Arnold, Moss — **Chi-Reflexology : Guidelines for the Middle Way**. Specialist Chi-Reflexology: combination of Reflexology and Traditional Chinese Medicine (TCM)

Bayley, Doreen — **Reflexology Today.** Bayley School of Reflexology approach from United Kingdom

Booth, Lynne — **Vertical Reflexology.** Reflexology done standing. New approach and chart.

Byers, Dwight — **Better Health with Foot Reflexology**, Ingham Publishing, Florida, 1986. The most widely used text. Practical, concrete and layman's approach. Simply written.

Carter, Mildred — **Helping Yourself with Foot Reflexology.** Very early US Reflexologist, studied with Eunice Ingham, and went off and did her own thing; of historical interest.

Cosway-Hayes, Joan — **Reflexology for Every Body: Book and Video.** The book that now tends to be the textbook of a lot of trainings. Good textbook and simple approach. Canadian Reflexology.

Crane, Beryl — **Professional Reflexology for Everyone.** Extensive text. Extremely detailed. Recommended as a reference book.

Dougans, Inge with Ellis, Suzanne — **The Art of Reflexology: A New Approach Using the Chinese Meridian Theory**, 1992. Useful for combining Reflexology and Chinese meridians, as Inge is the first to do this, that is combine meridians from Touch for Health with Reflexology.

Enzer, Susanne — **Maternity Reflexology** and **Reflexology : A Tool for Midwives.** Specialist Maternity Reflexology books. If interested in Maternity, excellent works, and there are other publications now available.

Gillanders, Ann — **Family Guide to Reflexology**. Another United Kingdom training institution's approach.

Grinberg, Avi — **Holistic Reflexology**. Israeli: physically reading the feet. Pioneer. Book now difficult to get.

Hall, Nicola M — **Reflexology: A Better Way to Health**; and **Reflexology for Women**. Another United Kingdom training institution's approach.

Ingham, Eunice D. with Revision by Byers, Dwight C. — **The original Works of Eunice Ingham: Stories the Feet can Tell Thru Reflexology and Stories the Feet Have Told Thru Reflexology,** 1992. Grandmother of Reflexology; worth reading for basics, origins and see Eunice's heart was in the process and that it was alive for her.

Issel, Christine — **Reflexology: Art, Science and History** USA, 1993. Very good for the history and theory of Reflexology and its varieties.

Kaiser, Scharmann, & Poyck-Scharmann — **Hand Reflexology**. German Hand Reflexology book. Covers Incan ancient Foot Reflexology.

Kunz, Kevin & Barbara — **The Complete Guide to Foot Reflexology**. US Reflexology couple.

MacKereth, Peter (Editor) — **Clinical Reflexology**. A compilation on Reflexology within the medical health care industry. Thus Clinical Reflexology, the title.

Marquardt, Hanne — **Reflex Zone Therapy of the Feet** and **Reflexotherapy of the Feet**. Early German Reflexologist. Her approach.

Norman, L with Cowan, T. — **Feet First** and **The Reflexology Handbook: A Complete Guide**. Very good for the basics (home use) and for its wholistic approach.

Stormer, Chris — **Language of the Feet: What Feet Can Tell You**, 1995. Pioneer in Reflexology and Foot Reading. Good for emotional aspects of reading the feet.

Stormer, Chris — **Reflexology: The Definitive Guide**. Excellent: Good practical resource book for professional Reflexologists. Lists problems, reflexes and more.

Williamson, Jan — **Guide to Precision Reflexology**. Specialist book on Indian system, charkas and Linking techniques. Gentle approach.

Wills, Pauline — **The Reflexology Manual Colour Reflexology**. UK Reflexologist who also works with Indian Chakra system and Colour.

REFLEXOLOGY RESOURCES

The best person in Australia for anything to do with Reflexology is Russell McAllister, publisher of Reflexology World Magazine. Russell also has Reflexology books and other resources available. His details are below. Reflexology World Magazine is highly recommend as it is the only independent reflexology publication in the world, and is an international Reflexology magazine. All other magazines are either tied to a particular training institution and/or professional organisation.

Reflexology World Magazine, Russell McAllister
www.reflexologyworld.com

APPENDIX E:
REFLEXOLOGY AROUND THE WORLD

REFLEXOLOGY IN AUSTRALIA

The history of Reflexology in Australia is quite modern. For example, the Reflexology Association of Australia (RAA; now RAoA) was formed in 1989 in Victoria and New South Wales in 1990, and the oldest known Reflexologist in Australia was one Fergi Hastrich, a chiropractor and naturopath working in Burwood, New South Wales in the 1960s. Fergi studied Reflexology overseas in Germany and then returned to Australia.

There are two major professional organisations that recognise Reflexology in Australia: the Australian Traditional Medicine Society (A.T.M.S.) and the Reflexology Association of Australia. ATMS is the most professional and oldest national organisation in Australia. They are a national umbrella organisation for all natural therapies, and professionally represents all natural therapies to the general public as well as officially with the various State and Federal government bodies.

WEBSITES IN AUSTRALIA:

ATMS — www.atms.com.au
National RAoA — www.reflexology.org.au
Reflexology World — www.reflexologyworld.com

Moss Arnold: Australian College of Chi-Reflexology —
www.chi-reflexology.com.au

INTERNATIONAL REFLEXOLOGY

Reflexology is found in nearly every country of the world. This in itself is an amazing fact in that it has occurred within a relatively short space of time, some forty odd years, and no more than one hundred years. There is at least one Reflexology organisation in most countries and sometimes there are more. For example, there are a multitude of Reflexology organisations in the United Kingdom, with the AoR (Association of Reflexologists) being the largest. Also there are some professional organisations that are actually called training institutions, so it is difficult to be completely accurate and up-to-date with this information, but at least it is a starting point.

For international enquiries the best starting point is the ICR (International Council of Reflexologists) or Russel McAllister.

Overseas Organizations' Websites:

International Council of Reflexologists —
www.icr.reflexology.org
Association of Reflexologists (AoR) —
www.aor.org.uk
FDZ Danish Reflexology Association —
www.fdz.dk
Reflexology Association of America —
www.reflexology-usa.org
Reflexology Association of Canada —
www.reflexologycanada.com
South African Reflexology Society —
www.users.lia.net/sareflex

INDEX

AUSTRALIAN COLLEGE OF CHI-RELFEXOLOGY

College Products

www.chi-reflexology.com.au

Chi-Reflexology: Guidelines for the Middle Way   by Moss Arnold

A unique and original illustrated Text which combines the Chinese Philosophy, including Traditional Chinese Medicine (TCM) Theory, and Acupressure with Reflexology. Topics covered include:

* Perspective of the Feet
* The Chinese Philosophy
* Balance and Imbalance
* Solar Plexus Revisited
* The Two Chinese Clocks
* Pressure and Pain
* Acupressure in Reflexology
* Reading the Chi of the Feet
* Holding the Person, Holding the Feet
* Wholistic Approach
* Chi: Energy of the Universe
* Yin and Yang Theory
* Acu-points & Meridians of the Foot & Leg
* Reflexions: Mirrors of the Chi of the Body
* The Five Phases Theory
* Chi-Reflexology: Five Phases Applications

Chi-Reflexology is an approach that can either be combined with Reflexology and all Natural Therapies, or used exclusively to achieve balance and well-being.

Chi-Reflexology : Guidelines for the Middle Way – The Video

A 53-minute colour video of the practical techniques of Chi-Reflexology, including:

* Perspective of the Feet
* Relaxation/Openings Techniques
* Balancing Organ Chi Sequence
* Acupressure in Reflexology – Treatment Techniques
* Balancing Organ, Meridian Chi & Integration Sequence
* Balancing Chi, Meridian, Elements & Integrating Sequence
* Holding the Person, Holding the Feet
* Meridian & Acu-point Work

Allow Moss, in his unique, friendly & relaxed style, to take you on a step by step journey through the Chi-Reflexology practical techniques that he has developed. Designed as a companion to his book and Foot Chart, the video will enhance your practical understanding of the approach.

Chi-Reflexology Foot Chart   by Moss Arnold

A unique and original Foot Chart of the energy or Chi of the body through the feet! The Chart links the Chinese Philosophy including Traditional Chinese Medicine (TCM) and Acupressure with Reflexology. Included on the Chart are the Reflex points of each Organ's Chi found on the sole; the spine and limbs of the body; and the "Reflexions" of the Acu-points; and in FULL COLOUR!

Products Order Form

Please send me –
Number of Copies

BOOK – **"Chi-Reflexology: Guidelines for the Middle Way"**
    Australian $38.00   Overseas $48.00 includes GST & P&H   ....

DVD – **Chi-Reflexology**
    Australian $38.00   Overseas $48.00 includes GST & P&H   ....

FOOT Chart – **Chi-Reflexology**
    Australian $38.00   Overseas $48.00 includes GST & P&H   ....

DISCOUNTS

a) **Book and DVD** (15% discount)
    Australian $66.05 Overseas $81.60 includes GST & P&H   ....

b) **DVD and Chart** (15% discount)
    Australian $66.05 Overseas – $81.60 includes GST & P&H   ....

c) **Book, DVD & Chart** (20% discount)
    Australian $94.15 Overseas $115.20 includes GST & P&H   ....

Bulk Orders – upon request   *All prices include GST and postage & handling*

Name ....

Address ....

.... Postcode ....

Telephone (H) .... (W) ....

PAYMENT BY –

Cash / Cheque / Money Order / Credit Card   **TOTAL COST** ....

CREDIT CARD DETAILS

Visa   Mastercard   OR   Bankcard   ONLY   (Please circle)

Card number _ _ _ _ / _ _ _ _ / _ _ _ _ / _ _ _ _

Expiry date _ _ / _ _

Name on card..

Signature...

Date _ _ / _ _ / _ _ _ _

    PLEASE NOTE: Your signature and the date section must be completed.

Mail to: The Principal
           Australian College of Chi-Reflexology
           PO Box 4071
           Winmalee NSW 2777

Reflexology
Basics of the Middle Way

Moss Arnold

		Qty
	AU$24.99	.....
Postage within Australia	AU$6.00	.....
	TOTAL★ $_____ ★	
	All prices include GST	

Name: ....Phone:...............................

Address: ....

....

Email: ....

Payment: ❑ Money Order   ❑ Cheque   ❑ Amex

❑ MasterCard   ❑ Visa

Cardholder's Name: ....

Credit Card Number:

___ ___ ___ ___   ___ ___ ___ ___   ___ ___ ___ ___   ___ ___ ___ ___

Signature: ....

Expiry Date: __ __ / __ __

Allow 10 days for delivery.

Payment to: Better Bookshop (ABN 14 067 257 390)
PO Box 12544
A'Beckett Street, Melbourne, 8006
Victoria, Australia
sales@brolgapublishing.com.au

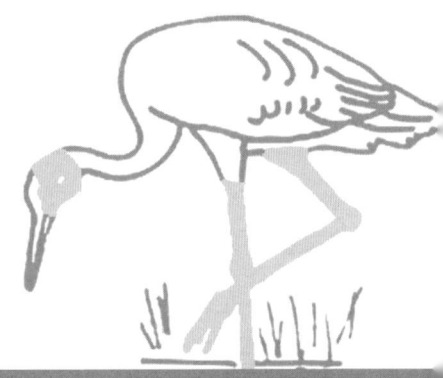

BE PUBLISHED

Publishing through a successful
Australian publisher.
Brolga provides:
- Editorial appraisal
- Cover design
- Typesetting
- Printing
- Author promotion
- National book trade
distribution, including
sales, marketing and
distribution through Pan
Macmillan Australia.

For details and inquiries, contact:
Brolga Publishing Pty Ltd
PO Box 12544
A'Beckett St VIC 8006

Phone: 03 9614 3205
Fax: 03 9614 3250
bepublished@brolgapublishing.com.au
markzocchi@brolgapublishing.com.au
ABN: 46 063 962 443